Prof Ramani's Spinal Series

Current Trends in Surgical Management of

Lumbar Canal Stenosis

Editor-in-Chief

PS Ramani MD

Senior Neuro Spinal Surgeon
Lilavati Hospital and Research Centre
Bandra Reclamation, Bandra (W)
Mumbai

Co-Editors

Sumeet Pawar MD

Associate Consultant
Department of Pediatric Neuro and Spinal Surgery
Narayana Health SRCC Children's Hospital
Mumbai

JKBC Parthiban MD

Consultant Neurosurgeon
Kovai Medical Center and Hospital
Coimbatore, Tamil Nadu, India

Shradha Maheshwari MD

Incharge
Department of Neurosurgery
Dr RN Cooper Hospital and HBT Medical College
Mumbai

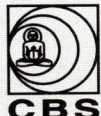

CBS

CBS Publishers & Distributors Pvt Ltd

New Delhi • Bengaluru • Chennai • Kochi • Kolkata • Mumbai

Bhopal • Bhubaneswar • Hyderabad • Jharkhand • Nagpur • Patna • Pune • Uttarakhand • Dhaka (Bangladesh)

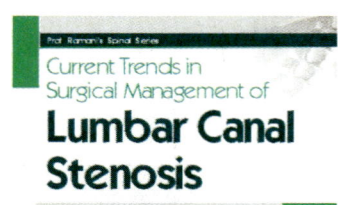

ISBN: 978-93-88327-56-5

First Edition: 2019

Published by Satish Kumar Jain and produced by Varun Jain for

CBS Publishers & Distributors Pvt Ltd
4819/XI Prahlad Street, 24 Ansari Road, Daryaganj, New Delhi 110 002, India.
Ph: 23289259, 23266861, 23266867   Fax: 011-23243014   Website: www.cbspd.com
e-mail: delhi@cbspd.com; cbspubs@airtelmail.in.
Corporate Office: 204 FIE, Industrial Area, Patparganj, Delhi 110 092
Ph: 4934 4934   Fax: 4934 4935   e-mail: publishing@cbspd.com; publicity@cbspd.com

Branches

- **Bengaluru:** Seema House 2975, 17th Cross, K.R. Road,
  Banasankari 2nd Stage, Bengaluru 560 070, Karnataka
  Ph: +91-80-26771678/79   Fax: +91-80-26771680   e-mail: bangalore@cbspd.com
- **Chennai:** 7, Subbaraya Street, Shenoy Nagar, Chennai 600 030, Tamil Nadu
  Ph: +91-44-26680620, 26681266   e-mail: chennai@cbspd.com
- **Kochi:** 42/1325, 1326, Power House Road, Opposite KSEB Power House,
  Ernakulam 682 018, Kochi, Kerala
  Ph: +91-484-4059061-65   Fax: +91-484-4059065   e-mail: kochi@cbspd.com
- **Kolkata:** 6/B, Ground Floor, Rameswar Shaw Road, Kolkata-700 014, West Bengal
  Ph: +91-33-22891126, 22891127, 22891128   e-mail: kolkata@cbspd.com
- **Mumbai:** 83-C, Dr E Moses Road, Worli, Mumbai-400018, Maharashtra
  Ph: +91-22-24902340/41   Fax: +91-22-24902342   e-mail: mumbai@cbspd.com

Representatives

- **Bhopal**   0-8319310552
- **Nagpur**   0-9021734563
- **Dhaka (Bangladesh)** 01912-003485
- **Bhubaneswar**   0-9911037372
- **Patna**   0-9334159340
- **Hyderabad**   0-9885175004
- **Pune**   0-9623451994
- **Jharkhand**   0-9811541605
- **Uttarakhand**   0-9716462459

Printed at Goyal Offset Printers, GT Karnal Road, Industrial Area, Delhi, India

Foreword

It is an immense honor for me to write the Foreword to Professor Ramani's latest publication *Current Trends in Surgical Management of Lumbar Canal Stenosis*. Lumbar canal stenosis is defined as any type of narrowing of the spinal canal, nerve root canals, or intervertebral foramen to cause compression of cauda equina and exiting nerve roots, and degenerative process is the most common cause of this condition. Without doubt, this clinical entity is one of the most frequent subjects in the practice of spinal neurosurgery, and there are several factors to be considered in the decision-making process of each patient, such as operative or conservative, with or without fusion, and conventional or minimally invasive approach. Minimally invasive microsurgical bilateral decompression by unilateral approach is still regarded as one of the relevant gold standards in its surgical treatment, and its derived techniques with tubular retractor or endoscope have recently been introduced to attract spinal neurosurgeons. A fusion by one of several varieties is carried out in patients having instability. Minimal access procedures with percutaneous pedicle screw fixation have become extremely popular in recent times. There has been a rapid progress in techniques and tools giving the surgeon a variety of options and I am certain that this is the right time to publish this book to highlight this common disease. At the outset, I would like to congratulate Prof Ramani and the contributors on their endeavor to provide updated knowledge of lumbar canal stenosis to the readers.

Following the excellent introduction by the editor, the first four chapters describe epidemiology, anatomy, and pathogenesis of lumbar canal stenosis. A better understanding of these fundamental subjects is expected to build the foundation for the following articles. The next two chapters describe important issues related to correct diagnosis, which help the readers to understand symptomatic features and neurological

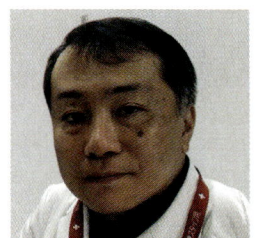

findings of this clinical entity, and their correlation between the radiological studies including standing dynamic radiographs, computerized tomography, and magnetic resonance imaging.

Finally, the remaining articles provide information on management of lumbar canal stenosis, including biomechanical considerations, treatment options such as fusion and minimally invasive approach, and complications and outcomes. It is quite evident that surgical treatment is effective for lumbar canal stenosis in halting the symptomatic progression, but its decision making depends on an adequate assessment of the risks and benefits of each available option. The book concludes with the discussion by the editor to disclose currently confronting problems and then to provide a future direction in management of lumbar canal stenosis. By reading this book with careful attention, the readers are expected to acquire the standardized diagnostic procedure and indication criteria for each treatment modality. Further fruitful learning by visiting and spending some time in specialized spinal centers or referring their difficult patients to the spine experts, the young spinal surgeons can observe the actual clinical course of this intriguing disease.

The contents compiled here cover contemporary and evidence-based information on lumbar canal stenosis, and I believe this comprehensive textbook contributes to improve our daily practice, resulting in better outcome of our patients. At the conclusion I would like to express my sincere gratitude to Prof Ramani for this opportunity to share such an outstanding work with the readers from all over the world.

Dr Yoshitaka Hirano MD
Spine Section, Department of Neurosurgery
Southern Tohoku Research Institute for Neuroscience
Tohoku, Japan

Contributors

Abdul Hafid Bajamal
Department of Neurosurgery
Faculty of Medicine of Airlangga University
Dr Soetomo General Hospital
Surabaya, Indonesia

Achal Gupta
Department of Neuro Spinal Surgery
Lilavati Hospital and Research Centre
Mumbai

Ahmed Nouby
Fellow in Training in Spinal Surgery
Luxor, Egypt

Amitesh Dubey
Department of Neurosurgery
NSCB Medical College
Jabalpur, MP, India

Anil Pande
Institute of Neurosciences
Apollo Hospitals
Chennai

Apurva Prasad
Department of Neuro Spinal Surgery
Lilavati Hospital and Research Centre
Mumbai

Arjun Dhar
Department of Neuro Spinal Surgery
Lilavati Hospital and Research Centre
Mumbai

Arvind Kulkarni
Mumbai Spine, Scoliosis and Disc Replacement Centre
Bombay Hospital Institute and Medical Research Centre
Mumbai, India

Brian T David
Department of Neurosurgery
Rush University Medical College
Chicago, IL-USA

Eko Subagio
Department of Neurosurgery
Faculty of Medicine of Airlangga University
Dr Soetomo General Hospital
Surabaya, Indonesia

Gordan Grahovac
Department of Neuro and Spine Surgery
King's College, London, UK

Irfan Malik
Department of Neuro and Spine Surgery
King's College, London, UK

Jitendra Jain
Pain Physician
Spine and Pain Clinic
Lilavati Hospital and Research Centre
Mumbai, India

JKBC Parthiban
Consultant Neurosurgeon
Kovai Medical Center and Hospital
Coimbatore, Tamil Nadu, India

Kavya Kaushik
Department of Imaging
Jaslok Hospital and Research Centre
Mumbai

Kumar Abhinav
Department of Neuro Spinal Surgery
Lilavati Hospital and Research Centre
Mumbai

Mazda Turel
Department of Neurosurgery
Rush University Medical College
Chicago, IL-USA

Mena G Kerolus
Department of Neurosurgery
Rush University Medical College
Chicago, IL-USA

Mewara N
Mumbai Spine, Scoliosis and Disc Replacement Centre
Bombay Hospital Institute and Medical Research Centre
Mumbai, India

Mohammed Suheel
Department of Neurosurgery
Aberdeen Royal Infirmary
Foresterhill, Aberdeen
Scotland, UK

Muhammad Faris
Head of Spine Division
Department of Neurosurgery
Faculty of Medicine of Airlangga University
Dr Soetomo General Hospital
Surabaya, Indonesia

Nidhikumar Patel
Institute of Neurosciences
Apollo Hospitals
Chennai

Patel A
Mumbai Spine, Scoliosis and Disc Replacement Centre
Bombay Hospital Institute and Medical Research Centre
Mumbai, India

PD Kulkarni
Department of Neuro and Spine Surgery
King's College, London, UK

Pragnesh Bhatt
Consultant
Department of Neurosurgery
Aberdeen Royal Infirmary
Foresterhill, Aberdeen, Scotland, UK

PS Ramani
Senior Neurospinal Surgeon
Lilavati Hospital and Research Centre
Bandra Reclamation, Bandra (W)
Mumbai

Richard G Fessler
Department of Neurosurgery
Rush University Medical College
Chicago, IL-USA

Ritu Kakkar
Consultant
Department of Imaging
Jaslok Hospital and Research Centre
Mumbai

Ruparel S
Mumbai Spine, Scoliosis and Disc Replacement Centre
Bombay Hospital Institute and Medical Research Centre
Mumbai, India

Shailendra Ratre
Department of Neurosurgery
NSCB Medical College
Jabalpur, MP, India

Shraddha Sinhasan
Consultant
Department of Imaging
Jaslok Hospital and Research Centre
Mumbai

Shradha Maheshwari
Incharge
Department of Neurosurgery
Dr RN Cooper Hospital and HBT Medical College
Mumbai

Shrinivas B Desai
Consultant and Head
Department of Imaging
Jaslok Hospital and Research Centre
Mumbai

Siddharth Ghosh
Institute of Neurosciences
Apollo Hospitals
Chennai

Sudhendoo Babhulkar
Junior Consultant
Department of Neurosurgery
Nanavati Superspeciality Hospital
Mumbai

Sumeet Pawar
Associate Consultant
Department of Pediatric Neuro and Spinal Surgery
Narayana Health SRCC Children's Hospital
Mumbai

Vijay Parihar
Department of Neurosurgery
NSCB Medical College
Jabalpur, MP, India

Yoshitaka Hirano
Spine Section
Department of Neurosurgery
Southern Tohoku Research Institute for Neuroscience
Koriyama, Japan

YR Yadav
Department of Neurosurgery
NSCB Medical College
Jabalpur, MP, India

Yunus Kuntawi Ali
Department of Neurosurgery
Faculty of Medicine of Airlangga University
Dr Soetomo General Hospital
Surabaya, Indonesia

Preface

Times are changing. I have written several books which contain knowledge on lumbar canal stenosis but as time passes technology is advancing in leaps and bounds. New concept results in change of tools as well as implants to be used in spinal surgery. Operative techniques are changing so fast that I fear a time will come when young doctors training in spinal surgery will not know what a laminectomy procedure was in the past. This is not to downplay the fact and I can say this authority that laminectomy as a decompressive procedure for lumbar canal stenosis has stood the test of time and has indeed earned the reputation of being a gold standard on which other techniques can be compared. What is more important is the fact that long-term outcome of this procedure is available and they are not unfavorable in the least.

All the same life is moving very fast. Today's operative techniques are minimally invasive and more comforting to the patient. Gone are the days when patient after a discoidectomy procedure spent more than 10 days in the hospital. He was then discharged with loads of restrictions and there was no chance that he could return to his original job one day, if it involved hard work. I feel happy to say that today's operative procedures are aimed to send the patient back to his original job, however, hard it may be. Long bedrests have become a thing of the past and it is replaced with early mobilization, muscle toning and building exercises, keeping the body in shape and remain healthy for many more years to come. This is the greatest advantage of today's spinal surgery in an era where people have no time to rest. Competition is fierce and job is always competitive. Unless one falls in line he may be left behind. Such concepts have made spinal surgery popular once again.

When I surveyed my surgical data I realized that in recent years the incidence of surgical procedure for lumbar canal stenosis has taken over the incidence for prolapsed lumbar intervertebral disc. It has reason. Medicine has helped to improve longevity. Today, India banks on young population. Tomorrow may be different and one may have to face the reality of looking after aged population as it happens in many western civilized countries today. The incidence of lumbar canal stenosis will increase tremendously. Surgery for lumbar canal stenosis will become the most frequent and popular surgery and once patients know that it is minimally morbid, the incidence of surgical procedures for lumbar canal stenosis will increase further resulting in development of yet newer surgical techniques. As a routine, the hospital stay then could last a few hours only.

With these thoughts in mind, I felt that establishing a strong base for this concept is essential. A comprehensive book like this should help the young doctors to lay a sturdy foundation for the topic of lumbar canal stenosis. The advantage of having a separate book is the fact that one has not to search for his answer from a mix of several topics. This is a handbook and one can carry it anywhere so that it is available easily to refer.

Today's trend of young doctors is to search on the net. One gets to see latest papers. The greatest drawback of recently published papers is the fact that it contains a personal series rather than the in-depth knowledge on the topic. This book is aimed to provide in-depth knowledge on one topic which is popular today so that the young spinal surgeons can familiarize with the topic before they venture into doing surgical procedures.

I have still maintained a chapter on laminectomy as unless one understands it completely, he should not venture into newer techniques. The most popular technique of today is endoscopic discectomy and/or fusion in LCS followed by percutaneous techniques of pedicle screw insertion or interbody cage insertion. One can appreciate such concepts better on the backdrop of open laminectomy.

Chapters on MISS techniques including percutaneous techniques which are most prevalent today will give a boost to read this book further.

Included in this book is a chapter on precautions to maintain sagittal balance of the spine while using implants so that long-term outcome should be satisfactory. Most spinal surgeons have vague knowledge on this topic. It is important for them to familiarize with this section so that a patient can stand in erect posture for many years to come after surgery. After all standing erect has indeed been evolution.

I have laid a stress on basic knowledge. Without a good base on this issue one cannot expect to do successful surgery. Spinal surgery today is the most popular surgical branch. There is no neurosurgeon who is not doing spinal surgery and a new trait of only spinal surgery is evolving fast. I am a convert as during my time purity in this field did not exist. It is interesting to note that the visiting card of the surgeon make a mention on competence in spinal surgery and yet patients travel hundreds or even thousand miles in search of a good spinal surgeon. The answer lies in inadequate basic knowledge.

I sincerely hope that this book will prove to be a popular reading among young spinal surgeons. I strongly believe that net is not everything. Those who read books, they will attain maturity quickly.

PS Ramani
Senior Consultant, Neuro Spinal Surgeon

Contents

Lumbar Canal Stenosis: Introduction and Historical Background

PS Ramani

INTRODUCTION

Today lumbar canal stenosis (LCS) is a well-recognized, very common and disabling entity. It was present in the past but its recognition came much later. In a study in India by Chahal et al[4] in 1978 it was found that majority of the adults in the 4th decade of life suffered from back pain due to spondylotic degenerative changes of the facet joints and thickening and incurling of ligamentum flavum.

It is a degenerative disorder generally regarded as part of the aging process. Progressive and disabling symptomatology leads to significant compromise of activities of daily living.[8] Even after surgery, it is unfortunate, that over a period of time the functional quality of life is affected because of progression of disease. It is surprising to know in recent articles[1,2,6,7,9, 11–13,15,17,22,32] that neither the current surgical options nor decompression with fusion[10,28] are able to adequately address the full pathophysiology of lumbar canal

stenosis.[24,25] Recently Spine Patient Outcome Research Trial (SPORT) has reported re-operation rates of 13% at 4 years follow up.[3]

In the past the diagnosis depended on indirect findings of bulbous spinous processes, diminished interlaminar space on plain X-rays and hour glass constriction on coronal view of iophenydol (myodil myelogram). Basically the pathology involves cauda equina compression and some investigators in the past tried to establish the severity by measuring the antero-posterior diameter of less than 15 mm to confirm the diagnosis as well as severity. It is common in lumbar canal stenosis to get complete obstruction of thecal sac in both AP and LAT views of a myelogram (myelographic block) (Fig. 1.1). In fact the block can be reversed by assuming flexion posture suggesting the clinical diagnosis of LCS. Advent of MRI has provided better understanding and more objective evaluation of the pathology.

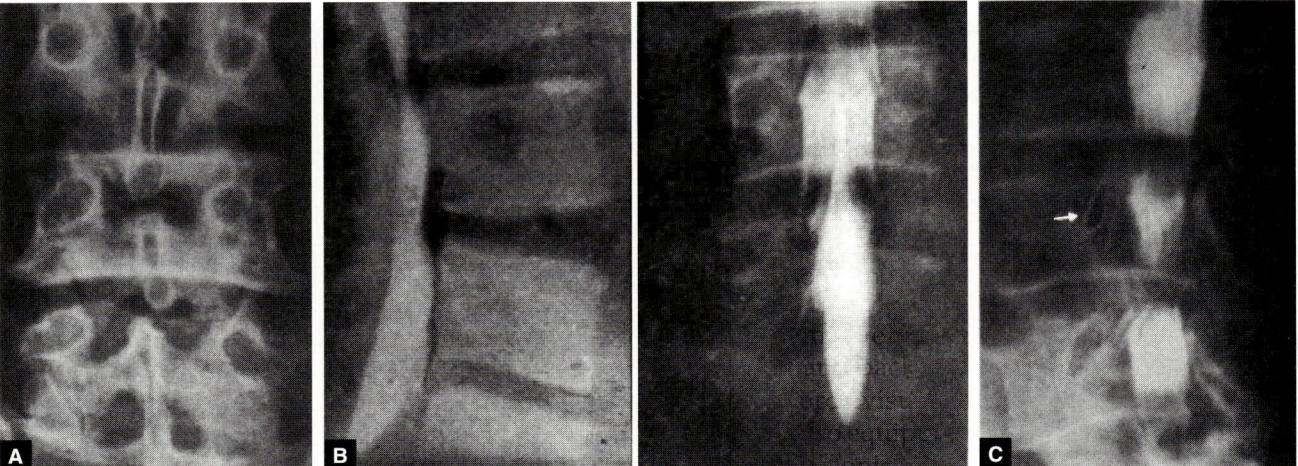

Fig. 1.1A to C: (A) Plain X-ray showing bulbous spinous processes, obliteration of interlaminar space and coronal orientation of facets in spinal stenosis; (B) Myelogram showing hour glass defect due to facet hypertrophy without any evidence of disc prolapse; (C) Myelogram showing multiple spinal stenosis

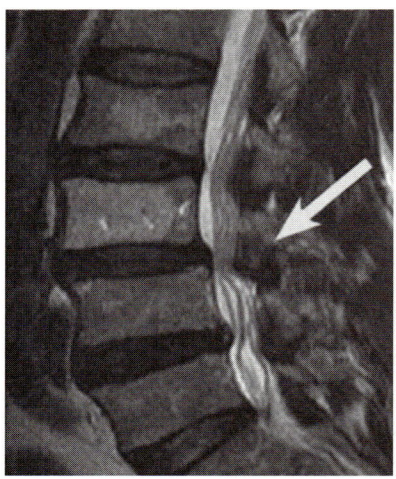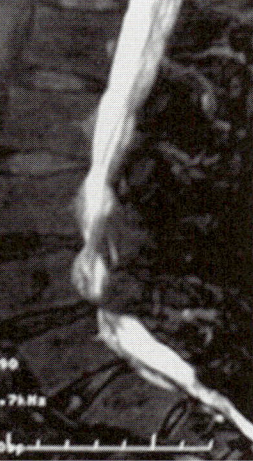

Fig. 1.2: MRI sagittal view showing lumbar canal stenosis in the elderly (lateral recess stenosis)

Lumbar canal stenosis is thus a degenerative process causing hypertrophy of bones and narrowing of spinal canal and intervertebral foramina causing compression of cauda equina and exiting nerve roots (Fig. 1.2). The correct management depends on accurate delineation of severity and extent of cauda equina compression. Two factors contribute to stenosis. (i) Spondylotic changes and (ii) Narrowing of the canal causing thecal sac compression.[18] Usually it is common at more than one level but the level L4/5 is most common and next common is L3/4. Prolapse of intervertebral disc is not a part of the syndrome although it can be associated with stenosis.

It can be seen from the above description that LCS starts and progresses as a result of abnormal micromotion in the interverbral disc and the facet joints. It is necessary to understand the motion segment of the spine.

Historical Background

The beginning of the 14th century saw emergence from the dark age to Renaissance period of free thinking. It was born in Italy and then spread to Europe and other parts. Several people fled from the dark age of belief in God to the new era of free thinking and humanism. One of them was Hippocrates who fled from Constantinople after its fall to Turks in 1453.[29] Although, he did not write specifically much on lumbar canal stenosis, he did have interest in spine and described several other ailments.

The write up on spine came from Egypt. Imhotep (2686 BC approx.) is the original author and he has described 48 spinal cases and these scriptures were acquired by Edwin Smith at the beginning of the 19th century[23] and now they are known as Edwin Smith Papyrus. It is only in 1803 that Portal specifically described the concept of lumbar canal stenosis. More

information came forwards through the writings of several authors in the subsequent years. In the years 1954 and 1955, Hank Verbiest from Holland[30,31] first recognized the clinical and surgical significance of stenosis in the lumbar canal. By then lumbar spinal surgery had well established. Epstein later described the pathological changes in the articular facets in both congenital and acquired spinal stenosis and gave description of compression of nerve roots in the intervertebral foramina. Much to my delight it was Ciric[5] who gave detailed account of narrowing of the lateral recesses causing compression of cauda equina and exiting nerve roots in the intervertebral foramina. Appreciation of exact pathology in LCS the operative techniques changed over time.

Fabricus Hildrain was the first to describe the technique of laminectomy for LCS in the 17th century.[23] Clerk et. al.[6] in 1969 recommended removal of enough bone during laminectomy to widen the lateral recesses. The concept of excision of medial portion of posterior facet was then described by several authors like Ciric,[5,11] Epstein,[14] Schatzer,[26] Schesinger[27] and Hopp[19] They also expressed concern for preserving pars in an attempt not to create instability.

By this time Junghans[20] had described the concept of motion segment and the surgeons, impressed by the concept, felt obliged to preserve the posterior motion segment while excising the compressive pathology. The present author then described and popularized the concept of IDSS (internal decompression for spinal stenosis) preserving the posterior functioning elements of the motion segment.

The process of stenosis passes through the phase of instability before settling to the phase of fixed deformity. The concept of IDSS has become all the more important in the present era of minimally invasive endoscopic or microscopic or endo-microscopic procedures.

In the present concept of minimally invasive spinal surgery (MISS) the endoscope allows bilateral decompression through unilateral approach. In 1983 Forst and Hausman introduced modified arthroscope into the intervertebral disc space and Kambin, famous for Kambin's triangle, showed the first endoscopic view of herniated nucleus pulposus in 1988.[16,21]

Normal Motion Segment

The 2 facet joints and the intervertebral disc along with interlaminar, interspinous and supraspinous space form the motion segment (Fig. 1.3). The concept of motion segment was first described by Junghans.[20] The brunt of abnormal motion is born by the bones in the absence of tensile strength which is present in the ligaments.

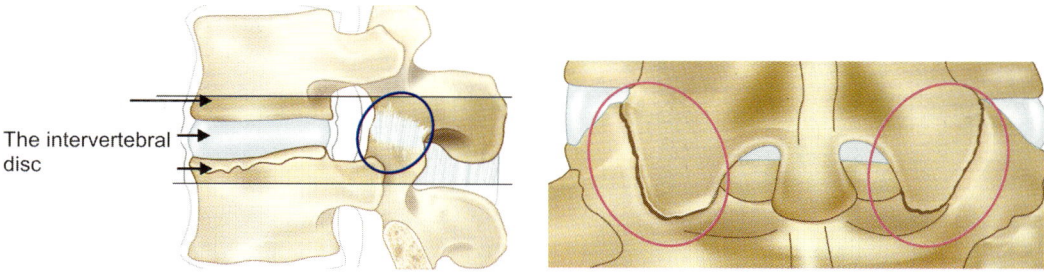

Fig. 1.3: The normal motion segment of the spine. It consists of the intervertebral disc and the adjacent vertebrae; the 2 facet joints; the capsule around the joints and interlaminar, interspinous and supraspinous ligaments

Factors Contributing to the Development of Lumbar Canal Stenosis

Besides degenerative process there are several other factors which contribute to its development.

1. Congenital narrow lumbar canal (not common)
2. Congenital short pedicles.
3. Degeneration causing hypertrophy and tropism in facets.
4. Settlement of disc space.
5. Upward migration of superior facet.
6. Associated prolapse of intervertebral disc.
7. Thickening and in curling of the ligamentum flavum.
8. Chronic calcified disc.
9. Formation of osteophytes along the vertebral margins.
10. Formation of synovial cyst.
11. Presence of degenerative spondylolisthesis.

Lateral Recess Stenosis

LCS can cause narrowing of the canal in the centre or laterally. Since the main culprit is facet joints, LCS is more common due to stenosis in the lateral recesses (Fig. 1.5). Narrowing of lateral recesses reduces the available space in the canal and in the intervertebral foramen.

Parameters to Define Stenosis

The bony spine develops quite fast and soon after birth with the result that by one year the mid-sagittal diameter of the canal is practically the same and by 3 years the width of canal is settled.

The mid sagittal AP diameter is 1.5 cm from one year till 12 years. In adults it is 1.7 cm. The width is established at 3 years and remains so till 12 years at 1.8 cm. In adults it is 2.1 cm. The third important parameter is the cross sectional area of the dural sac which in adults is 130 mm^2.

Lumbar canal stenosis can be severe or absolute or moderate or relative and mild.

Measurements

Mid-sagittal diameter (Fig. 1.4)
- 15 mm or more—normal
- 13 and 15 mm—mild
- 10 to 13 mm—moderate
- Less than 10 mm—severe

Lateral recess
- 5 mm or more—normal
- 4 to 5 mm—mild
- 3 to 4 mm—moderate
- Less than 3 mm—severe

Transverse area of the dural sac (Fig. 1.6)
- 130 mm or more—normal
- 120 to 130 mm—mild

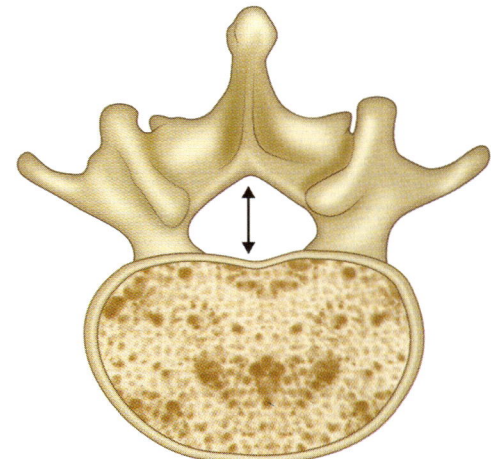

Fig. 1.4: Mid-sagittal diameter of the bony canal

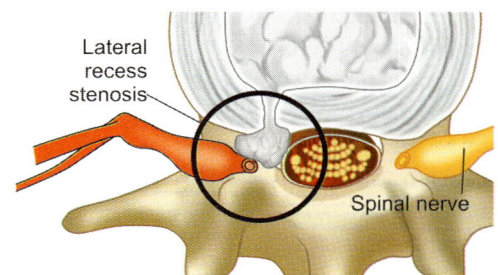

Fig. 1.5: Lateral recess of the bony canal (stenosis due to PIVD)

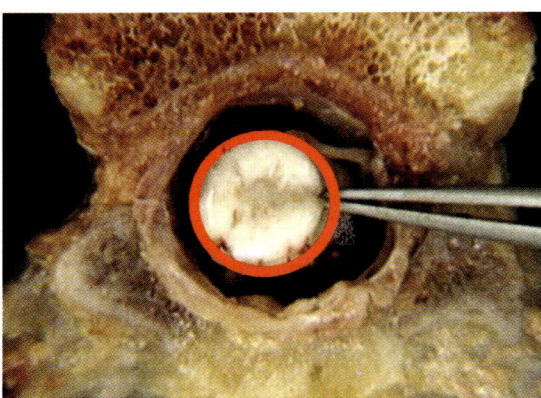

Fig. 1.6: Transverse diameter of the dural sac

- 100 to 120 mm—moderate
- Less than 100 mm—severe

Location of Stenosis

Stenosis can be at three areas.
1. *In the canal or central.* It is not so common in degenerative LCS stenosis.
2. *Lateral recess*: Most common in adults in degenerative disorder.
3. Most of the times lateral recess stenosis is associated with foraminal stenosis and it is mandatory to decompress the intervertebral foramen without causing instability in all such cases coming for surgery. The procedure involves excising extra portion of ligamentum flavum along with excision of capsule from undersurface of the superior facet. When ultrasound swiveling curette blade is available, the undersurface of bone compressing the exiting nerve root can be safely scrapped off to further decompress the nerve root.

Pathophysiology of degenerative process: Usually degeneration first starts in the disc space and leads to changes in the disc in chronological order as follows.
- Degeneration in the disc
- Settlement of disc space
- Narrowing of the foramen both at the top and bottom.
- Ligament flavum is incurled and buckled.

There is increased stress on the facets leading to abnormal micro motion resulting in facetal hypertrophy, osteophyte formation and medial rotation of posterior facet called tropism and upward migration of the tip of anterior facet.

Obligatory posterior disc bulge with associated osteophyte formation along the edges of the two vertebral bodies.

The facet joint being an important element in this process, needs further explanation.

Stress on the facet joint produces inflammation in the capsule causing sinovitis which is a painful process adding to backpain.

The cartilage in the facet joint then starts degenerating and getting thinned out. The capsule then becomes loose setting the stage for abnormal motion. This is known as **unstable phase in facet degeneration** and when surgical intervention is undertaken at this stage, the segment needs to be stabilized or fused. But this phase coming for surgery is not common.

Formation of osteophytes causes autostabilization in the segment and is known as **stable phase in facet degeneration**. When surgical intervention is undertaken there is no obligation for stabilization or fusion. This is the most common form of lumbar canal stenosis asking for surgery.

Principle of Management

The main culprit is abnormal motion in the facet joints. Philosophically if there was a process of halting this process, the problem of LCS would have been quickly solved. Attempts have been made either to fix the joint with screws or separate the joint surfaces by interposing a spacer or debriding the cortical bone and spreading a chrono granules strip (ChronOS) over it to achieve fusion and thus prevent abnormal motion but the results have not so far confirmed its success.

Dilemma

The standard principle of management has been liberal laminectomy, excision of ligamentum flavum, excision of any osteophytes, and opening the foramen by excising the capsule on the under surface of anterior facet and the procedure has given long term lasting relief from back pain. But recent studies show the procedure can create instability in the spine necessitation fusion.

Conclusion

The 31 vertebral units are joined together by three joints in each motion segment to constitute the spine which is flexible and can move in any direction except the sacrum and coccyx where the relevant units of vertebrae are fused together and do not have motion. The three joints are the two facet joints and the intervertebral disc as described earlier in motion segment. Slightest trauma or degeneration to one joint affect the whole motion unit and the slightest trauma to intervertebral disc immediately causes stress in facet joints.

Lumbar canal stenosis includes (i) central canal stenosis, (ii) lateral recess stenosis and (iii) foraminal stenosis. Prolapsed intervertebral disc could be associated with LCS but is not a part of syndrome.

REFERENCES

1. Alexander E. Significance of small lumbar canal. Cauda equine compression syndrome due to spondylosis. J. Neurosurg 1969; 31:513–519.
2. Appleby A, Joffe R, Arjona V. Intermittent ischaemia of the cauda equine due to stenosis of lumbar canal. J Neurol Neurosurg Psychiat 1966;29:315–318.
3. Budithi S, Dhawan R, Cattell A, et al. Only walking matters—assessment following lumbar stenosis decompression. Eur Spine J 2017;26: 481–487.
4. Chahal AS et. al. Lumbar canal stenosis; Paraplegia; Vol 20; 1982; 288–295.
5. Ciric I, Michael AM. The lateral recess syndrome. Neurosurgery ed. Wilkins, Rengachary. 2279–82.
6. Clark K. Significance of small lumbar canal. Cauda equine compression syndrome due to spondylosis. J. Neurosurg 1969;31: 495–98.
7. Cloward RB. Spinal Stenosis. Treatment by posterior lumbar interbody fusion. Spine. 1987;1:457–516.
8. Davis RJ, Errico TJ, Bae H, Auerbach JD. Decompression and Coflex interlaminar stabilization compared with decompression and instrumented spinal fusion for spinal stenosis and low-grade degenerative spondylolisthesis: two-year results from the prospective, randomized, multicenter, Food and Drug Administration Investigational Device Exemption trial. Spine (Phila Pa 1976) 2013;38:1529–39.
9. Delamarter RB. Sherman JE, Carr J. Lumbar spinal stenosis secondary to calcium pyrophosphate crystal deposition. Clin Orthop 1993;289: 127–130.
10. Deyo RA, Mirza SK, Martin Bl et al, Trends, major medical complications and charges associated with surgery for lumbar spinal stenosis in older adults. JAMA 2010;303:1259–1265.
11. Dodge LD, Bohlman HH, Rhodes R. Concurrent lumbar spinal stenosis and peripheral vascular disease. Clin Orthop 1988;141–148.
12. Donovan MJ, Gargano FP, Vining DQ, et al. A comparison of radiographic methods of diagnosis of constrictive lesions of the spinal canal. J Neurosurg 1978;49:360–368.
13. Ehni G. Significance of the small lumbar canal. Cauda equine compression syndrome due to spondylosis. J Neurosurg 1969;31:507–12.
14. Epstein JA, Epstein BS, Rosentahl AD, et al. Sciatica caused by nerve entrapment in the lateral rescess. J Neurosurg 1973;36:584–89.
15. Forsth P, Olafsson G, Carlsson T, et al. A randomized, controlled trial of fusion surgery for lumbar spinal stenosis. N Engl J Med 2016;374:1413–23.
16. Forst R, Hausmann B: Nucleoscopy—a new examination technique. Arch Orthop Trauma Surg1983;101:219–21.
17. Ghogawala Z, Dziura J, Butler WE, et al. Laminectomy plus fusion versus laminectomy alone for lumbar spondylolisthesis. N Engl J Med 2016;374:1424–34.
18. Hawkes CM and Roberts GM: Contemporary Neurology; Chap 1984;60; 564–74.
19. Hopp E, Tsou PM. Post decompression lumbar instability. Clin Orthop 1988;143–151.
20. Junghans J, Schmorl G. The human spine in health and disease. Published Grune and Stratton, NY. 2nd ed. 1977; 35–7.
21. Kambin P, Nixon JE, Chait A, et al. Annular protrusion: pathophysiology and roentgenographic appearance. Spine (Phila Pa 1976) 1988;13:671–675.
22. Modhia U, Takemoto S, Braid-Forbes MJ, et al. Readmission rates after decompression surgery in patients with lumbar spinal stenosis among medicare beneficiaries. Spine (Phila Pa 1976) 2013; 38:591–96.
23. Ramani PS, Sharma A. Brief history of spinal surgery. 1994;13–16.
24. Richter A. Schutz C, Hauck M, et al. Does an interspinous device (CoflexTM) improve the outcome of decompressive surgery in lumbar spinal stenosis? One-year follow up of a prospective case control study of 60 patients. Eur Spine J 2010;19:283–89.
25. Roder C, Baumgartner B, Berlemann U, Aghayev E. Superior outcome of decompression with an interlaminar dynamic device versus decompression alone in patients with lumbar spinal stenosis and back pain: a cross registry study. Eur Spine J 2015;24:2228–35.
26. Schatzer JT. Pennal GF. Spinal stenosis, a cause of cauda equine compression. J Bone Jt Surg. 1968;50(3):606–18.
27. Schlesinger PT. Falls G. Law lumbar nerve root compression and adequate operative exposure. J Bone JtSurg 1957;39:541–53.
28. Sigmundsson FG, Jonsson B, Stromqvist B. Outcome of decompression with and without fusion in spinal stenosis with degenerative spondylolisthesis in relation to preoperative pain pattern: a register study of 1,624 patients. Spine J 2015;15:638–46.
29. Udwadia FE. Man and Medicine. Oxford University Press. Chap 2000; 25:159–60.
30. Verbiest H. A radicular syndrome from developmental narrowing of the lumbar vertebral canal. J Bone Joint Surg 1654;36B:230–237.
31. Verbiest H. Further experience on the pathological influence of a developmental narrowing of the lumbar vertebral canal. J Bone Joint Surg 1955;37B:576–81.
32. Weinstein JN, Tosteson TD, Lurie JD, et al. Surgical versus nonsurgical therapy for lumbar spinal stenosis. N Eng J Med 2008; 358:794–810.

2

Historical Landmarks in the Development of Degenerative Lumbar Canal Stenosis

PS Ramani

Lumbar canal stenosis was first observed in 1880 in Egyptian mummies.[6] The aging spine is but natural phenomenon as age advances. The degenerative process produces bending of the spine and kyphotic deformity resulting in aged people walking bending forwards.

Patient found relief on bending forwards (bony canal becomes long and the nerve). In 1893 English surgeon Lane did surgery in lumbar canal stenosis to decompress cauda equina and the patient obtained relief.[5]

In 1900 Sachs and Frenkel described a successfully operated patient and observed that before surgery.

The patient could walk with some comfort by bending forwards but after surgery he could walk comfortably in erect position. The canal is stretched along with nerve roots in flexion but in extension they are shorted and crowded superseded by in curling of ligamentum flavum and prolapsed disc.[8]

During this period the motion segment of spine was described by Junghans and he felt that any degeneration in one part will produce instability.[3]

The concept was followed further by R. Roy Camille when he divided the spine into three columns as follows.[7]

Anterior column: Anterior and posterior long. Ligaments, the vertebra and intervertebral disc.

Middle column: The two facet joints and the laminae.

Posterior column: Spinous processes and intra and supraspinous ligaments.

He too opined like Junghans that degeneration in one column will produce degenerative changes in all columns of the biomechanical construct.

A Danish radiologist CI Baastrup in 1933 described Baastrup disease. But he observed only the posterior column and went on to describe the grades in the development starting with breakdown in the interspinous ligament with abutment, enlargement, sclerosis and formation of bursa resulting in deformity which he called "Kissing Spine".

He described four types:
- Type I: End to end touching of spinous processes.
- Type II: Hypertrophy of spinous processes.
- Type III: Ball and socket formation.
- Type IV: Oblique lie.

He opined that loss of lordosis happened due to disc degeneration and hypertrophy in the spinous processes.[1]

The degenerated facet joints were further classified into four types by Grogan but Fujiwara graded them depending on formation of osteophytes.

The concept of biomechanical columns and degeneration was scientifically first described by Kirkaldy and Willis in 1978.[4]

He described three joint complex being intervertebral disc and the two facet joints, i.e. anterior and middle column. He ignored the posterior column.

In 2014, Bam Bang Darwono from Jakarta in Indonesia has proposed a new classification called Jakarta 2014 classification including all the three columns and has suggested appropriate treatment including stabilization depending on the grade and extent of degeneration.[2]

Conclusion

It is concluded that degeneration in any column has a tremendous bearance on other 2 columns and therefore the surgical strategy should be such that decompression and stabilization will address to keep all 3 columns healthy.

REFERENCES

1. Baastrup C.I. Pathological changes in the spinous processes of lumbar vertebrae.; Acta Radiol; 1933;14; 52–54.

2. Bam Bang Darwono: Personal communication. Paper in press.

3. Junghans J, Schmorl G. The human spine in health and disease. 2nd Ed. NY:Grune and Straton:1971;35–7.

4. Kirkaldy Willis et. al. The concept of degeneration in the vertebral columns; Spine 1978;3(4); 319.

5. Lane WA. Case of spondylolisthesis associated with progressive paraplegia: Laminectomy. Lancet 1893;1: 991.

6. Portal A. Cours d' AnatomieMedicaleou Elements de I'Anatomie de I'Homme. Vol 1; Paris: Baudouin, 1803.

7. Roy-Camille R, Saillant G, Mazel C. Plating of thoracic, thoracolumbar and lumbar in juries with pedicle screw plates. Orthop. Clin. N. Am.;1986;Jan17(1):147–59.

8. Sachs B, Fraenkel J. Progressive ankylotic rigidity of the spine (SpondyloseRhezomelique). J NervMent Dis. 1900;27:1–15.

Epidemiology of Lumbar Canal Stenosis

Ahmed Nouby, PS Ramani

INTRODUCTION

Despite the fact that lumbar canal stenosis (LCS) is one of the most commonly diagnosed pathological conditions, very little is known about the epidemiology of stenosis in the general population. The main reason for the dilemma is the fact that till today no co-relation has been found between patient's symptoms and radiological findings as many patients with gross radiological findings are proved to be asymptomatic. This is a big hindrance for population survey in any area.

Another difficulty in performing any epidemiologic analysis is the absence of universally accepted diagnostic criteria for Lumbar canal stenosis.[8] Magnetic resonance imaging (MRI) and computed tomography (CT) are the most frequently utilized diagnostic modalities in clinical practice, but strict measurements defining the presence of clinically significant canal, subarticular, or foraminal narrowing do not exist, for example, Fanuele et al.[7] reported a prevalence of 13.1% among 17,744 patients. This was a large study utilizing a multicenter clinical database without providing criteria for diagnosis of LCS. Typically, the preliminary diagnosis is based on clinical symptoms and signs.

Researchers tried to classify lumbar canal stenosis as an attempt to unify the criteria upon which the diagnosis can be made. One classification is according to the etiology into congenital (developmental) and acquired (degenerative).[2] Another is according to the degree of stenosis as judged by AP diameter of bony canal into relative (≤12 mm) and absolute (≤10 mm).

Another group of researchers have described cross-sectional area (<70 mm^2) of spinal cord.[14] For lateral recess stenosis height and depth of the lateral recess and for foraminal stenosis the foraminal diameter were typically investigated. Of all such investigations the highest rated quantitative criterion has been the antero-posterior diameter of the osseous canal.

In spite of increasing use of diagnostic imaging, the association of spinal stenosis radiographic findings with symptoms remains unclear. LCS is one of the most common indications for spinal surgery today and, therefore, a clear understanding of its prevalence in the community and its association with symptoms is greatly needed.

Lumbar Canal Stenosis and Age

Age range: Middle-aged and elderly population.

LCS is the most common cause in patients above 65 years needing spinal surgery.[6]

The exact prevalence of LCS is still unknown. It is estimated that more than 200,000 adults are affected by LCS in the United States,[13] and will rise to 64 million elderly adults by the year 2025,[14] but roughly it is around one in 1,000 patients per year, over the age of 65 years.[10]

In one study the prevalence of congenital LCS did not change with age (p = 0.455 for relative LCS, and P = 0.601 for absolute LCS). However, as expected, the prevalence of acquired LCS increased with age (p = 0.015 for relative LCS, and P = 0.034 for absolute LCS). The prevalence of relative and absolute LCS increased from 16.0 to 38.8% and from 4.0 to 14.3% between age group 40 and 60 years. In another study, the prevalence of radiographic stenosis in a sample of patients 60–69 years old was 47% for relative stenosis and 19% for absolute stenosis, but it was only a radiological finding. It did not mean that the patient was symptomatic. Symptomatic stenosis typically present in patients in the fifth to seventh decade of life.

Lumbar Canal Stenosis and Sex

Some researchers made an attempt to correlate sex to the incidence of lumbar canal stenosis but their analysis did not prove their assumption.[11,12] Among 11,283 cases studied, no statistically significant differences were found.[4]

Types of Lumbar Canal Stenosis

Putting together all types of stenosis (congenital or acquired), the prevalence of relative LCS was 23.6% and of absolute LCS 8.4%.

Splitting the group, the Framingham Study[9] found that congenital relative lumbar canal stenosis was 4.7% and absolute lumbar canal stenosis was 2.6% and acquired relative lumbar canal stenosis was 22.5% and absolute LCS was 7.3% in a population study aged 60–69 years.

Consistent with previous reports and consensus opinion, the results demonstrate that the prevalence of acquired LCS increases with age.

Lumbar Canal Stenosis and Different Levels

It occurs most frequently at L4–L5 level, followed by L5–S1 and L3–L4 levels. However, one study concluded that LCS is more prevalent at L5 than L4 and that individuals with AP canal diameters ≤12 mm, particularly at L5 have a statistically significant association between LCS and occurrence of LBP, odds ratio (OR = 0.3) (95% CI: 0.4–0.7).

In yet one more, the authors reported that the L5 root was involved in 91%, S1 in 63%, L1 to L4 in 28%, and S2 to S5 in 5%. Only 35% of their patients had single root involvement, the others having multiple roots involvement.[1]

Lumbar Canal Stenosis and Clinical Presentation

Lumbar canal stenosis can be asymptomatic or symptomatic.

Prevalence in asymptomatic individuals over 55 was distributed as follows: 21–30% for moderate radiographic stenosis and 6–7% for severe. Haig and colleagues[3] using a cut-point of 11.5 mm found 23% prevalence of LSS in 31 asymptomatic individuals. In an MRI study of 67 individuals who had never had LBP, sciatica, or neurogenic claudication. Boden and colleagues[15] found LCS in one percent of individuals younger than 60, and 21% in individuals over 60 years old. Wiesel and colleagues[5] reported that among 52 asymptomatic individuals over 40 years of age, 50% of CT scans were abnormal with the most common diagnosis being lumbar canal stenosis and facet degeneration.

The general incidence of symptomatic stenosis ranging from 1.7 to 8%.[1] The clinical hallmark finding of LCS is neurogenic intermittent claudication, presenting as intermittent pain or paresthesia in the legs brought on by walking and standing, and classically relieved with flexion. However, other symptoms are also frequent. It has been reported[1] that 95% of patients with LCS presented with back pain, 91% claudication, 71% leg pain, 33% weakness, and 12% voiding disturbances.

REFERENCES

1. Amundsen T, Weber H, Lilleas F, Nordal HJ, Abdelnoor M, Magnaes B. Lumbar spinal stenosis: clinical and radiologic features. Spine 1995; 20:1178–86. 5.
2. Arnoldi CC, Brodsky AE, Cauchoix J, Crock HV, Dommisse GF, Edgar MA, et al. Lumbar spinal stenosis and nerve root entrapment syndromes. Definition and classification. ClinOrthopRelat Res. 1976:4–5.
3. Boden SD, Davis DO, Dina TS, Patronas NJ, Wiesel SW. Abnormal magnetic-resonance scans of the lumbar spine in asymptomatic subjects. A prospective investigation. J Bone Joint Surg Am. 1990;72:403–408.
4. Ciol MA, Deyo RA, Howell E, et al. An assessment of surgery for spinal stenosis: time trends, geographic variations, complications, and reoperations. J Am GeriatrSoc 1996;44:285–90. (Ref not found)
5. De Villiers PD, Booysen EL. Fibrous spinal stenosis: a report on 850 myelograms with a water soluble contrast medium. ClinOrthop 1976; 115:140–4.
6. Deyo RA, Gray DT, Kreuter W, et al. United States trends in lumbar fusion surgery for degenerative conditions. Spine (Phila Pa 1976) 2005;30:1441-5; discussion 1446–7.
7. Fanuele JC, Birkmeyer NJ, Abdu WA, Tosteson TD, Weinstein JN. The impact of spinal problems on the health status of patients: have we underestimated the effect? Spine. 2000;25:1509–1514.
8. Gunzburg R, Keller TS, Szpalski M, Vandeputte K, Spratt KF. A prospective study on CT scan outcomes after conservative decompression surgery for lumbar spinal stenosis. J Spinal Disord Tech. 2003;16:261–67.
9. Haig AJ, Geisser ME, Tong HC, Yamakawa KS, Quint DJ, Hoff JT, et al. Electromyographic and magnetic resonance imaging to predict lumbar stenosis, low-back pain, and no back symptoms. J Bone Joint Surg Am. 2007;89:358–66.
10. Jansson KA, Blomqvist P, Granath F, Nemeth G. Spinal stenosis surgery in Sweden 1987–1999. Eur Spine J. 2003;12:535–41.
11. Kalichman L, Cole R, Kim DH, et al. Spinal stenosis prevalence and association with symptoms: the Framingham Study. Spine J 2009;9:545–50.
12. LaBan MM, Imas A. "Young" lumbar spinal stenotic: review of 268 patients younger than 51 years. Am J Phys Med Rehabil. 2003;82:69–71.
13. Lurie J, Tomkins-Lane C. Management of lumbar spinal stenosis. BMJ 2016;352:h6234.
14. Steurer J, Roner S, Gnannt R, Hodler J. Quantitative radiologic criteria for the diagnosis of lumbar spinal stenosis: a systematic literature review. BMC MusculoskeletDisord. 2011;12:175. doi: 10.1186/1471-2474-12-175.
15. Wiesel SW, Tsourmas N, Feffer HL, Citrin CM, Patronas N. A study of computer-assisted tomography. I. The incidence of positive CAT scans in an asymptomatic group of patients. Spine. 1984;9:549–51.

Anatomical Determinants of Lumbar Spine

Arjun Dhar, PS Ramani

INTRODUCTION

The lumbar spine, located between the sacrum and thoracic regions of the vertebral column, typically consists of five vertebrae. These five vertebrae generally increase in size from the superior to the inferior lumbar spine and are larger than both the cervical and thoracic vertebrae. Similar to size, the weight-bearing ability of lumbar vertebrae is often greater, resulting in a higher incidence of pain following injury. From a mechanical point of view, the weight-bearing or structural capacity of the vertebrae depends on both material properties (bone mineral content, trabecular bone tissue density, and apparent density) and geometric properties (size, orientation, and connectivity of bone elements) (Fig. 4.1).

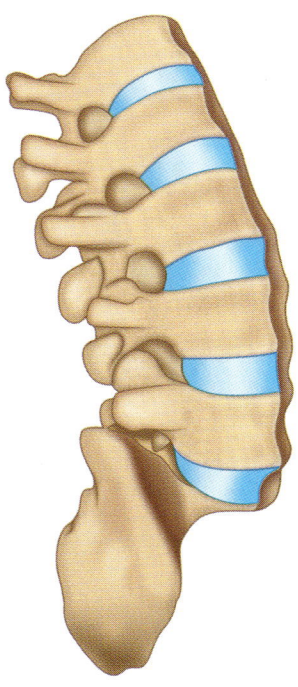

Fig. 4.1: The lumbar spine

Features of a Lumbar Vertebra

1. They are large in size
2. Absence of costal facets
3. The body is wider transversely
4. Vertebral canal is elliptically round to triangular, larger than in thoracic segment of spine
5. Pedicles are short
6. Spinous process is horizontal
7. The anterior facet joint faces posteromedially
8. The posterior facet joint faces anterolaterally

Mechanical Properties

Mechanical properties not only vary from vertebra to vertebra or level to level, but also can vary dramatically within a given vertebral body. Trabeculae tend to be denser, rod-like structures in the inferior and superior sections in contrast to the less dense, plate-like trabeculae that are associated with the central region of the lumbar vertebral centrum.

The anterior column, or centrum, of human vertebrae is comprised of only a very thin cortical shell (less than 2 mm), which is virtually indistinguishable from the trabeculae that comprise the bulk of the vertebral centrum.

The superior facet joint in the lumbar vertebrae are oriented anterolateral to the inferior articular facets of the vertebra above and are directed dorsomedially. From L1 to L5, the pedicles become larger in diameter and become more medially oriented.[6,7]

Ligaments Stabilizing the Anterior and Posterior Elements of Lumbar Spine

Several ligamentous structures stabilize the bony elements of the vertebrae.

The supraspinous and interspinous ligaments connect the spinous processes, while the intertransverse ligaments segmentally connect the transverse processes. The ligamentum flavum passes between the ventral side of the lamina to the superior lip of the next caudal lamina. The ligamentum flavum has a midline raphe, providing a convenient plane through which the canal may be entered. The broad anterior longitudinal ligament runs the length of the spinal column, intimately integrated with the periosteum of the anterior vertebral body, while the posterior longitudinal ligament lies along the posterior aspect of the vertebral body, adhering strongly to the intervertebral discs.

Vertebral Body

The posterior aspect of both vertebral bodies have both a mediolateral and superoinferior concavity. Only the opposing ends of L5 and S1 bodies demonstrate no mediolateral concavity and hence they and their intervening intervertebral disc have an elliptical outline in transverse section rather than usual kidney shape. There is no complete cortical bony end plate covering the vertebral body ends, there is only a peripheral rim of compact bone. Rest of the end of vertebral body made up of cancellous bone is in direct apposition with hyaline cartilage end plates (Fig. 4.2 and Table 4.1).

Vascular supply of vertebral body: There is a network of periosteal arteries joining the arteries of adjacent vertebrae on the anterolateral and posterior surfaces. These are prominent between the fourth and fifth lumbar arteries. There are three types of intraosseous arteries: Equatorial, metaphyseal and peripheral. Each supplies a separate zone. The peripheral arteries are short, branch early and have centripetally directed terminal branches; they supply the outer collar of the vertebral body. The equatorial and metaphyseal arteries are morphologically similar, having straight unbranching stems, pre-terminal coils and centrifugal terminal branches. The equatorial arteries supply the central core of the vertebral body subjacent to the nucleus pulposus, and the metaphyseal arteries supply an annular zone between the other two types.[4]

The shape of the bony canal is elliptical at L1 and L2, triangular at L3 and becomes trifoliate in shape L5. This change in shape is attributable to the progressive shortening of lower lumbar pedicles (Fig. 4.3).

The Pedicle

The dimension, location, orientation and shape of pedicle varies substantially at different vertebral levels. It is generally not recognized that changes in pedicle morphology are primary determinants of spinal canal shape, configuration of lateral recesses and the three dimensional anatomy of intervertebral foramina (Fig. 4.4 and Table 4.2).

- The pedicle of the lumbar vertebrae are short and strong
- Arise posterolaterally from each vertebra
- Superior vertebral notch is shallow

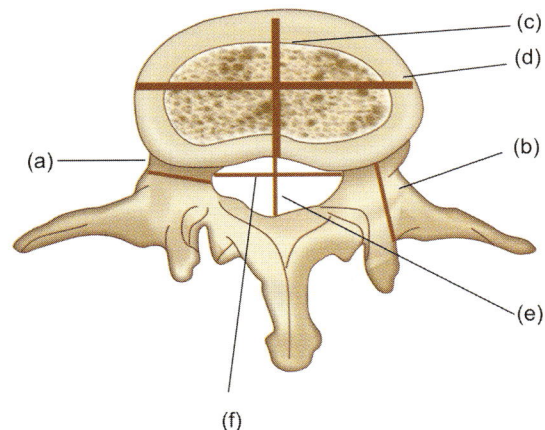

Fig. 4.2: Dimensions showing in particular the AP and transverse diameter of the vertebral body. (a) Pedicle width; (b) Pedicle length; (c) AP diameter of vertebral body; (d) Transverse diameter of vertebral body; (e) AP diameter of bony canal and (f) Transverse diameter of bony canal

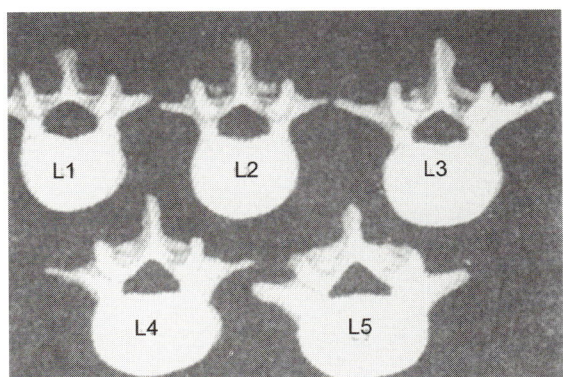

Fig. 4.3: The bony spinal canal

Table 4.1: Measurements of vertebral body									
Anteroposterior	32.41	+4.87	30.58	+2.09	32.07	+1.86	33.19	+2.59	37.28	+5.04
Transverse	40.61	+3.82	40.16	+2.88	41.28	+2.21	44.31	+2.07	51.46	+6.44

Table 4.2: Measurements of transverse and AP diameters of the vertebral canal									
Transverse	22.46	+1.35	22.80	+2.14	23.98	+2.09	26.38	+2.43	29.78	+3.50
AP	16.75	+0.7	15.85	+1.1	15.09	1.2	15.46	+1.0	16.36	+1.0

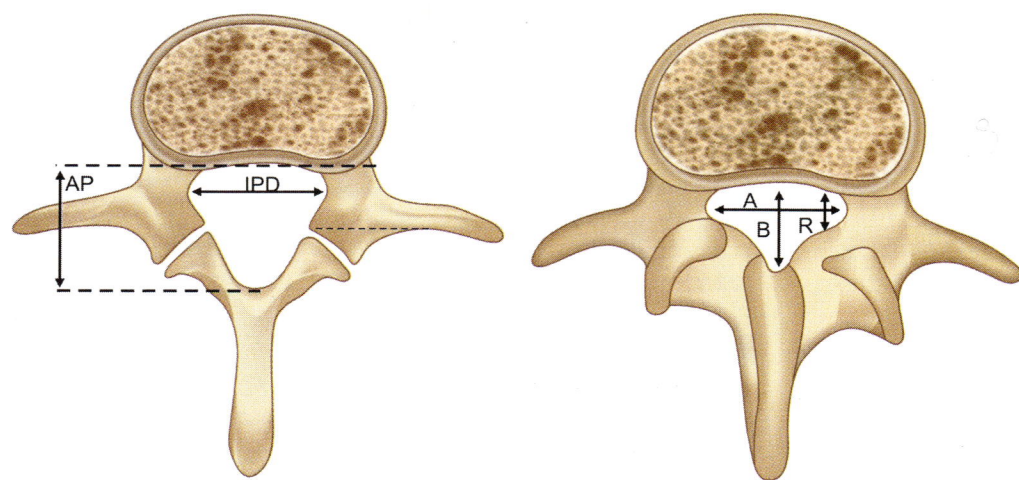

Fig. 4.4: Shape of bony canal. AP represents the anteroposterior diameter. IPD represents the interpedicular distance or horizontal diameter. Note the change in the canal changes to trifoliate shape as we move down from L1 to L5. A: Interpedicular distance, B: AP diameter of canal, R: Angle of lateral recess

- The inferior vertebral notch is deep
- Progressively shortened from L1–S1
- It supports posteriorly superior and inferior articular processes; laterally the transverse process; medially the lamina
- The interpedicle distance increases from L1 to L5.

The changes in pedicle morphology is nature's adaptation to the increasing load bearing demands of the pedicle. The width of the pedicles increases as we go down, hence increasing the mediolateral dimension of the intervertebral foramen. The interpedicle distance increases at lower lumbar levels. This contributes to formation of lateral recesses by contributing to the encroachment of superior articular process over the posterolateral aspect of the spinal canal. The posterior end of the lower lumbar pedicles are farther away from the midline. The inferior surface of the pedicles are farther away from the midline conforming to the obliquity and congruency of the sacroiliac joint. The anteroposterior dimension of the pedicles of lower lumbar vertebra decreases at their superior margin which causes the superior articular process to create lateral recesses.[13]

Functions of the Pedicle

- It forms the lateral support for the tripod made by vertebral body anteriorly and facet joints posterolaterally.
- It forms weight transmitting strut between vertebral arch posteriorly and vertebral body anteriorly.
- Helps to transmit load both gravitational and muscle induced.

Pedicular width: Transverse diameter of the pedicle measured from both external cortexes of the pedicle. Transverse width of the pedicle is the anatomic parameter that mostly affects the feasibility of screw placement.

Pedicular length: Measured by a horizontal line from the posterior border of the vertebral body at the level of the upper border of the pedicle to the posterior border of the upper articular facet (Fig. 4.5 and Table 4.3).

Pedicle height is measured by joining two cortical surfaces vertically.

Pedicles are intimately related inferomedially to the nerve roots in the lateral recess and the dorsal root ganglion in the upper part of the intervertebral foramen. The superomedial and inferolateral aspects of the pedicles are separated from the neural structures.

Surgical Landmarks for Insertion of Pedicle Screws

Roy-Camille point: It is the point of intersection of a vertical line through the facet joint and a horizontal line through the middle of insertion of transverse process.[12]

Steffee point: It is the point of convergence of mammillary ridge on the superior articular facet, the ridge on the pars inter-articularis and ridge on the transverse process.

Weinstein point: Lateral and inferior corner of the inferior articular facet.[14]

Ramani point: 1 mm inferior and lateral to the Weinstein point. More useful in L4 lumbar vertebra.

The transverse angulation of a pedicle determines the medial angulation required for placement of a pedicle screw. From L1 down to S1 the transverse angle gradually increases approximately 5 degrees per level. The angle at S1 is approximately 20 to 25 degrees. The pedicle of L5 is not straight and is angled medially by 30 degrees.

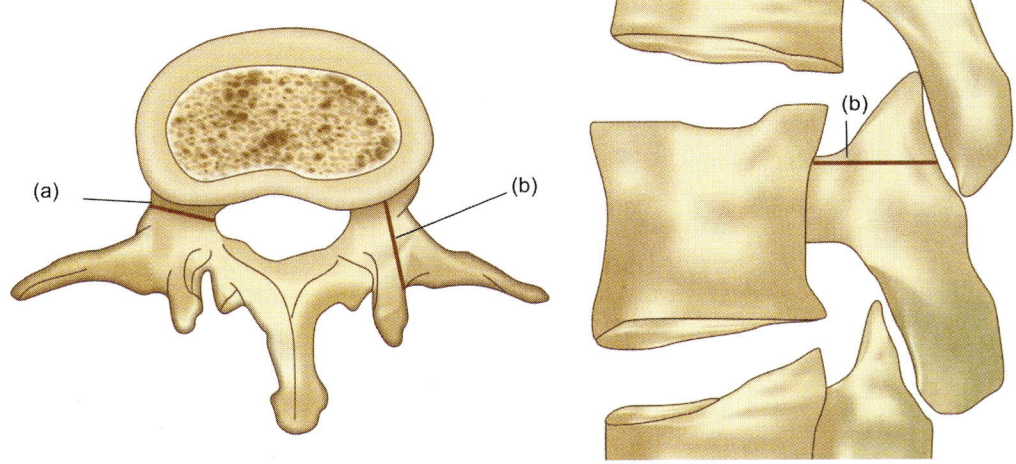

Fig. 4.5: Pedicle width (a) and pedicle length (b)

Table 4.3: Measurements of pedicle in lumbar spine										
Width	7.81	+1.30	8.26	+1.42	9.57	+0.99	10.79	+0.59	14.36	+1.85
Length	20.92	+2.62	19.86	+2.93	17.57	+2.12	16.67	17.23	17.23	+1.35

Bony Lateral Recess

Bounded laterally by pedicles. Medial boundary by an anteriorly directed plane constructed from the obtuse angle bend made by superior and inferior ligamentum flavum on the anterior aspect of lamina. Anteriorly by the posterior aspect of the vertebral body. The posterior boundary of the upper portion of lateral recess is formed by lower part of superior articular process while the posterior boundary of the lower portion by the pars inter-articularis. Since the lower part of the lamina slopes posteriorly, this also contributes to the increasing antero-posterior dimension of the lower lateral recess (Fig. 4.6).

Lateral recess are frequently present at L3 and L4, consistently present at L5 and usually present at S1 (Tables 4.4 to 4.6).

Lateral recess angle <30 degrees suggests stenosis.

Table 4.4: Measurements of height of lateral recess					
	L1	**L2**	**L3**	**L4**	**L5**
Mean	3.44	3.24	2.92	2.36	2.6

Table 4.5: Measurements of angle of lateral recess (standard values)					
	L1	**L2**	**L3**	**L4**	**L5**
Mean	25.88	24.94	24.64	23.44	23.12

Table 4.6: Lateral recess height	
5 mm	Normal
4–5 mm	Narrow
3–4 mm	Stenotic
2–3 mm	Severely stenotic

Laminae

From L1 to L5, the laminae show an increasing medio-lateral dimension increasing the stability of the tripod system. Only the upper part of the laminae enters into formation of posterior wall of osteo-ligamentous spinal canal. The lower part of each canal slopes posteriorly where ligamentum flavum is attached to the midlamina anteriorly. Surgical removal of this part of ligamentum aids in complete exposure of contents of spinal canal.

Articular Facets

As the anteroposterior dimension of superior margin of the pedicle is shorter than its inferior margin and because of the posterior slope of the lower part of the lamina, the superior articular facets are situated anteriorly than the inferior facets, hence forming the posterior wall of intervertebral foramen and upper part of the bony lateral recess. This statement does conclude that any hypertrophic degenerative changes involving the superior facet can contribute to the stenosis of lower part of the intervertebral foramen and the upper part of the lateral recess.

3 mm was defined as the criterion for defining lateral recess stenosis.

The posterior margins of both superior and inferior articular facets are farther from midline than their anterior margins at all lumbar levels which causes superior facets to face posteromedially and inferior facets to face anterolaterally. The orientation changes from sagittal to coronal from upper to lower lumbar levels. This coronal orientation is indeed a blessing for all humans as it directs vertebral loads across the sacro-

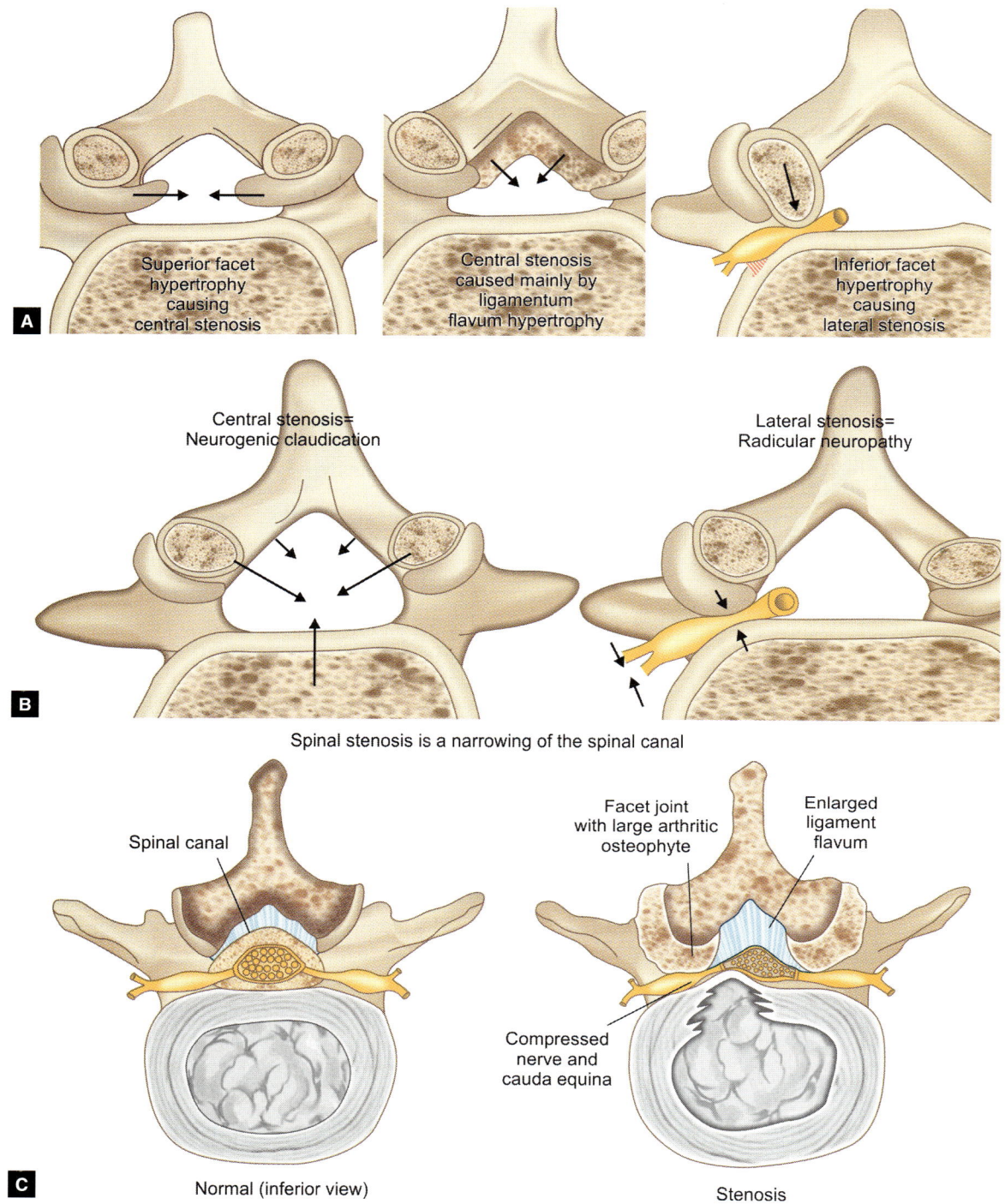

Fig. 4.6A to C: Stenosis in the central part of the canal as well as the lateral recesses

iliac joint to the acetabulum and also resists forward displacement of L5 on S1.

It is interesting to note that shortness of both pars interarticularis and pedicles at L5–S1 level reduces the moment arm (lever) of the forces applied to these supporting surfaces. However, the failure of pars interarticularis of L5 in spondylosis occurs because of its relative orientation being at right angles to the direction of forces applied against the inferior facet.

Average angles of facet joints relative to the spinous process as an aid to the insertion of transfacetal screws Table 4.7).

Table 4.7: Angle of facet joint				
Level	L1–L2	L2–L3	L3–L4	L4–L5	L5–S1
Angle	25 (15–47)	28 (17–51)	3 (15–57)	48 (13–70)	53 (36–70)

Surgical Landmark for Transfacetal Screws

The trajectory of transfacetal screws starts at the junction of the pars interarticularis and the inferior facet. The goal is to ultimately place the screw perpendicular to the joint surface, with final purchase into the bone of the adjacent pedicle through the superior articular process. Each level has a different orientation of the facet surface.

The Intervertebral Foramen

Bounded superiorly by inferior margin of pedicle of higher vertebra, anteriorly upper half by posterior aspect of higher vertebral body while the lower half by the posterior aspect of disc and small contribution by the posterior aspect of lower vertebral body, posteriorly the upper part is formed by the pars interarticularis while lower portion by the superior articular process of the lower vertebra.

Contents of the intervertebral foramen are the exiting nerve root with the dural sleeve, lymphatic channels, segmental artery, communicating veins between internal and external venous plexi, recurrent meningeal (sinu-vertebral) nerves, adipose tissue, ligaments.

The IVF from L1 to L4 is more the shape of an inverted pear, and at L5, it is more oval. The superior-inferior dimensions of the IVF are greatest at L2–L3. This length decreases as we move caudally, with the shortest lengths found at L5–S1. The anterior-posterior (AP) dimensions change from 7 mm at L1–L2 to 9 mm at L5–S1 (Table 4.8).[1,9]

Surgical Landmarks for Transforaminal Endoscopic Approach

Kambin triangle: It is a safe area described by the author for access to the herniated disk lies between the exiting and traversing nerve root. Kambin described this triangular safe zone in 1991 (Fig. 4.7) as being the annular zone bordered anteriorly by the exiting root, inferiorly by the end plate of the lower lumbar segment, posteriorly by the superior articular process of the inferior vertebra, and medially by the traversing root.

Intervertebral Disc (Fig. 4.8)

The IVD is a vital component of the joint system present at each spinal level. This system allows for the range of motion permitted at each segment. Each IVD works in conjunction with the paired dorsal zygapophyseal joints

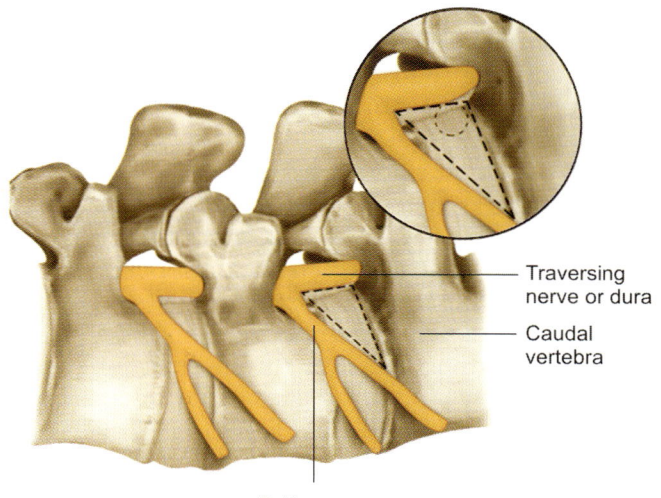

Fig. 4.7: Safe triangular zone of Kambin

Labels: Traversing nerve or dura; Caudal vertebra; Exiting nerve

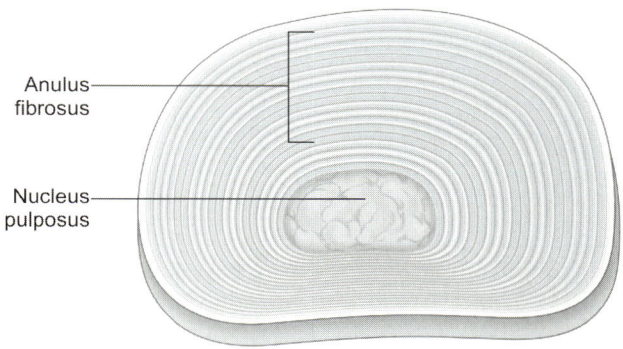

Fig. 4.8: Normal intervertebral disc

Labels: Anulus fibrosus; Nucleus pulposus; Intervertebral disc

to form a "three-joint complex." The function of the individual components of this complex are intimately related, as are their effects on one another during the degenerative process.

The bulk of the disc is made up of a central nucleus pulposus (NP) and the surrounding anulus fibrosus. The NP is 80% water, with proteoglycans contributing to 50% of its dry weight. The NP is rich in type II collagens. The outer AF is a tougher, less flexible component, composed primarily of densely packed type I collagen fibers. The inner AF is a softer, less dense, and more cartilaginous component, composed primarily of type II collagen fibers. Interface between the bony vertebral body and the disc itself. Their composition is similar to the disc; that is, made up of proteoglycans, type II collagen, and water. The end plates range from 0.5 to 1.5 mm in thickness. They are thinnest at the center where they interface with the NP.[10]

The most significant biochemical change in the degenerating disc is the net loss of proteoglycan[8,11]

In the young disc, aggrecan is the predominant proteoglycan. In the mature adult disc, only 10% of the

Table 4.8: Measurements of intervertebral foramen	
Height	>29 mm normal
	22–29 mm narrow
	<22 mm severely narrow
Width	2–3 mm narrow

proteoglycan is aggregated and these aggregates are smaller and have a higher keratan sulfate composition compared with their younger equivalents.[3,5] These degenerative features of disc proteoglycans may make them less effective in creating the swelling pressure necessary to resist compressive forces.

The gross structural and biochemical changes associated with early degeneration lead to changes in the intervertebral disc's mechanical properties, which make it less capable of performing its necessary functions. The discs become increasingly stiff and appear to undergo a transition from "fluid-like" behavior to "solid-like" behavior with increasing degeneration.[2]

Alterations in disc viscoelasticity, decreased Poisson's ratio as well as decreased radial permeability, which transforms the anisotropic hydraulic permeability of the normal disc to a more isotropic permeability in degenerated discs result in abnormal motion segments. The four stages of disc herniation are degeneration, prolapse, extrusion and sequestration.

Nerve Root

The nerve roots exit the spinal canal at the level of the corresponding pedicle. The L4 nerve root crosses the L3–L4 disk space and exits the spinal canal beneath the L4 pedicle before crossing the L4–L5 disk space. After exiting the foramen, the L4 nerve root crosses the L4–L5 disk space at its lateral margin. Paramedian disk herniations affect the lower spinal nerve root, so an L4–L5 disk herniation would result in compression of the L5 nerve root. A foraminal disk herniation or an extraforaminal or far lateral disk herniation at L4–L5 would compress the L4 nerve root.

Surgical Landmark and Applied Anatomy

The nerve root lies inferolaterally beneath the ligamentum flavum and the superior lamina. Muscles overlying lamina, facet and interlaminar space must be removed. Laminectomy and medial facetectomy performed. Ligamentum flavum is removed in layers. Inspect the nerve carefully before discectomy, and clearly visualize the lateral edge of the nerve root to avoid durotomy and nerve injury. The epidural space around the nerve root is dissected free of any adhesions to the ventral epidural space or the herniated disk to allow for mobilization and retraction of the nerve root, if necessary. Free fragments of disk may be located beneath the exiting nerve root, either caudally or rostrally, in relation to the interspace. If a disk fragment is found, it should be removed before retraction of the nerve root to prevent injury to the root by retracting a root that is already mechanically deformed and compressed by a herniated disk fragment.

REFERENCES

1. Epstein BS, Epstein JA, Lavine L: The effect of anatomic variations in the lumbar vertebrae and spinal canal on cauda equina and nerve root syndromes. Am J Roentgenol Radium TherNucl Med 1964;91:1055–1063.
2. Iatridis J, Setton L, Weidenbaum M, et al: Alterations in the mechanical behavior of the human lumbar nucleus pulposus with degeneration and aging. J Orthop Res 1997;15:318.
3. Inerot S, Axelsson I: Structure and composition of proteoglycans from human annulus brosus. Connect Tissue Res 1991;26:47.
4. JF Ratcliffe. The arterial anatomy of the adult human lumbar vertebral body: a microarteriographic study. J Anat. Aug; 1980;131: 57–79.
5. Johnstone B, Bayliss M: The large proteoglycans of the human inter-vertebral disc: changes in their biosynthesis and structure with age, topography, and pathology. Spine (Phila Pa 1976) 1995;20:674.
6. Kostuik JP. Surgical approaches to the thoracic and thoracolumbar spine. In: Frymoyer JW, Ducker TB, Hadler NM, et al., eds. The adult spine: principles and practice, 2nd ed. Philadelphia: Lippincott-Raven.1997;1437–70.
7. Kramer DL, Booth RE, Albert TJ, et al. Posterior lumbar approach. In: Albert TJ, Balderston RA, Northrup BE, eds. Surgical approaches to the spine. Philadelphia: WB Saunders.1997;173–92.
8. Lyons G, Eisenstein S, Sweet M: Biochemical changes in intervertebral disc degeneration. BiochimBiophys Acta 1981;673:443.
9. Magnuson PB: Differential diagnosis of causes of pain in the lower back accompanied by sciatic pain. Ann Surg 1944;119(6):878–91.
10. Min JH, Jang JS, Jung B, et al: The clinical characteristics and risk factors for the adjacent segment degeneration in instrumented lumbar fusion. J Spinal Disord Tech 2008;21(5):305–09.
11. Raj P: Intervertebral disc: anatomy-physiology-pathophysiology-treatment. Pain Pract 2008;8:18.
12. Roy-Camille R, Saillant G, Mazel C: Internal fixation of lumbar spine with pedicle screw plating. Clin. Orthop. 1986;203:7–17.
13. Schneck CD. The anatomy of lumbar spondylosis. Clin. Orthop. 1985;193:20–37.
14. Weinstein JN, Spratt KF, Spengler D, et.al. Spinal pedicle fixation: reliability and validity of roentgenogram based assessment and surgical factors on successful screw placement. Spine. 1988;13:1012–1018.

Applied Anatomy of Lumbar Canal Stenosis

Muhammad Faris, Yunus Kuntawi Aji, Abdul Hafid Bajamal, Eko A Subagio

INTRODUCTION

Lumbar canal stenosis is defined as narrowing of the lumbar spinal canal (central stenosis), foramen (foraminal stenosis), or lateral recess (lateral recess stenosis) which causes compression of spinal nerve roots that produces symptoms of neurogenic claudication or radiculopathy with inability of the patient to walk long distance and with sensation of heavy legs and progressive lack of strength.[1,3,4,6] Lumbar canal stenosis is commonly associated with disk degeneration. However, degenerative spinal stenosis evidenced on imaging is significant only if clinically symptomatic. The most frequent physical findings are limited lumbar extension (66–100%), sensory deficit (32–58%), muscle weakness (18–52%), straight leg raising (10–90%), absent knee reflexes (10–50%), and absent ankle reflexes (50–68%). Lumbar canal stenosis more common after the fifth decade, men are more affected than women.[1] CT and MRI with axial acquisitions allow to accurately measure the amplitude of the canal.[9]

ANATOMY

Lumbar vertebrae are the largest vertebral bodies, typically increase in the diameter caudally and are greater in transverse width relative to anteroposterior diameter.[8] The L1–L2 vertebral bodies have greater depth dorsally, whereas the L4–L5 vertebral bodies have greater depth ventrally. The two subregions are balanced by the L3 vertebral body, which provides a transitional point between the two. Vertebral body angulation and translation are affected by these locoregional differences in anatomy during flexion and extension.[8] These variations produce changes in intervertebral disc height and foramen cross-sectional area, which are functionally linked to motion during flexion and extension. The variations may be associated with susceptibility at lumbar regions for disc herniation, canal stenosis, and other pathology. The vertebral bodies move closer ventrally and further apart dorsally during flexion, which increases the dimensions of the spinal canal; the opposite occurs during extension.

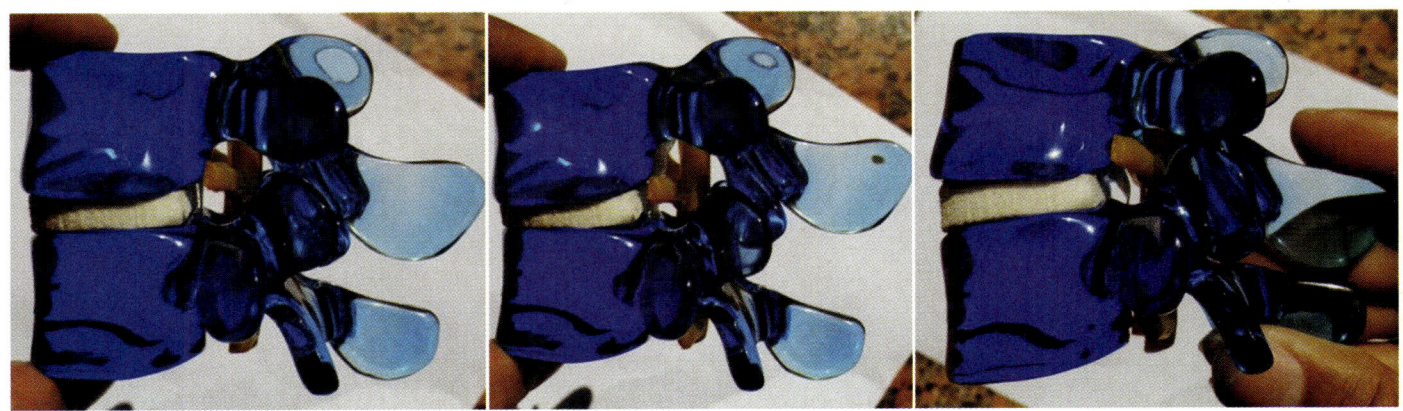

Fig. 5.1: The positioning of the lumbar spine can greatly affect spinal canal volume

Classification

Lumbar canal stenosis can be classified into two major categories: congenital/developmental and acquired.[1–3,5,6,9] Congenital stenosis is usually due to developmental disturbance. Most of them are primarily central canal stenosis.[1] Some of the characteristics are early clinical presentation, multilevel involvement, fewer degenerative changes on imaging, and subtle anatomical changes compressing the thecal sac.[1]

Acquired stenosis is most common in the sixth decade. It might be due to degenerative stenosis (central stenosis, lateral stenosis, or foraminal stenosis), degenerative spondylolisthesis, combined, iatrogenic, post-traumatic, and other etiology such as Paget's disease and achondroplastic.[1–3]

There are three variations of the spinal canal: A round/oblong canal, an ovoid canal, and a trefoil/triangular canal.[3] The lateral recesses of the trefoil canal can render the lumbar roots particularly vulnerable to compression by a herniated disc. The trefoil canal is seen in 15% of spinal canals and predisposes to lateral recess stenosis (Fig. 5.2).

According to whether the vertebral foramen width is increasing, constant or decreasing throughout the lumbar region, the following morphological patterns can be identified. Pattern I: The width of the canal increased from L1 to L2 then narrowed at L3 and re-widened again from L3 down to L5. Pattern II: The width of the canal increased gradually from L1 down to L5. Pattern III: The width of the canal remained constant from L1 to L2 lumbar vertebra, then it narrowed at the level of L3 to widen at L4 and L5. Pattern IV: The width of the canal narrowed from L1 to L2, then remained constant from L2 to L3 and finally widened down until L5. Pattern V: The width of the canal remained constant until the level of L4, then widened until L5. Pattern VI: The canal narrowed gradually from L1 reaching the narrowest diameter at L3, then widened down until L5.[4]

Pathogenesis

The sequences of the progressive age-related changes lead to the occurrence of a central or lateral stenosis. This suggested sequence of events highlights the relationship within the three-joint complex.[10]

Lumbar Canal Stenosis

In Indonesia lumbar canal stenosis is the most frequent indication for spinal surgery in patients older than

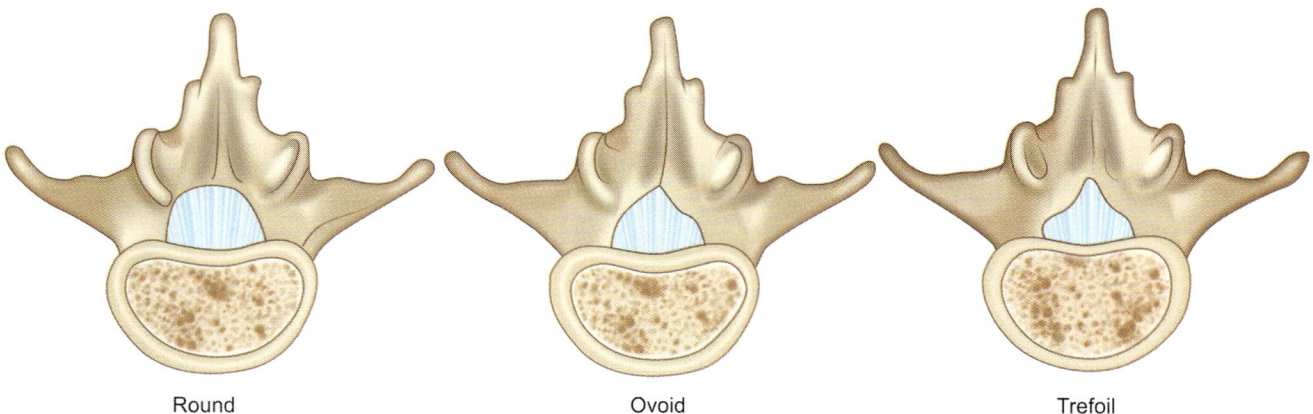

Round   Ovoid   Trefoil

Fig. 5.2: Three configurations of the spinal canal[3]

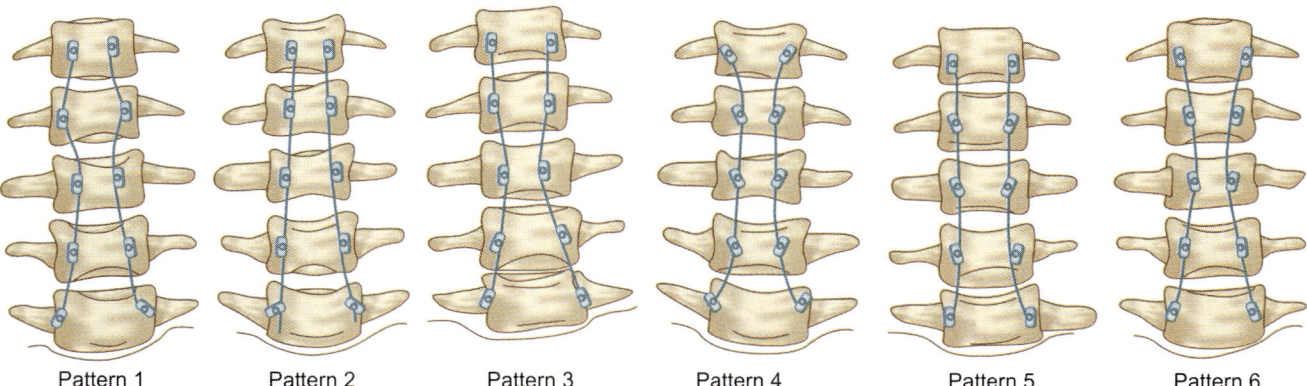

Pattern 1   Pattern 2   Pattern 3   Pattern 4   Pattern 5   Pattern 6

Fig. 5.3: Different morphological patterns of the lumbar vertebral canal[4]

65 years of age. In clinical medicine, lumbar canal stenosis is defined as buttock or lower extremity pain, which may occur with or without low back pain, associated with diminished space available for the neural and vascular elements in the lumbar spine. This definition includes two aspects: Morphological abnormalities and clinical manifestations, neurogenic claudication, caused by the somatic anomaly.[7]

From a radiological perspective, emphasizing the underlying structural anomaly, stenosis of the spinal canal with or without clinical manifestations is a more appropriate definition.[7] The condition underlying the clinical manifestations, as the term implies, is a stenosis of the spinal canal and it is well known that not all patients with a narrowing of the spinal canal, verified by an imaging procedure, suffer from neurogenic claudication. Various parameters were applied with regard to lumbar stenosis but none of them is satisfactory due to interindividual normal variation. These measures might be distinguished into determinants for central, lateral, and foraminal stenosis[7] (Figs 5.4 and 5.5).

Determinants for Central Stenosis

Different measurements are reported: Transverse and anteroposterior diameter of the osseous spinal canal, ligamentous interfacet distance (distance between the inner surface of flaval ligaments on a line connecting the joint space of the facet joints at the level of the intervertebral disc), and cross sectional area of the spinal canal.[7] Distances or areas were reported either in absolute numbers or in relative changes compared to specified reference measurements. Values for the anteroposterior diameter of the osseous spinal canal

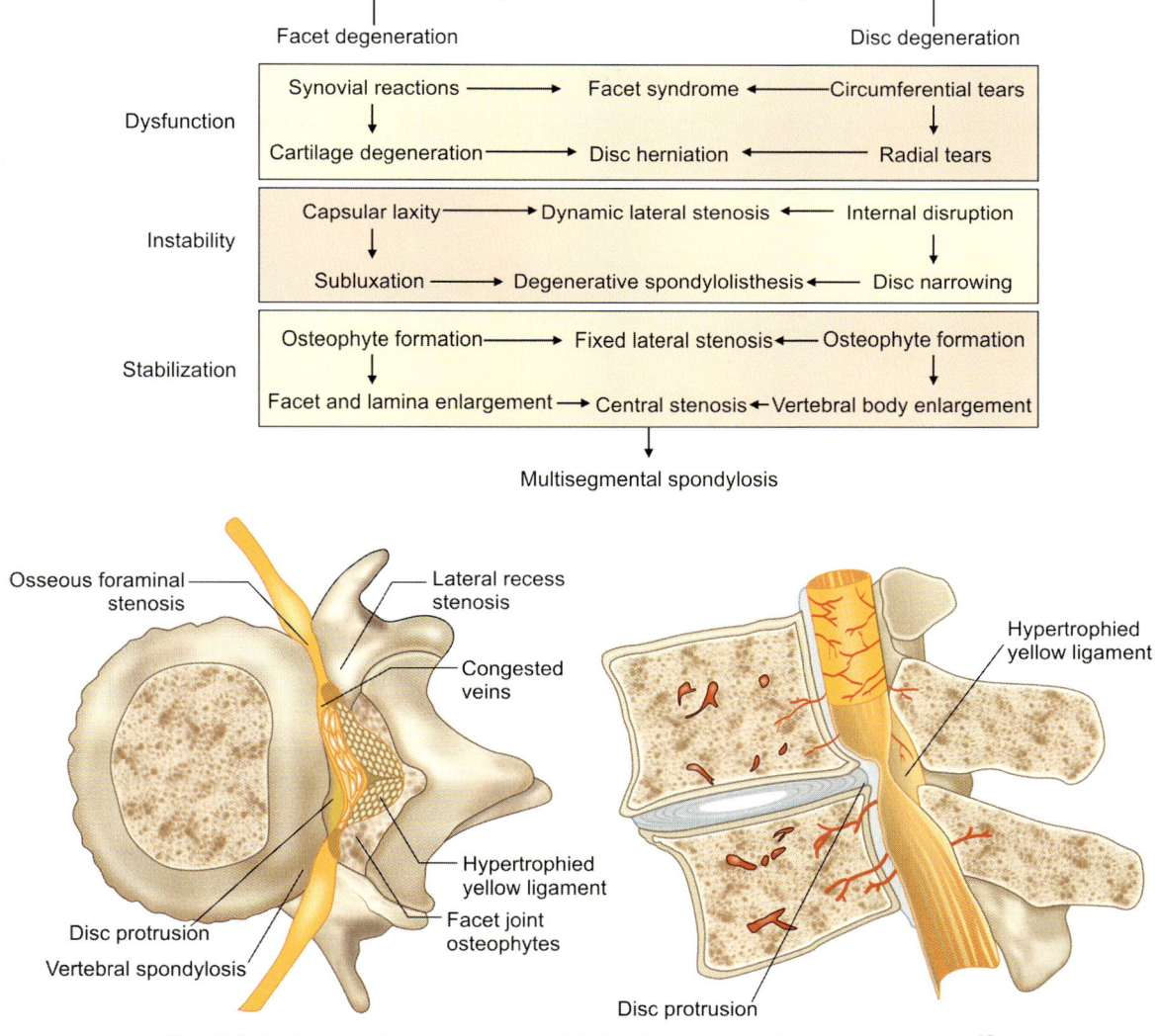

Flowchart 5.1: Degeneration of the three-joint complex[10]

Fig. 5.4: Pathomorphology of central, lateral recess, and foraminal stenosis[10]

were reported and stenosis is defined by some authors by a distance of less than 10 mm, by others below 7 mm. A cross-sectional area of the dural sac of less than 100 mm^2 indicated central stenosis.[7] Table 5.1 is determinants of central stenosis from various authors (Figs 5.6 to 5.11).

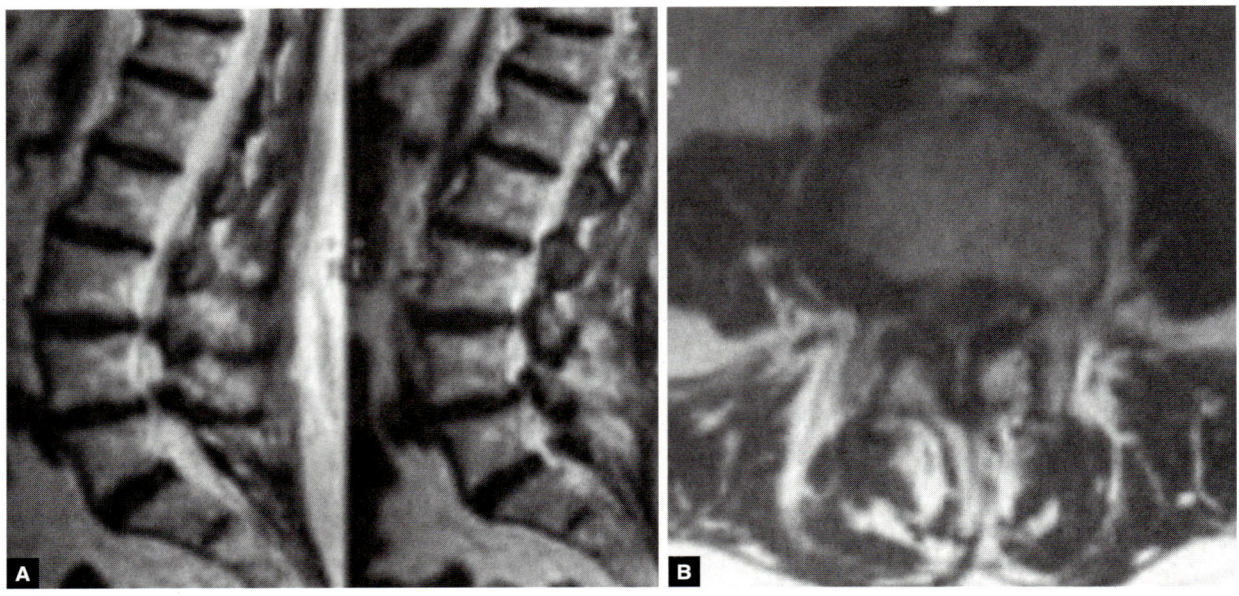

Fig. 5.5: (A) Sagittal image showing multiple level lumbar canal stenosis. (B) Axial image showing multifactorial lumbar canal stenosis[6]

Author	Site of measurement	Definition of stenosis
Table 5.1: Sites of measurement and definitions for central lumbar spinal stenosis[7]		
Fukusaki	Anteroposterior diameter of spinal canal	<15 mm
Koc		<12 mm
Bolender		<13 mm
Haig		≤11.95 mm
Lee		<15 mm (suggesting narrowing) <10 mm (usually diagnostic)
Ullrich		<11.5 mm
Verbiest		<12 mm (relative) <10 mm (absolute)
Kalichman	Anteroposterior diameter of dural sac	10–12 mm (relative) <10 mm (absolute)
Johnson		≤10 mm
Herzog	Mid-sagittal diameter of thecal sac	Compression of thecal sac area in % of normal mid-sagittal diameter: Grade 1: Anterior <15%, posterior <10% Grade 2: Anterior 15–30%, posterior 10–20% Grade 3: Anterior >30%, posterior >20%
Hamanishi	Cross-sectional area of dural tube or sac	<100 mm^2, at more than two of three intervertebral levels
Mariconda		<130 mm^2
Laurencin		Stenosis ratio: Cross-sectional area of dural sac of motion segment divided by stable segment cross-sectional dural sac area L3–L4 <0.66 L4–L5 <0.62 L5–S1 <0.73

(Contd.)

Author	Site of measurement	Definition of stenosis
Bolender		100–130 mm² (early stenosis)
		<100 mm² (present stenosis)
Schonstrom		75–100 mm² (moderate)
		<75 mm² (severe)
Ullrich		<145 mm²
Herzog	Ligamentous interfacet distance	L2–L3: <10 mm
		L3–L4: <10 mm
		L4–L5: <12 mm
		L5–S1: <13 mm
Wilmink		<11 mm
Koc	Transverse diameter of spinal canal	<15 mm
Ullrich		<16 mm

Table 5.1: Sites of measurement and definitions for central lumbar spinal stenosis[7] (*Contd.*)

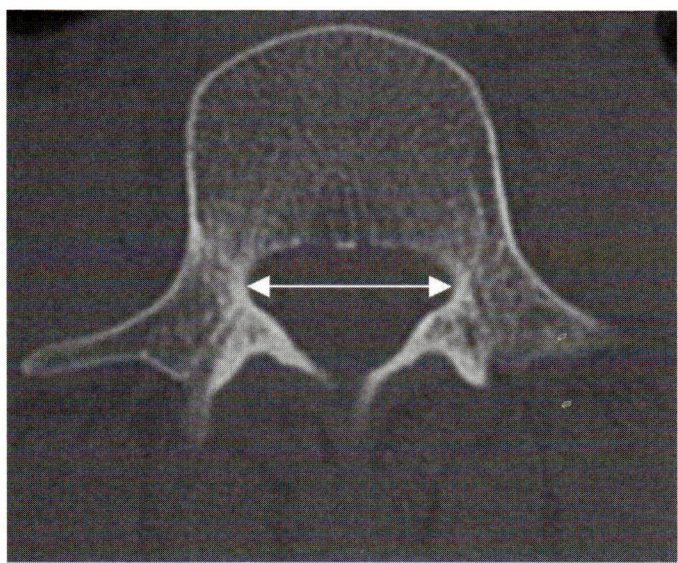

Fig. 5.6: The white arrow indicates the transverse diameter of the osseous spinal canal[7]

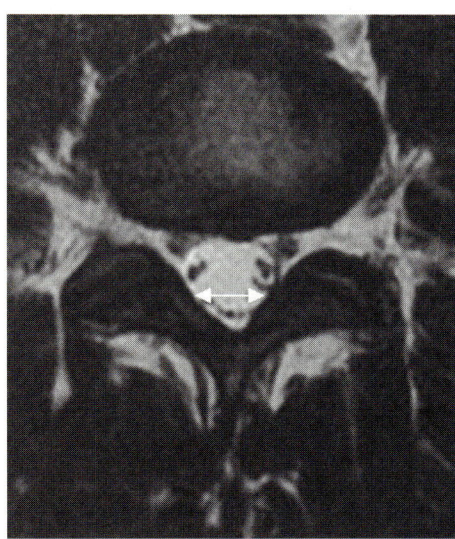

Fig. 5.8: The white arrow indicates the ligamentous interfacet distance measured between the inner surfaces of flaval ligaments on a line connecting the joint space of facet joints[7]

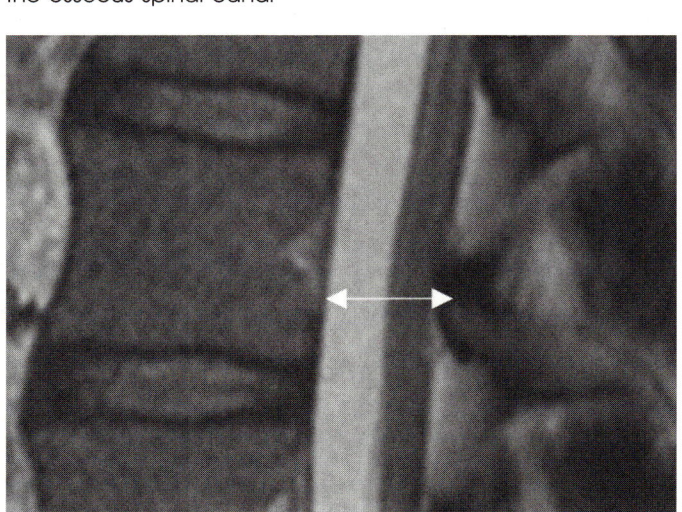

Fig. 5.7: The white arrow indicates the anteroposterior diameter of the osseous spinal canal[7]

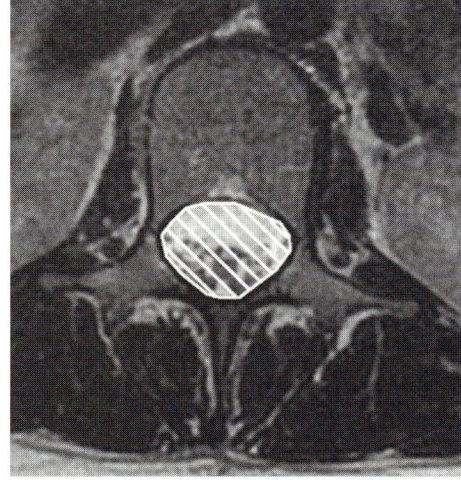

Fig. 5.9: Cross sectional area of the spinal canal is indicated by the white hatched area[7]

Table 5.2: Sites of measurement and definitions for lateral lumbar spinal stenosis[7]		
Author	Site of measurement	Definition of stenosis
Ciric	Lateral recess height	5 mm (normal)
		≤3 mm (highly indicative)
		≤2 mm (diagnostic)
Strojnik		≤3.6 mm
Dincer	Depth of lateral recess	>5 mm (normal)
		4–5 mm (group 3)
		3–4 mm (group 2)
		2–3 mm (group 1)
Mikhael		>5 mm (normal)
		3–5 mm (suggestive)
		≤3 mm (definitive)
Strojnik		<30°

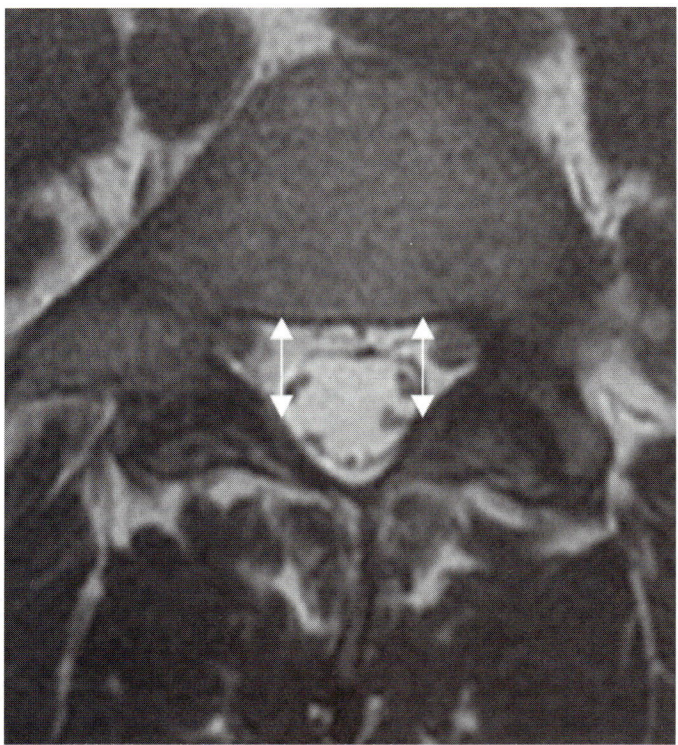

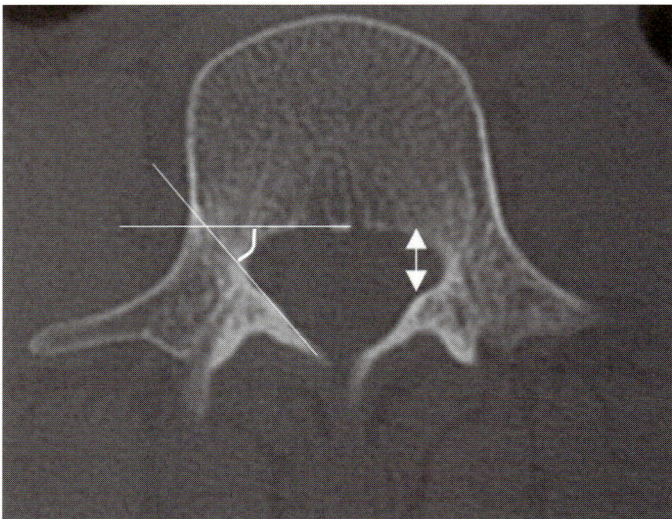

Fig. 5.11: The lateral recess angle is defined as the angle between the lines parallel to the floor and the roof of the lateral recess. The height of the lateral recess is defined as the shortest distance from the most anterior point of the superior articular process to the posterior border of the vertebral body[7]

Fig. 5.10: The white arrow heads mark the depth of the lateral recess is measured between the superior articular facet and the top part of the pedicle[7]

Determinants for Lateral Stenosis

Height and depth of the lateral recess, and lateral recess angle are criteria to describe lateral stenosis.[7] The depth of the lateral recess is measured between the superior articular facet and the top part of the pedicle. Recess height is specified as distance between the most anterior point of the superior articular facet and the posterior border of the vertebral body and the lateral recess angle as the angle between the lines parallel to the floor and

the roof of the lateral recess. A lateral recess height ≤2 mm and/or lateral recess depth ≤3 mm or a lateral recess angle <30° has been described as diagnostic for lateral recess stenosis.[7] Table 5.2 is determinants of lateral stenosis from various authors.

Determinants of Foraminal Stenosis

The only quantitative criterion was the diameter of the foramen. A diameter of 2 to 3 mm is considered to indicate stenosis.[7]

REFERENCES

1. AN HS, Singh K. Lumbar spinal stenosis. In: Synopsis of spine surgery. 3rd Ed. New York: Thieme; 2016;197–209.

2. AN HS, Andreshak TG. Spinal stenosis. In: Principles and techniques of spine surgery. Philadelphia: Williams & Wilkins. p. 443–60.

3. Botwin KP, Gruber RD. Lumbar spinal stenosis: Anatomy and pathogenesis. Phys Med RehabilClin N Am 2003;14;1–15.

4. El-Rakhawy M, El-Shahat AE, Labib I, Abdulaziz E. Lumbar vertebral canal stenosis: concept of morphometric and radiometric study of the human lumbar vertebral canal. Anatomy 2010;4; 51–62.

5. Ross JS, Bendok BR, McClendon J. Imaging in spine surgery. Philadelphia: Elsevier;. 2017;213–4.

6. Skyme AD, Selmon GPF, Apthorp L. Lumbar spinal stenosis. In: Common spinal disorders explained. London: Remedica; 2005; 47–51.

7. Steurer J, Roner S, Gnannt R, Hodler J. Quantitative radiologic criteria for the diagnosis of lumbar spinal stenosis: a systematic literature review. BMC Musculoskeletal Disorders. 2011;12:175;1–9.

8. Wardak Z, Lavelle ED, Lavelle WF. Functional anatomy of the spine. In: Benzel's spine surgery. 4th Ed. Vol.1. Philadelphia: Elseviere; 2017;47–9.

9. Weyreuther M, Heyde CE, Westphal M, Zierski J, Weber U. MRI atlas of orthopedics and neurosurgery. The Spine. Berline: Springer. 2006;102–4.

10. Zingg PO, Boos N. Lumbar spinal stenosis. In: Spinal disorders fundamentals of diagnosis and treatment. New York: Springer. 2008;513–37.

Pathogenesis of Lumbar Canal Stenosis

Achal Gupta, PS Ramani

INTRODUCTION

The vertebrae are joined together by three joints: Intervertebral disc and facet joints (two joints). Trauma or degeneration in one affects all the three joints and even the slightest degeneration in the intervertebral disc produces stress on the facet joints.

Spinal stenosis was defined in 1975 as any type of narrowing of the spinal canal, nerve root canals, or intervertebral foramina.[2]

Congenital Lumbar Canal Stenosis

Congenital lumbar canal stenosis is caused by growth disturbance of posterior parts of vertebrae during the prenatal period or early infancy. Premature fusion of the posterior elements leads to narrowing of the lumbar spinal canal commonly at L3, L4 and L5 vertebrae.[11] Short pedicles are typical seen in congenital variety of stenosis.[15] The pathology causes discrepancy in the canal size and the volume of neural elements leading to symptoms of stenosis at earlier age.[11, 15] A congenital spinal canal stenosis is typically seen in skeletal dysplasia such as achondroplasia or diastrophic dysplasia.[9,14] Narrowing of nerve canal can be enhanced by developmental abnormalities such as asymmetry of the facets and pedicles. These anomalies increase the length of canal resulting in stretching of nerve roots. The narrowing of the nerve root portion of the canal with nerve root entrapment may be recurrent or fixed.

Degenerative Lumbar Canal Stenosis

Degenerative lumbar canal stenosis includes: (1) Central stenosis (central spinal canal with the dural sac), (2) lateral stenosis (lateral recess at the level of facet joints) and (3) foraminal stenosis (narrowing is limited to neural foramina). The prevalence of the acquired form increases with age. Stenotic changes are most common at L4–L5 level, followed by L3–L4 and L5–S1 levels.[16]

The earliest change in the joint is synovitis. Later cartilage is destroyed and capsule becomes lax. Instability is created in the joint and it subluxates. The inferior facet moves upwards and forwards narrowing the lateral recess and the upper intervertebral foramen. The superior facet moves downwards and medially compressing the dural sheath and the lower nerve root, as it is about to exit from the lower foramen. Formation of osteophytes and hypertrophy of facets (Figs 6.1 to 6.4) leads to further encroachment of space in the central and lateral canals. Subluxation and hypertrophy leads to medial rotation of facet joints (coronal orientation, tropism), which is further aggravated by too much static stress on the already disrupted joint. The part of hypertrophy of superior facet may nearly bisect the spinal canal horizontally with inner edge almost approaching the midline. The tropism along with settlement of disc space further reduces the size of the most intervertebral foramina causing foraminal stenosis.

The earliest degenerative change in the intervertebral disc is biochemical. Later circumferential tears in the annulus coalesce to form radial tears. Internal disruption and disc resorption results in loss of disc height and the annulus bulges posteriorly into the canal as a result of settlement in the disc space. Loss of disc height leads to buckling of ligamentum flavum and thus, canal stenosis.[1,7] This process causes further encroachment on the already compromised lateral recess. Lateral spinal stenosis is the outcome of changes in the disc and the posterior joints. Osteophytes start forming on the back of the vertebral edges further embarrassing the nerve roots.[3–6, 10,17,18]

Foraminal stenosis is the overall outcome of hypertrophy and subluxation of facets, settlement of disc space and osteophyte formation on vertebral edges.[3,5]

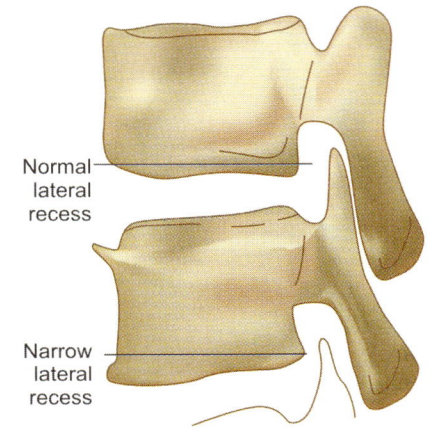

Normal lateral recess

Narrow lateral recess

Fig. 6.1

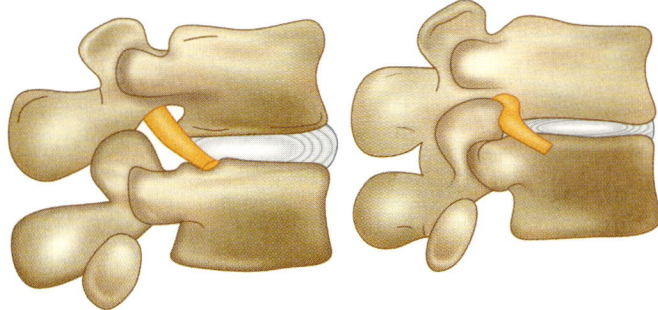

Fig. 6.2

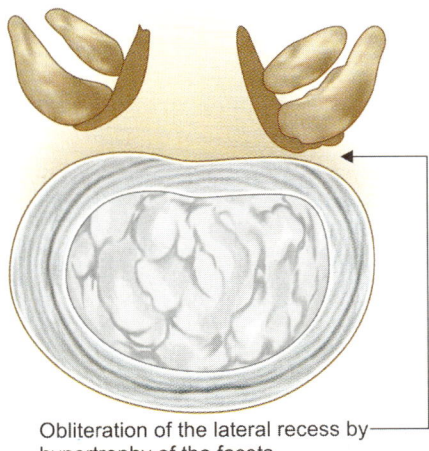

Obliteration of the lateral recess by hypertrophy of the facets

Fig. 6.3

Figs 6.1 to 6.3: Hypertrophy of facet causing narrowing of lateral recess, causing entrapment of the root in the foramen

Foraminal stenosis is an unavoidable sequelae of the settlement from chronic degeneration of the intervertebral disc.

The process of stenosis passes through the following stages:[13]

1. Transient Dysfunction

This is the beginning phase when possibly there is only synovitis in the facet joints. The patient's complaints

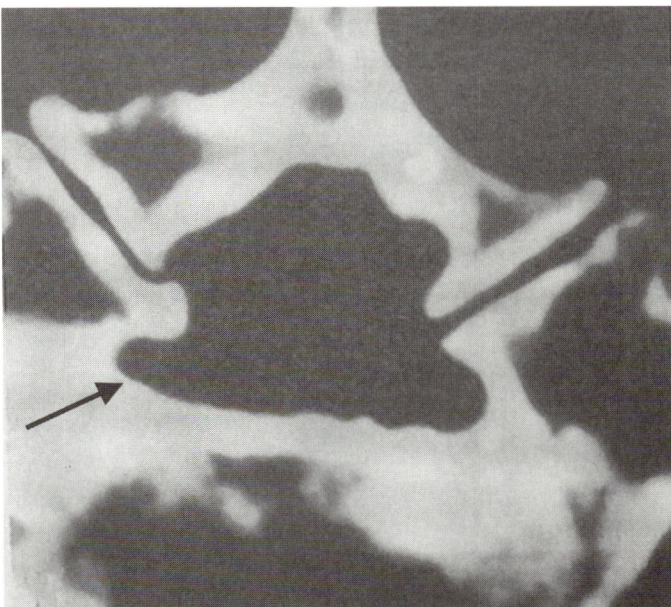

Fig. 6.4: CT scan axial cut showing hypertrophy of facet causing narrowing of the lateral recess

are mild and infrequent. Physical signs are absent. Radiological investigations are often normal and conservative treatment is successful. Surgery has no place in the management in this phase.

2. Instability

With the subluxation in the facet joints, there is abnormal movement at one or more levels. The superior facet moves upwards and downwards during flexion and extension movements and causes recurrent or intermittent entrapment of nerve roots. Patient's complaints become more severe and more frequent. He complains of morning stiffness and difficulty in getting out of bed. Radiological abnormalities start appearing. Conservative treatment should be tried, as the patient at this stage may not be willing for surgery. If symptoms become intractable, then surgery of posterior lumbar interbody fusion is indicated. The percentage of spinal stenosis patients, at this stage, coming for surgery is however very less.

3. Fixed Deformities

Majority of the patients fall in this group. As a result of severe degenerative changes into the posterior joints and the disc, the instability gives way to fixed deformity and reduced movements and fixed entrapment of nerve roots. Radiological changes are always present. Relief with conservative measures is not satisfactory. The surgical procedure of internal decompression for spinal stenosis is essential. Fusion is unnecessary in this phase.

Two Nerves at Risk

Two nerve roots are at risk at any one level. The nerve root exiting at this level is entrapped by upward migrated tip of the inferior facet and the inferior border of the pedicle (foraminal stenosis). The lower nerve root crossing the level is trapped in the lateral canal by the hypertrophied medial edge of superior facet. The curling in the ligament flavum under the thickened inferior facet causes severe compression of the lower nerve root.

Segmental instability, which can cause static and dynamic stenosis, is considered a cause of low back pain.[8] Recent researches show that typical symptoms of lumbar canal stenosis occur due to a combination of mechanical compression and disturbance of blood flow—either arterial ischaemia or venous congestion—in the cauda equina or individual nerve roots.[12]

REFERENCES

1. Altikaya N, Yildrim T, Demir S, et al. Factors associated with the thickness of the ligamentum flavum. Is ligamentum flavum thickening due to hypertrophy or buckling? Spine. 2011;18: 679–86.
2. Arnoldi CC, Brodsky AE, Cauchoix J, et al. Lumbar spinal stenosis and nerve root entrapment syndromes. Definition and classification. Clin Orthop Relat Res. 1976;115: 4–5.
3. Cric I, Michael AM. The lateral recess syndrome. Neurosurgery (ed.) Wilkins, Rengachary. 2279–82.
4. Ehni G. Significance of the small lumbar canal. Cauda equine compression syndrome due to Spondylosis. J Neurosurg. 1969;31: 507–12.
5. Epstein JA, Epstein BS, Lavine LS, et al. Lumbar nerve root compression at the intervertebral foramen caused by arthritis of the posterior facet. J Neurosurg. 1973;39:362–68.
6. Epstein JA, Epstein BS, Rosentahl AD, et al. Sciatica caused by nerve entrapment in the lateral recess. J Neurosurg. 1973;36:584–89.
7. Hansson T, Suzuki N, Hebelka H, et al. The narrowing of the lumbar spinal canal during MRI: the effects of the disc and ligamentum flavum. Eur Spine J. 2009;18: 679–86.
8. Inufusa A, An HS, Lim TH, et al. Anatomic changes of the spinal canal and intervertebral foramen associated with flexion-extension movement. Spine. 1996;21(21): 2412–20.
9. Jeong S-T, Song H-R, Keny SM, et al. MRI study of the lumbar spine in achondroplasia. A morphometric analysis for the evaluation of stenosis of the canal. J Bone Joint Surg Br. 88: 2006;1192–1196.
10. King KY, Kirkaldy Willis WH, Shannon R, et al. Anatomy, pathology and pathogenesis of lateral recess stenosis; Posterior lumbar interbody fusion ed by PM Lin. 1982;165–77.
11. Kitab SA, Alsulaiman AM, Benzel EC. Anatomic radiological variations in developmental lumbar spinal stenosis: a prospective, control-matched comparative analysis. Spine J. 14: 2013;808–15.
12. Kobayashi S. Pathophysiology, diagnosis and treatment of intermittent claudication in patients with lumbar canal stenosis. World J Orthop. 2014;5:134–145.
13. Ramani PS. Textbook of Spinal Surgery. Ist edition; volume 2; 2005; 574–576.
14. Remes V, Tervahartiala P, Poussa M, et al. Thoracic and lumbar spine in diastrophic dysplasia: a clinical and magnetic resonance imaging analysis. Spine J. 1992;17: 9–15.
15. Singh K, Samartzis D, Vaccaro AR, et al. Congenital lumbar spinal stenosis: a prospective, control-matched, cohort radiographic analysis, Spine J. 2005;5: 615–22.
16. Tomkins-Lane CC, Battié MC, Hu R, et al. Pathoanatomical characterstics of clinical lumbar canal stenosis. J Back Musculoskelet Rehabil. 2014;27:223–29.
17. Verbiest H. A radicular syndrome from developmental narrowing of the lumbar vertebral canal. J Bone Joint Surg 1954;36:230–37.
18. Wilson B. Significance of the lumbar canal: Cauda equine compression syndrome due to Spondylosis. Part 3; J Neurosurg 1969;31:499–506.

Lumbar Canal Stenosis: Radiological Features

Shrinivas B. Desai, Shraddha Sinhasan, Ritu Kakkar, Kavya Kaushik

INTRODUCTION

Lumbar spinal stenosis is a fairly common disease. The term 'stenosis' is derived from the Latin prefix "steno," meaning "narrowing."[1] It is defined as an anatomical or functional narrowing of the osteo-ligamentous vertebral canal and/or the intervertebral foramina causing direct compression or indirect compromise of dural sac, the caudal nerve roots and their vasculature, enough to cause symptoms or signs.[2]

We should be well acquainted with terminology of zones (central, subarticular, foraminal, extraforaminal and anterior zones) (Fig. 7.1) and levels (disc level, supra-pedicle level, pedicle level and infrapedicle level) for description of imaging abnormalities (Figs 7.2 and 7.3).

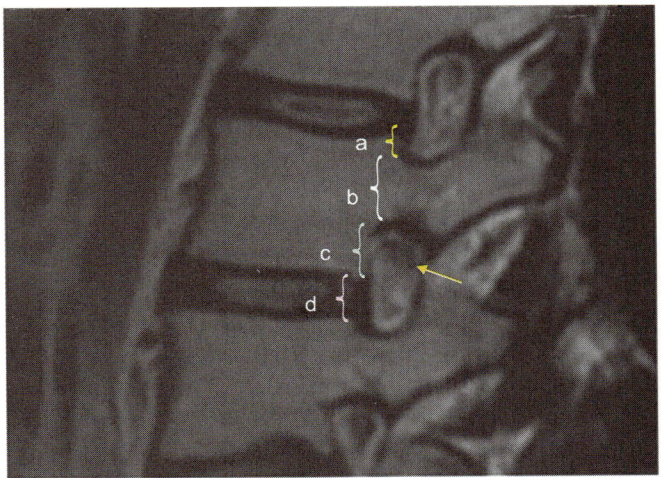

Fig. 7.2: T2-weighted sagittal image showing different levels. (a) Suprapedicular, (b) pedicular, (c) intrapedicular and (d) disc level

The goal of this chapter is to lay down accurate, easy and objective method for diagnosing lumbar canal stenosis on the basis of imaging.

IMAGING IN LUMBAR CANAL STENOSIS

Primary physicians of patients with lumbar pain expect to get appropriate information from imaging; whether stenosis is present or not; the location of the stenosis, anatomic structures (disc, ligamental, osseous) causing the narrowing and the degree of stenosis. The management of patients significantly depends on the details of this information.

Indication for radiologic examination and technique should be evaluated in every case. Uncomplicated acute low back pain or radiculopathy is a benign, self-limited condition that does not warrant any imaging studies. Imaging is considered in those patients who have had 4 to 6 weeks of medical management and physical

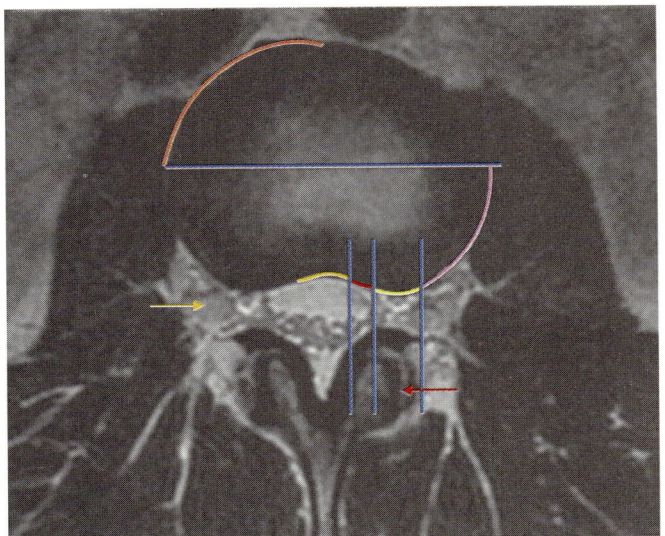

Fig. 7.1: T2-weighted axial image of lumbar spine. Yellow line represents central zone; red represents subarticular/paracentral zone; green represents foraminal/ posterolateral zone; pink represents extraforaminal/ far posterolateral zone and orange represents anterior zone. The red arrow point the facet joint and green arrow points the exiting nerve root

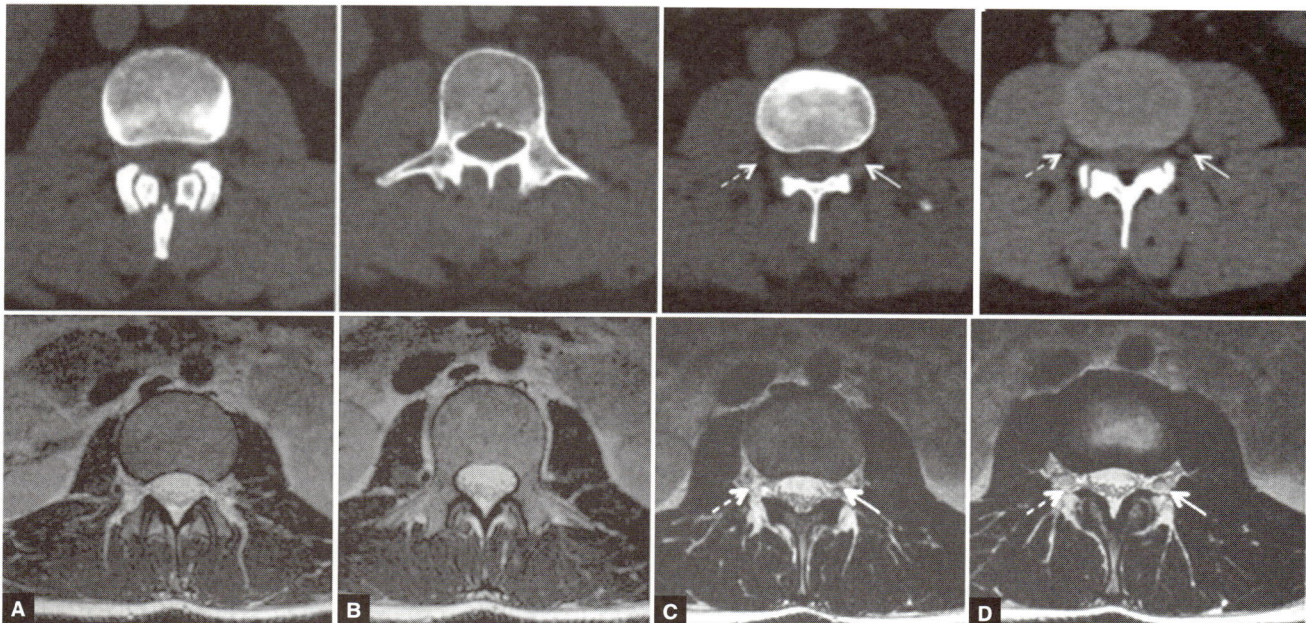

Fig. 7.3A to D: CT and T2 weight MRI axial images at different levels in lumbar spine. (A) suprapedicular; (B) pedicular (C) infrapedicular and (D) disc level. The straight arrow points towards isodense exiting nerve root and dotted arrow points towards hypodenseperineural fat

therapy that resulted in little or no improvement in their back pain. Imaging may be considered earlier if there is a history of malignancy, concern for infection, a fracture, symptoms of true myelopathy (progressive or severe neurologic deficits), clinical setting of cauda equina syndrome (urinary retention, fecal incontinence, motor deficit at multiple levels, and saddle anesthesia), or history of back surgery.

Degenerative changes are more common with increasing age. As these findings may be seen in both symptomatic and asymptomatic individuals, it is important that imaging findings be correlated with the physical exam.[3–6]

The main imaging modalities to evaluate back pain are plain radiographs, computed tomography (CT) and magnetic resonance imaging (MRI) in addition to CT myelogram and dynamic MRI which can be used in selected cases.

Plain Radiograph

Until a few years ago, X-ray was the only imaging modality for the spine in the upright position.

Spinal canal stenosis can be strongly suspected on plain radiographs which are performed on any patient with back pain. The interpedicular distance was the first feature to draw attention and later, the AP diameter of bony canal was considered to be more worthy. Verbiest had measured the sagittal diameters of spinal canal during surgery, at the level of the cephalad and caudal borders of the neural canal and calculated the ratio,

which is normally less than one and is equal or greater than one in a narrow canal.[7]

Plain films still play an important role in evaluation of the spine, because the examination is inexpensive and promptly available and gives a wide panoramic view of the spine. They can assess degenerative changes of disc height loss, vacuum phenomenon, osteophytes, and vertebral alignment (Fig. 7.4). Dynamic flexion—

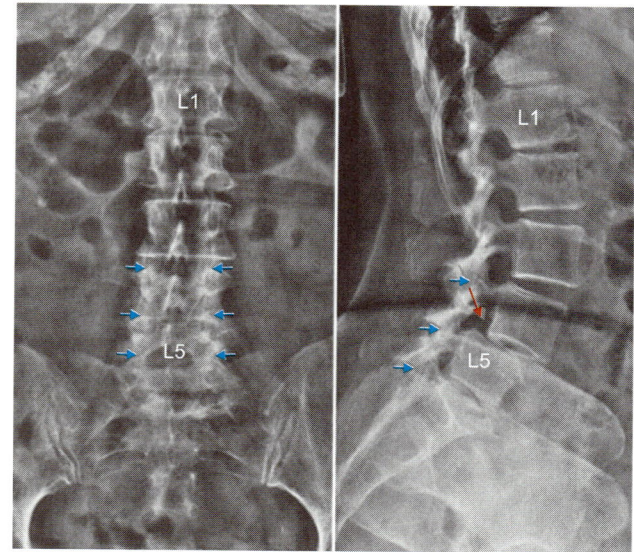

Fig. 7.4: X-ray AP and lateral lumbar spine reveals sclerosis of posterior elements and facet arthropathy (blue arrows) along with anterolisthesis of L4 over L5 vertebral body (red arrow). There is reduction in L4/L5 and L5/S1 disc spaces with vacuum phenomenon at L4/L5 level

extension radiographs can be obtained for additional information on instability.[8] Other causes of back pain, such as sacroiliac joint pathology, renal stones, or calcified aneurysmal dilatation of the aorta may be excluded by this modality. However, for accurate instability evaluation, plain films usually do not offer complete information. It shows its limitations for disc structures or when it is necessary to obtain measurements free from problems due to overlapping of anatomical images.[9]

Computed Tomography (CT)

CT is a better modality than plain radiograph in detecting disc herniation, spinal stenosis, as well as to exclude metastasis and infection. It also provides detailed bone anatomy for preoperative planning. Intervertebral discs and nerve roots appear isodense on CT in contrast to hypodense CSF and perineural fat, thereby providing contrast differentiation to aid canal and foraminal stenosis (Figs 7.3 and 7.5). Contrast-enhanced CT has been shown to provide improved visualization of disc pathology by evaluating for mass effect on the epidural venous plexus. Epidural enhancement surrounding a herniated disc can assist in its detection.[10]

Myelography

Myelogram can serve as an alternative for patients unable to have an MRI or who have had an inconclusive

MRI and CT. Although this is an invasive procedure, contrast in the subarachnoid space outlines the neural structures and is comparable to MRI in detecting stenosis and neural impingement. It has been shown to offer more information than MRI in presurgical diagnosis of symptomatic foraminal stenosis.[11,12] It is also a good modality to evaluate postoperative patients with metallic implants (Figs 7.6 and 7.7). Contrast CT myelogram is also useful in diagnosing CSF leak and nerve root avulsion.[13] However, due to potential complications, CT myelography is rarely performed and reserved for patients with contraindications to MRI or in whom subtle instability is suspected but not confirmed by other examinations.

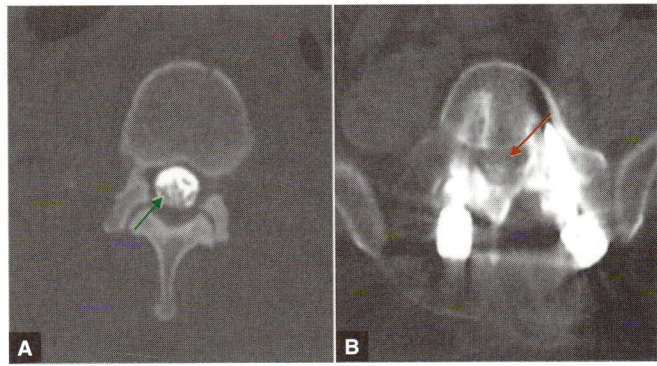

Fig. 7.6A and B: Axial CT myelogram images in lumbar spine. (A) Reveals normal spinal canal with hyperdense contrast and isointense nerve roots of cauda equine (red arrow). (B) Reveals postoperative epidural fibrosis causing severe lumbar canal stenosis. Pedicle screw fixation is seen at same level

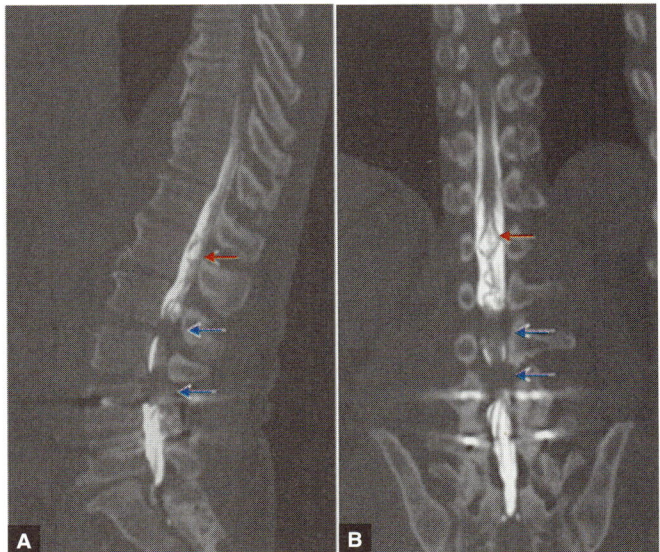

Fig. 7.7A and B: Lateral (A) and Coronal (B) CT myelogram images of dorsolumbar spine. Metallic fixation is seen at L4 and L5 levels. Severe lumbar canal stenosis is seen at L2/L3 and L3/L4 levels with effacement of hyperdense CSF space, compression of cauda equina and serpine/ redundant proximal nerve roots

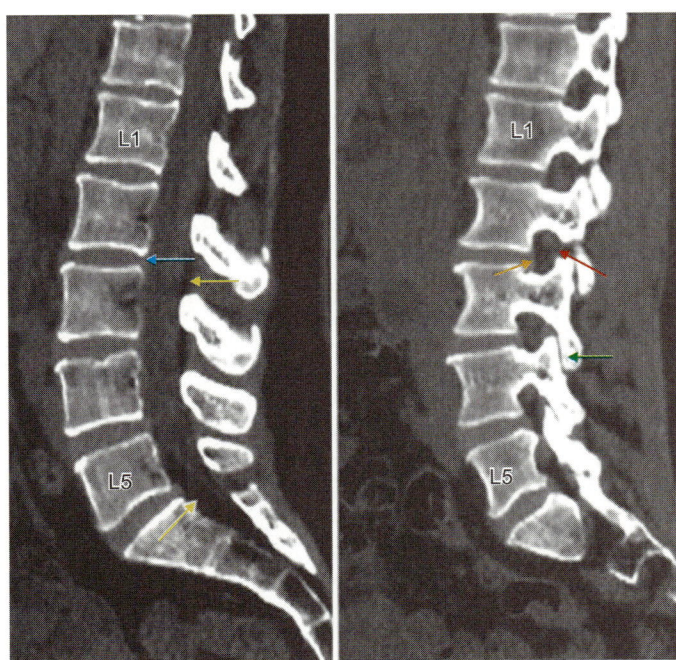

Fig. 7.5: Mid-sagittal and para-sagittal CT images of lumbar spine showing normal anatomy including intervertebral disc (blue); epidural fat (yellow); nerve root (red); perineural fat (orange) and facet joint (green)

Magnetic Resonance Imaging (MRI)

In the current scenario, MRI without contrast is generally considered the best initial test for most patients with low back pain who require advanced imaging. MRI is a more sensitive and specific modality as compared to plain radiographs and CT[14] (Fig. 7.8). It provides axial as well as sagittal views which can demonstrate normal and pathologic discs, ligaments, nerve roots, epidural fat, as well as the shape and size of the spinal canal. MRI is the standard imaging modality for detecting disc pathology due to its advantage of lack of radiation, multiplanar imaging capability, excellent spinal soft tissue contrast and precise localization of intervertebral discs changes.[15] It is the modality of choice for patients in whom lumbar canal stenosis is clinically suspected.[16]

The standard MR sequences obtained are sagittal T1-weighted, T2-weighted and STIR and axial T1-weighted and T2-weighted sequences (Figs 7.9 to 7.11). 'Disc through' T2 axial sequence with thin cuts at the level of disc is obtained for best visualization of disc pathology. In addition, contrast T1 weighted sequences may be obtained in case of infection, tumor or post surgical evaluation.[17] Figure 7.12 shows severe canal stenosis due to disc herniation and hypertrophic changes in ligamentum flavum causing lumbar canal stenosis.

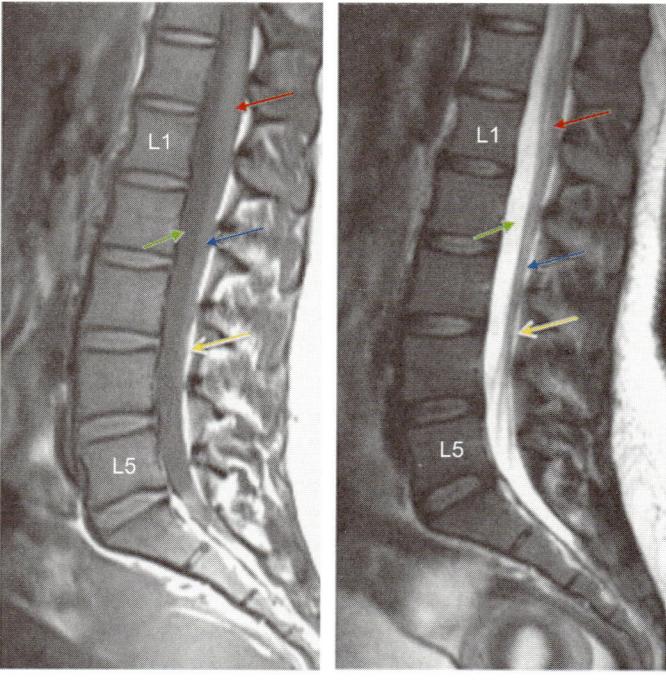

Fig. 7.9: Sagittal T1- and T2-weighted images showing normal structures. Conus (red arrow); cauda equina (blue arrow); epidural fat (yellow); CSF (green)

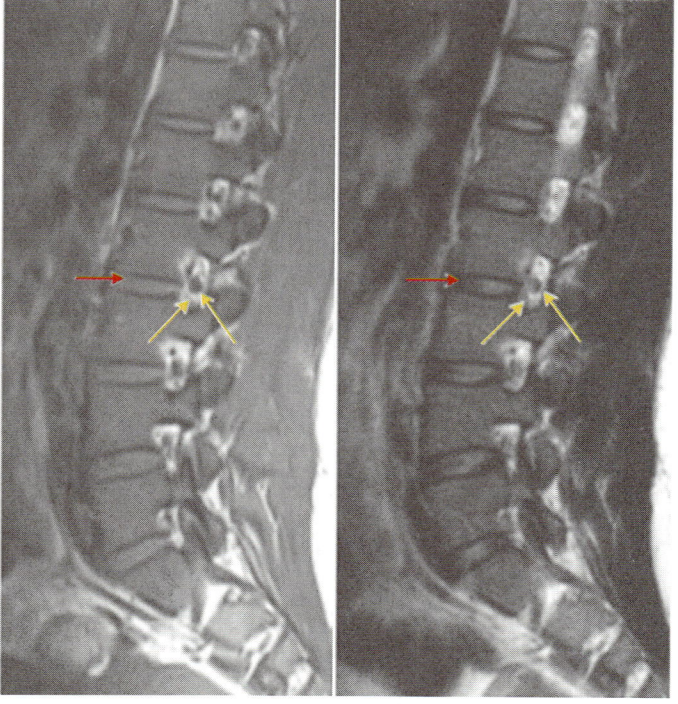

Fig. 7.10: Parasagittal T1 and T2 images showing normal structures. Disc (red arrow), exiting nerve root (yellow arrow) and perineural fat (dotted yellow arrow)

Fig. 7.8A and B: (A) Sagittal X-ray of lumbar spine. (A) Reveals bone anatomy, degenerative changes in the form of end plate sclerosis, anterior syndesmophytes, facetal arthropathy, concavity along L4 and L5 endplates and suspicious lower lumbar canal. (B) Sagittal T2-weighted MR image of lumbar spine of same patient reveals soft tissue details with severe lumbar canal stenosis, more marked at L4/L5 level (red arrow) due to disc bulge and ligamentum flavum hypertrophy, not appreciated on X-ray

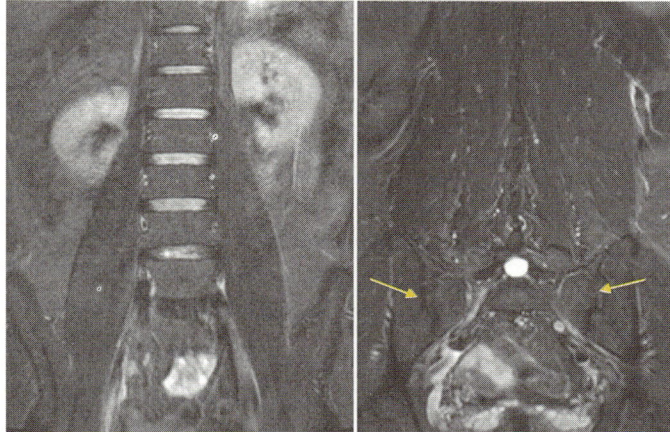

Fig. 7.11: Coronal STIR image showing normal lumbar spine and sacroiliac joints (yellow arrows)

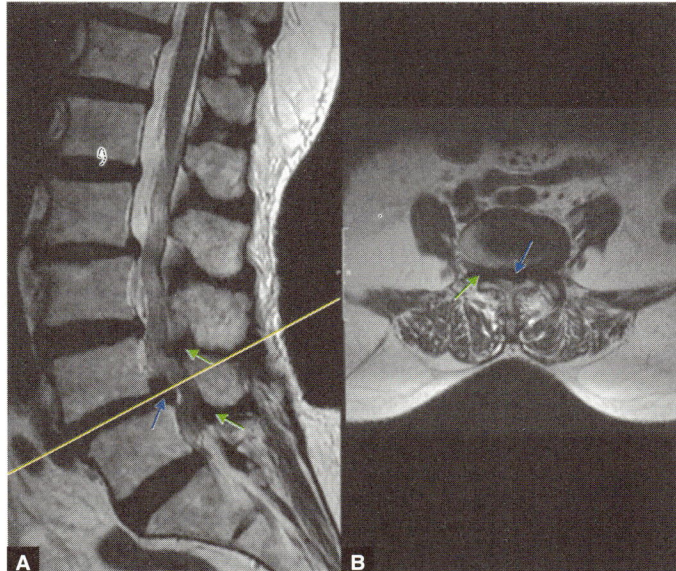

Fig. 7.12A and B: Sagittal (A) and axial (B) T2-weighted images showing severe canal stenosis at L4/L5 level due to disc herniation (blue arrow) and ligamentum flavum hypertrophy (green arrows) and compression of exiting nerve roots

Dynamic MRI

In patients with degenerative stenotic symptoms, sometimes, false negative MRI results lead to discordance between clinical and radiological findings. It is in such patients that axial loading (dynamic) MRI becomes a very valuable additional investigation to conventional supine MRI and may aid in assessing the degree of stenosis and spinal instability more accurately.

Additional levels of stenosis may be identified postapplication of axial load. The other valuable information obtained after the application of axial load is increase in the thickness of the ligamentum flavum, a known dynamic factor that contributes significantly to functional canal stenosis.

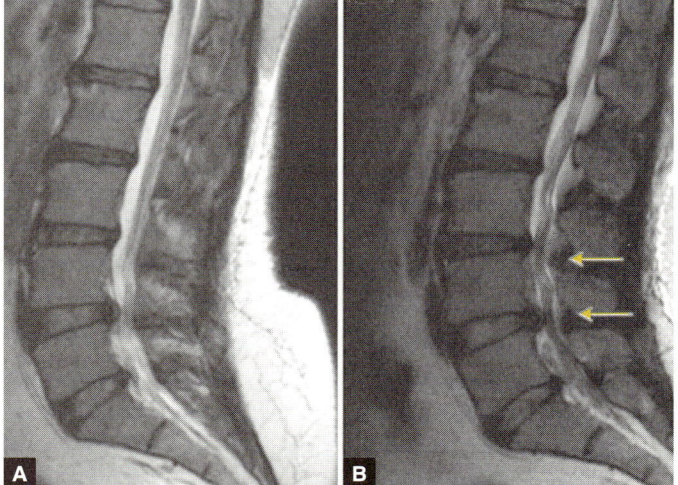

Fig. 7.13A and B: T2 weighted sagittal images at rest (A) and postaxial loading (B) reveals increase in canal stenosis at multiple levels, predominantly due to buckling of ligamentum flavum (green arrows)

A DSCA (dural sac cross-sectional area) more than 100 mm^2 is considered as normal, between 75 and 100 mm^2 is relative stenosis and less than 75 mm^2 is absolute stenosis.[18–21] A decrease in more than 15 mm^2 in the DSCA on the application of axial load is considered significant for dynamic canal stenosis (Fig. 7.13).

The imaging features may be roughly classified into two categories—qualitative and quantitative findings. Qualitative criteria for canal stenosis are discussed below.

QUALITATIVE CRITERIA

- Disc protrusion/extrusion/sequestration
- Hypertrophic facet joint degeneration
- Hypertrophy of ligamentum flavum
- Absent fluid around cauda equina
- Serpine and/or redundant nerve roots
- Perineural intraforaminal fat obliteration
- Perineural and synovial cysts
- Epidural lipomatosis.

The main causes of spinal canal and neural foraminal stenosis include disc herniation, facetal arthropathy and ligamentum flavum hypertrophy amongst others listed above.

Disc herniation is an important cause of spinal/foraminal stenosis. Disc bulge is extension of disc material for >25% circumference and 3 mm or less beyond the disc space. Disc herniation may either be a protruded disc where maximum diameter of herniated disc is less than at its base (from site of herniation to parent disc) or extruded disc, where maximum diameter of herniated disc is more than at its base

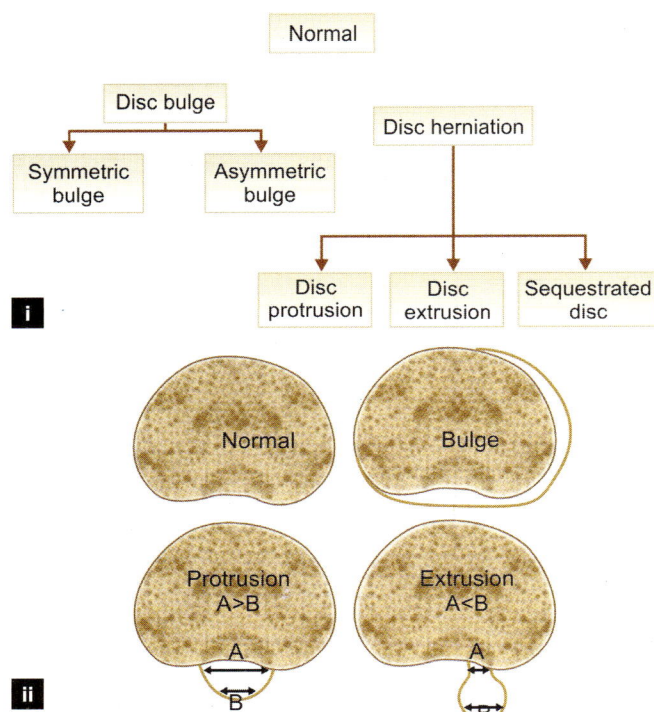

Fig. 7.14i and ii: Disc pathology with flowchart (i) and line diagram (ii) showing disc bulge, herniation, prolapse, extrusion and sequestration

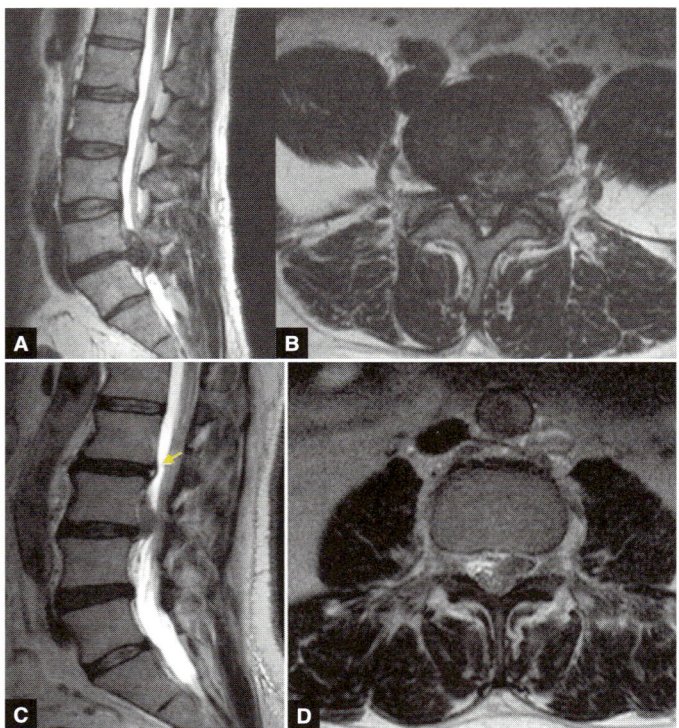

Fig. 7.15A to D: T2-weighted sagittal and axial images (A and B) showing T2 hypointense extruded disc material at L5/S1 level causing severe lumbar canal stenosis, complete effacement of T2 hyperintense CSF at that level and compression of cauda equina. T2-weighted sagittal and axial images (C and D) showing another patient with T2 hypointense extruded disc material at L3/L4 level with peripheral T2 hyperintensity suggestive of acute inflammatory changes. The disc has migrated cranially and leftward causing compression of left exiting L4 and traversing L5 nerve roots. There is in addition posterior annular tear seen in L2/L3 intervertebral disc (yellow arrow)

(Fig. 7.14i and ii). Sequestrated disc is where disc material loses its connection with parent disc and may migrate superiorly or inferiorly within the canal (Fig. 7.15).

Severe compression of cauda equina may lead to effacement of T2 hyperintense CSF within thecal sac and serpine/redundant proximal nerve roots (Figs 7.7 and 7.15).

Facetal and ligamentum flavum hypertrophy more often coexist. Facetal arthropathy refers to degenerative bony overgrowth that causes narrowing of lateral recess, neural foramen and spical canal. Ligamentum flavum hypertrophy is due to degenerative fibrosis which leads to encroachment on posterior CSF space within the thecal sac and resultant posterior narrowing of spinal canal (Fig. 7.16A and B).

Load-induced symptoms due to cauda equina encroachment seem more likely to be caused by bulging of the ligamentum flavum than protrusion of the disc[22] (Fig. 7.13). Even in cases of claudication, as symptoms are relieved by forward bending or stooping, stretching of ligamentum flavum seems like the cause rather than an increased protrusion of the disc.[11]

Epidural lipomatosis is a condition seen in obese individuals where there is hypertrophy of adipose tissue in epidural space, causing compression on the sac and thereby symptoms of lumbar canal stenosis.

Figure 7.17 depicts excessive T2 hyperintense fat in epidural space causing compression over thecal sac.

Synovial cysts result from degeneration of facet joints. Excessive fluid in the joint space projects into the lateral recess/neural foramen as a T2 hyperintense fluid filled cyst, causing stenosis and sometimes, nerve root compression.

Similarly, perineural cysts also reveal homogenously T2 hyperintense signal and may be seen along spinal nerve roots. They are commonly seen as incidental findings and are majorly asymptomatic, but sometimes they can cause compression of nerve root and present with neuralgia.

Effect on Neural Elements

T2W MR images provide detailed information of effects of spinal stenosis on neural elements.

Spinal canal stenosis may lead to effacement of CSF space, displacement/indentation cord or cauda equina or direct compression. Cord compression leads to T2

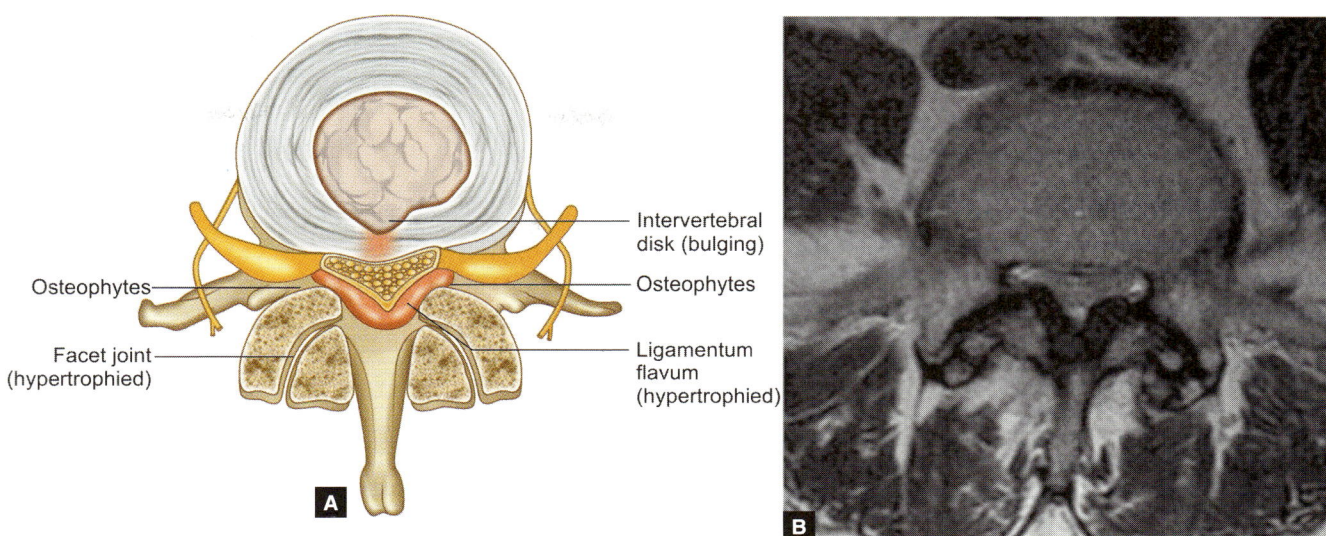

Fig. 7.16A and B: (A) Anatomical depiction of combination of central disc bulge, ligamentum flavum hypertrophy and facetal joint arthropathy. (B) Reveals T2 weighted axial image in a patient with claudication, showing similar findings—hypertrophy of ligamentum flavum and facetal joint arthropathy causing lumbar canal stenosis

hyperintense signal which suggests cord edema in acute stage and atrophy/myelomalacia in chronic stage. Compression of spinal canal may cause serpine appearance or redundancy of nerve roots above the level of compression as described earlier in the chapter (Fig. 7.7). Linear T2 hyperintense hydrosyrinx may be seen proximally in cases of severe compression (Fig. 7.18).

Foraminal stenosis can be observed by effacement of perineural T1 and T2 hyperintense fat within the foramen (Fig. 7.19). In lumbar spine, inferior portion of foramen is the first to become narrow followed by nerve bearing upper portion[24] Qualitative grading system for foraminal stenosis was described by Wildermuth et al,[25] which does not take into consideration the morphological changes in the nerve root. Hasegawa et al,[26] in a cadaveric study, showed that significant nerve root compression is commonly

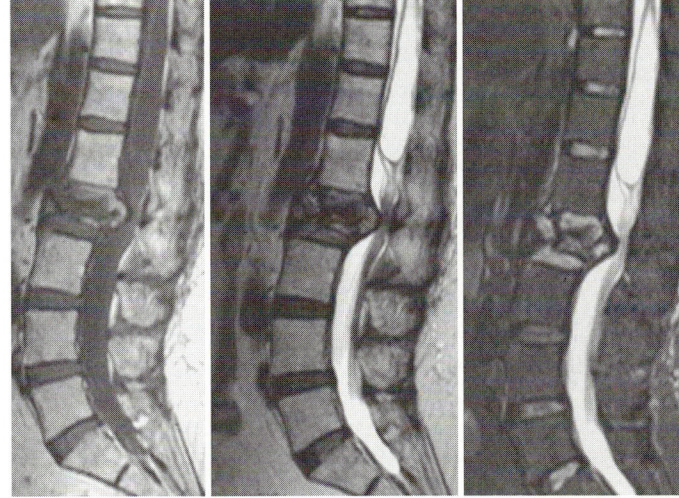

Fig. 7.18: Sagital T1-weighted, T2-weighted and STIR images showing solitary metastasis to L2 vertebral body with pathological fracture, retropulsion causing severe canal stenosis and compression of cauda equina. There is hydromyelia seen in the cord above the level of compression

associated with a foraminal height of 15 mm or less and a posterior disc height of 4 mm or less.

Disc space narrowing with overgrowth of ligamentum flavum and bone spurs, anterior to the facet joint capsule may lead to anteroposterior stenosis (transverse stenosis). Craniocaudal compression (vertical stenosis) of nerve root is caused by posterolateral osteophytes from the vertebral end plates protruding into the foramen along with a laterally bulging annulus fibrosis or herniated disc, compressing the nerve root against the superior pedicle. A combination of these two types of static changes in

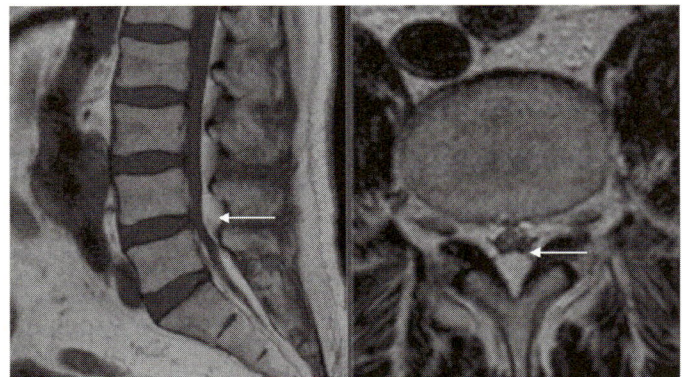

Fig. 7.17: T2 weighted sagittal and axial images of lumbar spine with excessive epidural fat deposition (blue arrow) consistent with epidural lipomatosis

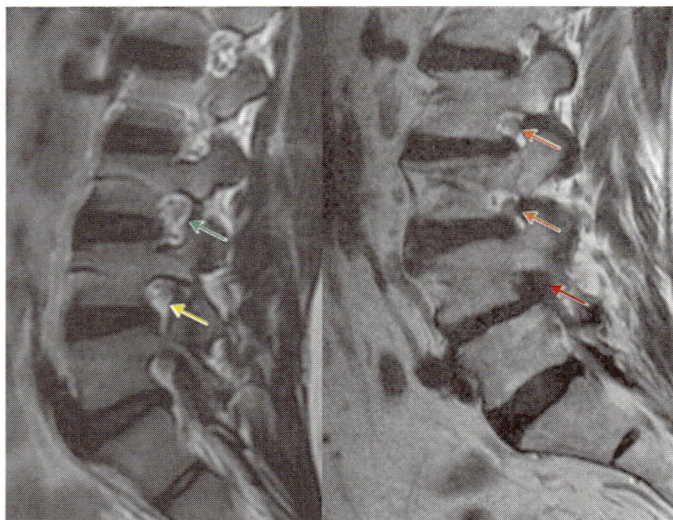

Fig. 7.19: T2W parasagittal images at the level of neural foramen showing Sheunghun Lee grading for canal stenosis: Normal (green arrow); Grade 1 (yellow arrow—mild effacement of perineural fat); Grade 2 (orange arrow—moderate effacement of perineural fat); grade 3 (red arrow—complete effacement of perineural fat with nerve root compression)

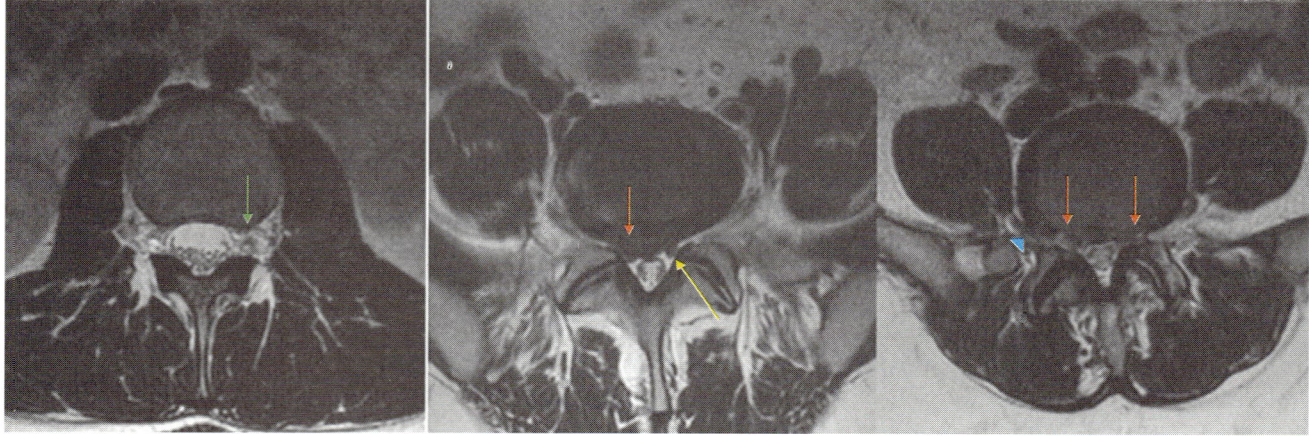

Fig. 7.20: Pfirrmann grading for disc herniation: Normal: Grade 1 (green arrow); Grade 2 (yellow arrow—abutment of the nerve root); Grade 3 (orange arrow—abutment with displacement); Grade 4 (red arrow—compression of nerve root)

foraminal volume may develop and cause severe circumferential stenosis.[24]

Seunghun Lee et al staging includes both perineural fat obliteration and nerve root morphology on the basis of sagittal MR images (Fig. 7.18). This system is more practicable for grading foraminal stenosis considering the frequency of radiculopathy caused by nerve root irritation: Grade 0 refers to the absence of foraminal stenosis; grade 1 refers to mild foraminal stenosis showing perineural fat obliteration in the two opposing directions, vertical or transverse; grade 2 refers to moderate foraminal stenosis showing perineural fat obliteration in the four directions without morphologic change, both vertical and transverse directions; and grade 3 refers to severe foraminal stenosis showing nerve root collapse or morphologic change.[23]

A higher incidence of foraminal stenosis is found in the left side and lower lumbar segments. According to previous reviews,[23,26] the most common roots involved are the fifth lumbar root, followed by the fourth, third, and second.

Pfirrmann et al divided disc herniation into 4 grades: Normal (grade I), contact of disc with nerve root without displacement (grade II), displacement of nerve root (grade III) and compression of nerve root (grade IV)[27] (Fig. 7.20).

Imaging has become an integral part of patient management of lumbar canal stenosis. With the introduction of new diagnostic methods and improvement in imaging modalities, there has been significant increase in diagnostic accuracy, thereby aiding in better patient outcome.

REFERENCES

1. C. Arnoldi, A. Brodsky, and J. Cauchoix, "Lumbar spinal stenosis and nerve root entrapment syndromes: definition and classification," Clin Orthop Relat Res, vol. 1976;115, pp. 4–5.

2. D. Bosworth, J. Filding, and L. Demarest, "Bonequist, of cases treated by arthrodesis," J Bone Jt. Surg Am, vol. 37, pp. 1955;767–786.

3. Imaging spinal stenosis By Kiran S. Talekar, MD; Mougnyan Cox, MD; Elana Smith, MD; and Adam E. Flanders, MD Applied Radiology-01–17.

4. Patel ND, Broderick DF, Burns J, et al. American College of Radiology ACR Appropriateness Criteria® Low Back Pain. Available at https://acsearch. acr.org/docs/69483/Narrative/American College of Radiology. Accessed 12/12/2016.

5. Chou R, Qaseem A, Owens DK, Shekelle P. Diagnostic imaging for low back pain: advice for high-value health care from the American College of Physicians. Ann Intern Med.;2011;154 (3):181–189.

6. Arana E, Kovac F, Royuela A., et al. Influence of nomenclature in the interpretation of lumbar disk countour on MR imaging: a comparison of the agreement using the combined task force and the Nordic nomenclatures. AJNR Am J Neuroradiol. 2011;32(6):1143–1148.

7. P. Gopinathan, "Lumbar spinal canal stenosis-special features," Journal of Orthopaedics, vol. 12, no. 3, 2015;pp. 123–125.

8. Kreiner DS, Shaffer WO, Baisden JL, et al. An evidence-based clinical guideline for diagnosis and treatment of degenerative lumbar spinal stenosis. Spine J. 2013; 13(7):734–743.

9. Giulia Michelini et al., "Dynamic MRI in the evaluation of the spine: state of the art," Acta Biomed, vol. 89, 2018;pp. 89–101.

10. Russell D, D'Angelo C, Zimmerman R, et al. Cervical disc hernation: CT demonstration after contrast enhancement. Radiology. 1984; 152(3): 703–712.

11. George McKay, Peter Alexander Torrie, Wendy Bertram, Priyan Landham, Stephen Morris, John Hutchinson, Roland Watura, and Ian Harding Myelography in the Assessment of Degenerative Lumbar Scoliosis and Its Influence on Surgical Management Korean J Spine. 2017 Dec; 14(4): 133–138.

12. Aota Y, Niwa T, Yoshikawa K, Fujiwara A, Asada T, Saito T. Magnetic resonance imaging and magnetic resonance myelography in the presurgical diagnosis of lumbar foraminal stenosis. Spine. 2007;32:896–903.

13. M. Gallucci, N. Limbucci, A. Paonessa, and A. Splendiani, "Degenerative Disease of the Spine," Neuroimaging Clinics of North America, vol. 17, no. 1. pp. 87–103, 2007.

14. J. G. Jarvik and R. A. Deyo, "Diagnostic evaluation of low back pain with emphasis on imaging," Ann. Intern. Med., vol. 137, no. 7, pp. 586–597, 2002.

15. P. Gopinathan, "Lumbar spinal canal stenosis-special features," Journal of Orthopaedics, vol. 12, no. 3, pp. 123–125, 2015.

16. Kreiner DS, Shaffer WO, Baisden JL, et al. An evidence-based clinical guideline for diagnosis and treatment of degenerative lumbar spinal stenosis. Spine J. 2013; 13(7):734–743.

17. Imaging spinal stenosis By Kiran S. Talekar, MD; Mougnyan Cox, MD; Elana Smith, MD; and Adam E. Flanders, MD Applied Radiology-01–17.

18. W. Reith, S. Bodea, M. Kettner, R. Mühl-Benninghausen, and A. Simgen, "Degenerative and age-related alterations of the spine," Radiologe, vol. 54, no. 11, pp. 1069–1077, 2014.

19. C. Arnoldi, A. Brodsky, and J. Cauchoix, "Lumbar spinal stenosis and nerve root entrapment syndromes: definition and classification," Clin Orthop Relat Res, vol. 115.

20. M. Chung, I. J. Dahabreh, and N. Hadar, "Emerging MRI Technologies for Imaging Musculoskeletal Disorders Under Loading Stress," 2011.

21. S. Goel, "Stress MRI for the assessment of lumbar canal stenosis in degenerative disc disease: comparison with routine MRI," in ECR, 2015, p. B-0302.

22. WT. Yoshiiwa, M. Miyazaki, N. Notani, T. Ishihara, M. Kawano, and H. Tsumura, "Analysis of the relationship between ligamentum flavum thickening and lumbar segmental instability, disc degeneration, and facet joint osteoarthritis in lumbar spinal stenosis," Asian Spine J., vol. 10, no. 6, pp. 1132–1140, 2016.

23. Neuroradiology Head and Neck Imaging A Practical MRI Grading System for Lumbar Foraminal Stenosis Seung hun Lee, Joon Woo Lee, Jin Sup Yeom, Ki-Jeong Kim, Hyun-Jib Kim, SooKyo Chung and Heung Sik Kang AJR April 2010, Volume 194, Number 4.

24. Hasegawa T, An HS, Haughton VM, Nowicki BH. Lumbar foraminal stenosis: critical heights of the intervertebral discs and foramina: a cryomicrotome study in cadavera. J Bone Joint Surg Am 1995; 77:32–38.

25. Wildermuth S, Zanetti M, Duewell S, et al. Lumbar spine: quantitative and qualitative assessment of positional (upright flexion and extension) MR imaging and myelography. Radiology 1998; 207:391–398.

26. Hasegawa T, Mikawa Y, Watanabe R, An HS. Morphometric analysis of the lumbosacral nerve roots and dorsal root ganglia by magnetic resonance imaging. Spine 1996; 21:1005–1009.

27. Pfirrmann C, Dora C, Schmid M, et al. MR image-based grading of lumbar nerve root compromise due to disk herniation: reliability study with surgical correlation. Radiology. 2004;230(2):583–588.

Clinical Presentation in Lumbar Canal Stenosis

Apurva Prasad, PS Ramani

INTRODUCTION

Lumbar canal stenosis is defined as a pathological narrowing of the vertebral canal and/or intervertebral foramen with ageing that leads to compression of the thecal sac and/or the nerve roots. The incidence of lumbar canal stenosis in the general population is between 1.7% and 8%, and it increases from the fifth decade of life onwards.[15] However, the senior author is of the opinion that in India it is seen at least 5 years earlier.[17]

Spinal stenosis is classified as either primary or secondary. The primary is caused by congenital abnormalities or a disorder of postnatal development,[3] and secondary (acquired stenosis) results from degenerative changes. It is also seen sometimes as a consequence of local infection, trauma or surgery. The components that contribute to acquired stenosis include the facets (hypertrophy, arthropathy), ligamentum flavum (hypertrophy), posterior longitudinal ligament (ossification of posterior longitudinal ligament [OPLL]), vertebral body (bone spurs) and intervertebral disc (prolapse). Congenital stenosis superimposed on degenerative changes can contribute to become symptomatic earlier in life.

Lumbar canal stenosis can be categorized as central and lateral forms, according to the anatomical area of the spine affected. Signs and symptoms are thought to result from vascular compromise to the vessels supplying the cauda equina (central stenosis) or from pressure on the nerve root complex (lateral stenosis) by the degenerative changes. Foraminal stenosis is more frequently seen at L4–L5 level compressing the L5 nerve root, as this foramen has the smaller foramen/root area ratio[9] resulting in sciatic pain and weakness in extensor hallucis longus muscle (EHL weakness) and sometimes tibialis anterior muscle (TA weakness).

Lumbar canal stenosis causes obliteration of normal lumbar lordosis and creates straightening of the lumbosacral angle. In most people, the posterolateral protrusion is common. It shifts the nerve root medially and to prevent irritation, the patient bends away from the side of pain (convexity of scoliosis on the side of pain).

The slowly progressive nature of degenerative changes has an important dynamic bearing. The available space in the central canal decreases in axial loading and extension of spine while it increases in axial distraction and flexion of spine.[18] The same dynamics also affect the foramen with flexion causing a 12% increase, and extension a 15% decrease, in surface area.[8]

Clinical Presentation

Ninety per cent of the population at some time or another suffer from back pain to warrant medical attention. An episode of lifting weight or unwarranted sudden bending or twisting brings on the pain.[15] However, most of the times the pain is musculofascial and the incidence is highest in the middle age. The pain resolves insiduously in the majority of patients. Only in the few, the pain persists.

The classical clinical presentation of lumbar canal stenosis is neurogenic claudication along with chronic low back pain with or without sciatica. It worsens on standing for longer periods, physical activity and lumbar extension. Usually there is a history of several years duration and may be associated with lower extremity weakness and numbness along the distribution of nerve roots or weakness in the relevant muscles.[11]

Coughing and sneezing increases intraspinal pressure and aggravates sciatic pain. Valsalva maneuver also aggravates sciatica. The shooting sciatic pain arises deep in the buttock and goes down the back of thigh into the posterior or posterolateral compartment of leg. From then on the 5th lumbar root pain may be felt on the dorsum of the foot or rarely in the great toe. Numbness rather than pain is felt more often in the great toe. The first sacral root pain stops at the ankle joint.

Symptoms of lumbar canal stenosis are more common in males in the 5th decade of life. They complain of discomfort in the thighs, calves, and feet when walking. Bilateral symptoms occur with a male: female ratio of 8:1, whereas the ratio in unilateral claudication is 3:1.[22]

Typically, symptoms are not present at rest, but after walking a short distance patients experience weakness, tiredness, or heaviness of the legs which gradually increases on continuing walking and causes them to stop.[19] Leg pain is often described as severe and radicular in distribution, and may be exacerbated with lumbar extension to the painful side (Kemp's test) (Fig. 8.1).[9]

The walking tolerance (when the patient stops) is usually twice the threshold distance when they first feel discomfort. While walking, the patient stoops forward, gradually reduces walking speed, and sometimes will stoop forward until he or she finally stops. These are maneuvers of the patient to compensate for symptoms and limiting distance of ambulation.

In patients with central stenosis, symptoms usually involve both the buttocks and both the posterior thighs in a non-dermatomal distribution. With lateral recess stenosis, symptoms are usually dermatome specific due to compression of a specific nerve root. Patients with lateral recess stenosis may have more pain during rest and at night, but their walking tolerance is better than patients with central stenosis. In addition, patients with symptomatic lumbar canal stenosis have a risk of falling.[12]

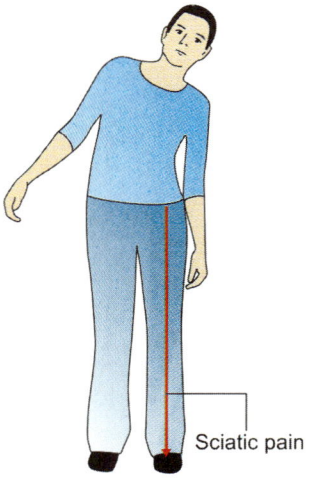

Fig. 8.1: Pain exaggerates on tilting to the painful side

Sciatic pain

Examination of the lower back shows straightening of the spine. Movements are restricted. Extension may be more limited than flexion.[23] Hamstring tightness is often found. The neurological examination typically is normal, and findings when present are usually mild focal motor weakness or sensory changes. Some of these signs may be increased immediately after the patient performs symptomatic exercises.[4] Straight leg raising test is variable. Jerks at ankle and knee may be absent or decreased in response. Half the patients have the feeling of decreased sensation.

In cases of severe lumbar canal stenosis, patients suffer from nocturnal leg cramps, rest pain and neurogenic bladder and bowel symptoms.[6]

LOW BACK PAIN

Back pain is usually the first symptom. The onset of back pain or lumbago is usually insidious with slow progress after twisting injury to the back. Often, the backache is mild to start with and is aggravated by exertion and relieved with rest. The pain is felt widely throughout the lumbar spine and the sacrum, usually bilaterally and feels deep. It spreads to sacroiliac joints and deep in the gluteal regions. The spine becomes stiff due to muscle spasm and movements become painfully restricted with the result that the patient turns in bed cautiously like a log of wood. He tries to move the whole body as a block rather than perform a movement. If muscle spasm is bilateral, then normal lordosis is obliterated and if it is unilateral, then scoliosis and list of the spine is produced. Rest relieves pain. Between episodes of acute pain, dull ache may persist in the back and tender spots can be elicited.

SCIATICA

Sciatica indicates a prolapsed disc along with lateral recess stenosis and the symptoms are distributed along the two involved nerve roots. The pain is deep in the muscles and the bone. Movements of the spine and maneuvers like coughing, sneezing aggravates the pain and it becomes increasingly intense, shooting like electric shock down the leg. Patient walks with limp keeping knee flexed, pelvis tilted and exaggerated lordosis.

NEUROGENIC CLAUDICATION

Claudication means to limp and be lame. The term was initially used to describe condition of limbs in vascular occlusive diseases.

In 1858, Charcot applied the term to describe the vascular occlusive condition in human beings. Dejerine (1911) introduced the term to describe spinal intermittent claudication. He described three cases in which activity was followed by limb weakness and appearance of pyramidal signs which disappeared with rest. The mechanism was thought to be exercise related spinal ischaemia resulting in weakness. T. Bergmark (1950) studied histopathology of the spinal cord of one of his patients who had died and showed destruction of anterior horn cells and demyelination of anterior pyramidal fibers, thus conclusively proving the existence of this entity in the spinal cord. Blau and Logue (1961) introduced the term further to describe intermittent claudication of the cauda equina.

Hank Verbiest can rightly be described as the father of neurogenic claudication. He established relationship between lumbar spondylosis and neurogenic signs and symptoms in the legs. In 1949, he described three cases of lumbar canal stenosis who were relieved by decompressive laminectomy. He then (1954) described congenital narrow lumbar canal and devised calipers to measure the canal at operation. As a result of this work most spinal surgeons now imply neurogenic claudication as lumbar canal stenosis.[1,2,5]

Based on this fact it can be assumed that sciatica is produced mostly by ischemia in the nerve root caused by compression.

Central canal stenosis classically presents as neurogenic claudication (NC), which is characterized by pain and weakness starting in the buttocks and thighs that becomes gradually worse in the orthostatic position and during walking, but improves after sitting down or leaning forward. Unilateral radicular symptoms may result from severe foraminal or lateral recess stenosis. Patients, typically aged more than 50 years, report insidious onset of neurogenic claudication. It can manifest as intermittent, crampy, diffuse, radiating to the thigh or leg with associated heaviness and paresthesias. The most common nerve affected is the L5, with associated weakness of extensor hallucis longus.[13]

Onset of symptoms during ambulation is believed to be caused by increased metabolic demands of compressed nerve roots that have become ischemic due to stenosis. This is the hallmark of neurogenic claudication.

The pain is relieved when the patient flexes the spine by leaning forwards or sitting. Flexion increases canal size by stretching the protruding ligamentum flavum and reducing the overriding laminae and facets. Enlargement of the foramina relieves the pressure on the exiting nerve roots and, thus, decreases the pain.

Lumbar spinal canal and lateral recess cross-sectional area increases with spinal flexion and decreases with extension. The cross-sectional area is reduced by 9%

with extension in the normal spine and 67% with severe stenosis. The "Penning rule of progressive narrowing" implies that the more narrowed the canal by stenosis, the more it narrows with spinal extension.[7,20]

Relief with sitting in lumbar canal stenosis contrasts with most non-specific low back pain which is commonly exacerbated by prolonged sitting. Patients with neurogenic claudication report that laying flat is often associated with less relief than while lying on the side (permitting lumbar flexion). The distance that can be walked before symptoms occur is more variable in those with neurogenic claudication compared with vascular claudication, and is increased by forward bending of the torso (increased thoracic kyphosis and decreased lumbar lordosis). As a consequence, patients adopt a position with hip and knee slightly flexed sometimes referred as "simian stance".

Examination of the lower back will reveal reduced mobility. Extension may be more limited than flexion. Hamstring tightness is often found. The neurological examination typically is normal, and findings when present are usually mild motor weakness or sensory changes. Some of these signs may be increased immediately after the patient performs symptomatic exercises. Absent or decreased ankle reflexes have been reported in about half of patients but this sign is frequently found in older patients without stenosis. Physical examination reveals normal pulsations, normal temperature of skin and no evidence of ischaemic changes.[10]

Neurogenic claudication must be differentiated from vascular claudication (VC), wherein, abnormalities of the arterial pulse along with trophic alterations aggravate symptoms on biking, uphill ambulation, and lumbar flexion.[8] Pain radiates downward in neurogenic claudication and, in contrast, it radiates upwards in vascular claudication (Table 8.1).

Table 8.1: Neurogenic *vs* vascular claudication		
Evaluation	Neurogenic claudication	Vascular claudication
Walking distance	Variable	Fixed
Provocative factor	Standing	Walking
Palliative factor	Sitting/bending	Standing
Walking uphill	Painless	Painful
Skin	No trophic changes	Loss of hair, shiny
Back pain	Common	Rare
Back movements	Limited	Free
Pain character	Numbness, proximal to distal	Cramping, distal to proximal
Peripheral pulsations	Present	Feeble/absent

Paraesthesiae

This is a subjective disturbance of cutaneous sensibility. It is fairly common if proper enquiry is made. It includes tingling, pins and needles and numbness. The skin over the area of distribution of nerve is unusually sensitive to light touch and pin prick. Paraesthesiae is usually felt peripherally over the foot or posterior calf often aggravated by pain.

Muscle Weakness

Slight degree of weakness evident on examination is usually not noticed by the patient. Foot drop is commonly observed by the patient as difficulty in clearing the ground while walking or climbing. Sudden fall may be due to knee giving way because of quadriceps weakness.

Disturbance of Sphincters

Inability to pass urine as a sole symptom of disc prolapse has been described. However, it is rare for the patient to present in this way. More often they have other associated symptoms of cauda equina compression including loss of sexual potency.

The Cauda Equina Syndrome[21,24]

It is an emergency; the severe pain is centered around the low back and the peri-anal region. Radicular symptoms may be masked. Difficulty in micturition or even frequency or retention with overflow may develop early. History of recent impotence may be elicited in males. Pain in the legs or sciatica is usually followed by numbness in feet and difficulty in walking. This syndrome is produced by large disc prolapse in the midline. It then compresses several nerve roots of the cauda equina. The centrally placed visceral fibers to the lower abdominal organs are most affected. Perianal numbness and loss of anal reflex characterize advanced cauda equina syndrome. This syndrome does not respond to the conservative line of treatment. It requires surgery and once the syndrome is diagnosed, the operation should be done expeditiously to avoid bladder complications.

The Conus Medullaris Syndrome[21]

Conus Medullaris syndrome occurs due to lumbar canal stenosis with disc prolapse at T12 to L2 vertebral levels and presents with combined UMN and LMN features. Patients present with sudden and bilateral low back pain and saddle anesthesia. Radicular pain is less severe but weakness and numbness in the legs is commonly found. Urinary retention and overflow incontinence with fecal incontinence may be present. Peri-anal numbness with dissociated sensory loss is common. It requires early surgery.

The Syndrome of Facet Hypertrophy and Tropism

The syndrome is not well understood by many. The author had described this in 1983.[22] It forms an important cause of backache. It is usually common in males and particularly those who are engaged in heavy labor. They have usually suffered from chronic backache for several years. They have degeneration in the disc followed by instability in the motion segment. This leads to chronic degenerative changes in the facet joints which become hypertrophied and coronally oriented. The ligamentum flavum is buckled under the hypertrophied facet and resultant lateral spinal stenosis compresses on the cauda equina and the nerve roots. Instability in the motion segment is the hallmark of this syndrome. They usually complain of morning stiffness and have difficulty in getting out of bed. There is pain deep seated in the lumbar region. The pain in both legs is not true sciatic type but vague. Walking for a while seems to loosen the back with diminution in the intensity of pain. Climbing becomes difficult and standing and sitting is painful.

On examination the back is found to be stiff. Lordosis is obliterated. There is no scoliosis. Spinal movements are painful and restricted. SLR and femoral stretch tests are negative. There is no wasting or weakness in the muscles. Localizing signs are often absent and X-rays along with myelography clinch the diagnosis. In spite of significant defect seen on the myelogram, prolapsed disc is usually absent.

PHYSICAL SIGNS

Stance and Gait

The pelvis of the patient is tilted usually to one side with the result that there is slight flexion of hip and knee joints and correction causes pain. The spine is tilted and there is scoliosis. Normal lumbar curve of the spine is usually obliterated and spinal movements are greatly restricted. There is hardly any rotational movement in the lumbar spine but attempts at rotation in the higher spine causes pain. The para-vertebral muscles are prominent due to spasm and the buttock on the affected side may be wasted. Standing tip-toe on the affected side is not possible due to pain and weakness of plantar flexion. Movements are slow. Trunk dips to the affected side and patient turns to one side as a whole like a block of wood rather than twisting.

Reflexes

The plantar response is usually normal. Presence or absence of ankle or knee jerks is of great importance. In compression of SI root the ankle jerk is absent. The knee jerk is diminished or absent if L3 and L4 roots are involved. When L5 root is involved, jerks are present. Anomalous reflexes may be due to multiple disc prolapses or to a previous healed disc lesion. It has been observed that an absent ankle jerk in prolapsed disc syndrome remains absent following surgical treatment of the prolapse disc.

Tension Signs

This term was introduced by O'Connel in 1951[14] to describe those tests which aggravated root pain by increasing stretch or tension in them. Two tests which are important are described here.

1. Straight Leg Raising (SLR or Lasegue's Test)

This is performed with patient lying supine and is well relaxed (Fig. 8.2). The leg is slowly raised with knee remaining extended. The leg is raised by the examiner by placing his hand under the heel. In young children the leg can be raised to beyond 90 degrees. In young adults it can be raised up to 90 degrees and in elderly patients up to about 75 degrees. In cases of prolapse of 4th or 5th lumbar disc, elevation of leg produces pain. Limitation of straight leg raising correlates with severity of the disc prolapse and SLR improves as acuity of disc pain becomes less. The test should be performed slowly with the confidence of the patient. The test can be refined by raising the leg to just short of causing pain and then passively flexing the head or dorsi-flexing the foot. Both these maneuvers will bring on the pain.

2. Femoral Stretch Test

This test applies tension to the upper lumbar roots and is useful in neurogenic claudication. The patient lies in the lateral position with affected side facing above with knee and hip slightly flexed. It has two components. The hip is first extended thus creating tension in the

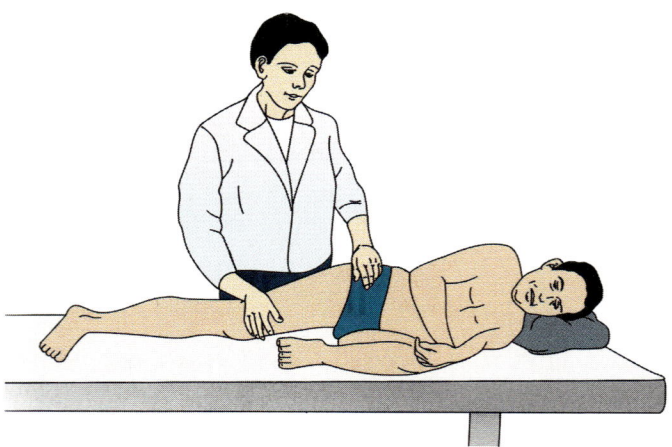

Fig. 8.3: The lumbar spine must be held rigid, if necessary, by flexing the lower hip. The upper hip is extended. A rotary strain is produced on the pelvis. The sacro iliac joint produces pain. In case of higher lumbar disc prolapse, the pain is felt anteriorly on the thigh

ileopsoas and hence traction on the upper lumbar nerve roots (Fig. 8.3). The knee is then progressively flexed to increase the tension in the femoral nerve. The pain is felt in front of the thigh.

Differential Diagnoses

Besides degeneration in lumbar spine, the other problems to be considered include:[16]

- Rheumatologic: Ankylosing spondylitis/spondylo-arthropathy, diffuse idiopathic skeletal hyperostosis (DISH).
- Infectious: Epidural, subdural, intradural abscess; diskitis; Pott disease.
- Metabolic: Osteomalacia, parathyroid disease, vitamin B_{12} or folic acid deficiency.
- Traumatic: Lumbar strain, lumbar compression fracture, spondylosis and spondylolisthesis.
- Developmental/congenital: Scoliosis.
- Vascular: Peripheral vascular disease (with vascular claudication), abdominal aortic dissection.
- Psychogenic: Conversion disorder, malingering.
- Others: Metastatic breast cancer, prostate cancer, Paget's disease.

REFERENCES

1. Bergmark G: Intermittent Spinal claudication. Acta Med. Scand Suppl 1950;246; 30–8.
2. Blan JN Logue V. Intermittent claudication of the cauda equina. An unusual syndrome resulting from central disc protrusion of the lumbar intervertebral disc. Lancet 1961;25;1081–1084.
3. Ciricillo SF, Weinstein PR. Lumbar spinal stenosis. West J Med. Feb 1993;158(2):171–7.
4. Crawshaw C, Kean DM, Mulholland RC, et al. The use of nuclear magnetic resonance in the diagnosis of lateral canal entrapment. J Bone Joint Surg Br 1984;66:711–5.

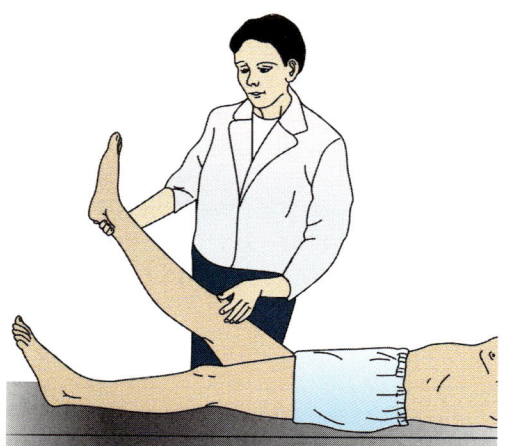

Fig. 8.2: Straight leg raising test is an important physical sign in backache and sciatica. The leg must be raised slowly with the knee extended

5. Dejerine J: La Claudication intermittente de la moelle eopiniere, Presses Med 1948;19:981–85.

6. Dodge LD, Bohlman HH, Rhodes RS. Concurrent lumbar spinal stenosis and peripheral vascular disease: a report of nine patients. Clin Orthop Relat Res. 1988;(230):141–48.

7. Hai Y. Classification, natural history and clinical evaluation lumbar spine; Herkowitz HH, Dvorak JJ, Bell G, et al. Philadelphia: Lippincott Williams & Wilkins;pp. 2004;464–71.

8. Inufusa A, An HS, Lim TH, Hasegawa T, et al. Anatomic changes of the spinal canal and intervertebral foramen associated with flexion-extension movement. Spine 1996 Nov 1;21(21):2412–20.

9. Jenis LG, An HS. Spine update. Lumbar foraminal stenosis. Spine 2000; 25(3):389–94.

10. Johnsson KE, Rosen I, Uden A. The natural course of lumbar spinal stenosis. Acta Orthop Scand Suppl 1993;251:67–8.

11. Julie M, Fritz, Anthony Delitto, William C. Welch. Lumbar spinal stenosis: A review of current concepts in evaluation, management and outcome measurements. Archives of physical medicine and rehabilitation; volume 79; issue 6; 1998;p 700–8.

12. Kim HJ, Chun HJ, Han CD, et al. The risk assessment of a fall in patients with lumbar spinal stenosis. Spine (Phila Pa 1976); 2011;36:E588–E592.

13. Morishita Y, Hida S, Naito M, et al. Measurement of the local pressure of the intervertebral foramen and the electrophysiologic values of the spinal nerve roots in the vertebral foramen. Spine 2006;Dec 15;31(26):3076–80.

14. O'Connel JEA:(1951) Protrusions of the lumbar intervertebral discs. J. bone Joint surg; 1951;33;8–17.

15. Pedro Sa, Pedro Marques, Bruno Alpoim et al. Rev Bras Ortop. 2014;Jul-August; 49(4); 405–8.

16. Porter, Richard W. Spinal stenosis and neurogenic claudication; Spine; Vol. 21;issue 17;1996;p 2046–52.

17. Ramani PS. Backache and Sciaitica; Falcon Publishers, Mumbai; India; 1996;p 46–54.

18. Schönström N, Lindahl S, Willén J, Hansson T. Dynamic changes in the dimensions of the lumbar spinal canal: an experimental study in vitro. Journal of orthopaedic research;1989;7(1):115–21.

19. Seung Y. Lee, Tae-Hwan Kim, Jae Keun Oh, et al. Lumbar stenosis: A recent update by review of literature. Asian Spine J; 2015;9(5); 8181–828.

20. Takahashi K, Miyazaki T, Takino T, et al. Epidural pressure measurements. Relationship between epidural pressure and posture in patients with lumbar spinal stenosis. Spine 1995;Mar 15;20(6): 650–3.

21. Tandon PN, Sankaran B. Cauda Syndrome due to lumbar disc prolapse. Ind. J. Orthopaed 1967;1:112–115.

22. Turner JA, Ersek M, Herron L, et al. Surgery for lumbar spinal stenosis. Attempted meta-analysis of the literature. Spine 1992;17;1–8.

23. Ullrich CG, Binet EF, Sanecki MG, Kieffer SA. Quantitative assessment of the lumbar spinal canal by computed tomography. Radiology 1980;134:137–43.

24. Verbiest H. Neurogenic intermittent claudication in cases with absolute and relative stenosis of the lumbar intervertebral foramina and in cases with both entities. Clin Neurosurg; 1973;20:204–07.

Ignored but Important Signs in LCS: Sedimentation Sign and Cross-Sectional Area of Dura

PS Ramani

INTRODUCTION

Sedimentation sign on axial cut of an MRI of lumbar sign shows this sign. In the past when I had observed it, I found a significant correlation between the sign and the symptoms and signs of the patient. I have written about it elsewhere.

There are several parameters by which lumbar canal stenosis is judged. I have also maintained throughout that of all the parameters the cross-sectional area of dura at the maximum level of compression gives quantitative and objective judgement about the severity of lumbar canal stenosis. Both these signs put together can give the surgeon a fairly correct idea about the severity of the disease.

The Judgement

Today it is common knowledge, that degenerative lumbar canal stenosis in the elderly is the most common indication for spinal surgery.[1,8] In this disorder due to overgrowth of bone the lateral recesses are narrowed down and the dural sac in the centre of canal gets compressed. The patient starts getting symptoms but on examination there are not many signs to document in spite of the fact that patient's activity is restricted and he slows down.

The diagnosis is established only after doing an MRI and demonstrating narrowing of the canal and compression of the dural sac.[2,6]

The cross sectional area of the dural sac can be measured on axial cut of the MRI at the desired level (Fig. 9.1). In normal patients it is more than 100 mm^2. If it is less than 100 mm^2, it indicates stenosis. Such signs are necessary as at any given time it is impossible to correlate patent's symptoms with severity of the disease.[10,11]

Sedimentation Sign

Sedimentation sign is observed on axial cuts of MRI imaging (Fig. 9.2). In patients with no suspected lumbar

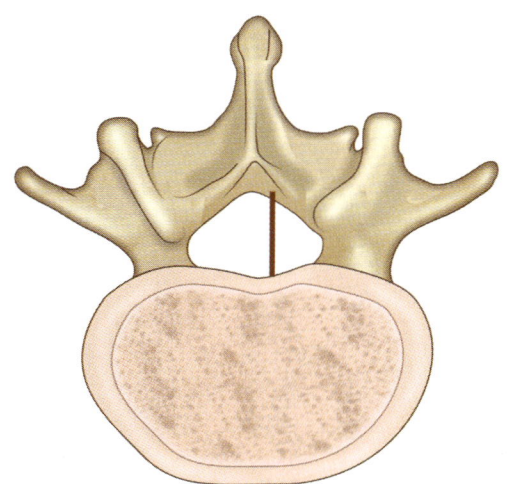
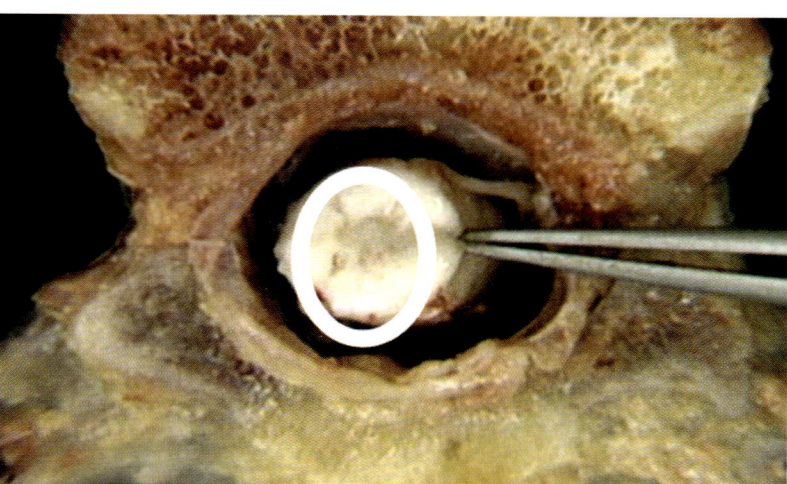

Fig. 9.1: Cross-sectional area of the dural sac (at least 10 mm^2 less than 100 mm^2) are definite objective criteria to determine lumbar canal stenosis

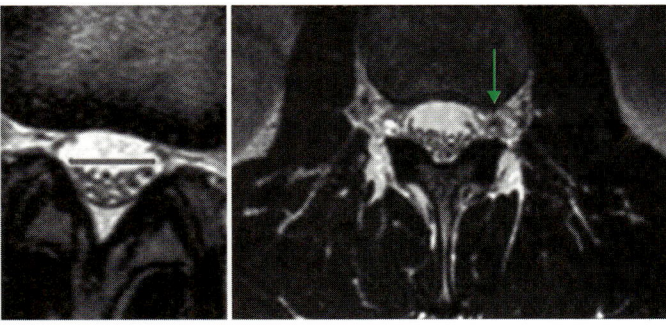

Fig. 9.2: In normal lumbar spine, all the nerve roots are sedimented posteriorly, beyond the diameter of the dural sac

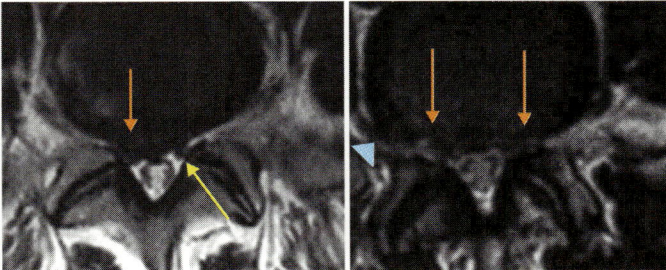

Fig. 9.3: In lumbar canal stenosis, there is absence of sedimentation sign

canal stenosis, owing to the gravitational force, the lumbar nerve roots sink to the dorsal portion of the dural sac (Fig. 9.2). Conversely, in patients with symptomatic LSS, such cauda equina nerve root sedimentation was rarely observed. A positive sedimentation sign is defined as the absence of sedimented nerve roots at the level above and below the stenosis in at least one cross-section magnetic resonance image (Fig. 9.3). Some investigators have found a strong correlation between the sedimentation sign and the symptoms of the patient.[1,9] One investigator has also found a strong correlation between symptoms and sedimentation signs as well as cross-sectional area of the dural sac[5] but it was in a selected group of patients considered for surgery.

Parameters

The parameters are defined as follows.

LCS: Backpain, neurogenic claudication and radiating pain.

Cross sectional area: Less than 100 cm^2.

Sedimentation sign: A positive sedimentation sign is defined as the absence of sedimented nerve roots at the level above and below the stenosis, in at least one cross-section magnetic resonance image.

Sedimentation sign is a precise tool for diagnosis of lumbar canal stenosis.[3]

It can be further confirmed by measuring claudication distance on treadmill and then ranged into different categories of severity. It can also be used for making a decision regarding type and extent of surgery.[4,12]

Similarly cross sectional area of dura has been well-correlated with severity of symptoms.[7]

Conclusion

The severity of lumbar canal stenosis can be well judged with objective criteria on sedimentation sign and cross-sectional area of the dura. The AP diameter of the bony lumbar canal is discussed elsewhere in the chapter on anatomical determinants. As far as the symptoms are concerned they are biased by the subjective feeling of the patient and may not correlate well with signs and therefore may not correlate well with RMDQ or ODI scores.

REFERENCES

1. Atlas SJ, Keller RB, Robson D, et al. Surgical and nonsurgical management of lumbar spinal stenosis: four-year outcomes from the maine lumbar spine study. Spine 2000;25:556–62.
2. Atlas SJ, Keller RB, Wu YA, et al. Long-term outcomes of surgical and nonsurgical management of lumbar spinal stenosis: 8- to 10-year results from the maine lumbar spine study. Spine 2005;30:936–43.
3. Barz T, Melloh M, Staub LP, et al. Nerve root sedimentation sign: evaluation of a new radiological sign in lumbar spinal stenosis. Spine 2010;35:892–97.
4. Barz T, Staub LP, Melloh M, et al. Clinical validity of the nerve root sedimentation sign in patients with suspected lumbar spinal stenosis. Spine J 2014;14:667–74.
5. Fazal A, Yoo A, Bendo JA. Does the presence of the nerve root sedimentation sign on MRI correlate with the operative level in patients undergoing posterior lumbar decompression for lumbar stenosis? Spine J 2013;13:837–42.
6. Fritz JM, Erhard RE, Delitto A, Welch WC, et al. Preliminary results of the use of a two-stage treadmill test as a clinical diagnostic tool in the differential diagnosis of lumbar spinal stenosis. J Spinal Disord Tech 1997;10:410–16.
7. Kanno H, Ozawa H, Koizumi Y, et al. Dynamic change of dural sac cross-sectional area in axial loaded MRI correlates with the severity of clinical symptoms in patients with lumbar spinal canal stenosis. Spine 2012;37:207–13.
8. Resende VAC, Teixeira A, Silva JBd, Neto AC, Leal FJF, Gouveia ARF, Miranda A. Lumbar spinal stenosis: sedimentation sign. Columna 2013;12:192–95.
9. Sangbong Ko. Correlations between sedimentation sign, dural sac cross-sectional area, and clinical symptoms of degenerative lumbar spinal stenosis. Eur Spine. J 2018;27(7):1623–28.
10. Sirvanci M, Bhatia M, Ganiyusufoglu KA et al. Degenerative lumbar spinal stenosis: correlation with Oswestry Disability Index and MR imaging. Eur Spine J 2008;17:679–85.
11. Speciale AC, Pietrobon R, Urban CW, et al. Observer variability in assessing lumbar spinal stenosis severity on magnetic resonance imaging and its relation to cross-sectional spinal canal area. Spine 2002;27:1082–86.
12. Staub LP, Barz T, Melloh M, Lord SJ, et al. Clinical validation study to measure the performance of the nerve root sedimentation sign for the diagnosis of lumbar spinal stenosis. ContempClin Trials 2011;32:470–74.

Unilateral or Bilateral Lateral Recess Stenosis: A Historical Perspective

PS Ramani

INTRODUCTION

The history of lateral recess stenosis is interesting. As such the history of spinal surgery is not very old.[2,4] Today (in 2018) lumbar canal stenosis in the elderly is so common that all spinal surgeons are talking about it. Degenerative lumbar canal stenosis starts in the lateral recess.[3] Hence the presentation of lumbar canal stenosis is with symptoms and signs of nerve root entrapment in the lateral canal. The degeneration is never symmetrical and symptoms of nerve root entrapment start unilaterally and as time passes it spreads to both sides. As time passes the degeneration becomes gross and spreads to medial part of the canal resulting in central degenerative lumbar canal stenosis.

During the early period when symptoms are unilateral. Lateral recess stenosis is unilateral. We do not see it often as most of the patients have a tendency to ignore back pain during the early period. By the time they reach the spinal surgeon the stenosis is always bilateral. But it is possible to get unilateral lumbar canal or lateral recess stenosis.

The Origin

Unilateral lumbar canal stenosis was first described by an Indian Dr PE Bilimoria in Mumbai.[1,8] He called it stenosis of one-half of the lumbar canal. In those days leave aside MRI, even CT scan was not available. He suspected the disease and then used high quality tomograms in sagittal plane and demonstrated narrowing of just one-half of the canal in the lumbar vertebra causing nerve root entrapment and symptoms.

The Interest

The period between 1978 and 1983 surgeon started talking about lateral recess stenosis, lumbar canal stenosis and their presentation specially in the elderly population. They used several methods to make the diagnosis.[3,7,5]

They used investigations such as radiculography by injecting water soluble dye but it was invasive. It did demonstrate the entrapment but not in all cases. But then they found computerized tomography (CT) scan more useful in demonstrating the lateral canal. But again it was not fullproof. Some investigators found it comparable with electromyography. In fact CT investigation of spine involved significant radiation dose to the patient. Surgeons were more happy using nuclear magnetic resonance (NMR) imaging as it is harmless to the patient and it is noninvasive. Multiplanar imaging was possible.

Magnetic Resonance Imaging (MRI)

The machinery was available in the later part of last century. Magnet being the mode of energy and being non-invasive it became quickly popular and remained the standard method to investigate patients of lumbar canal stenosis till today. It is a good investigations giving details of nerve roots and soft tissue. Today MRI is the word of mouth among most surgeons as well as patients with many patients presenting to the surgeon with MRI films.

However, coronal imaging still does not clearly demonstrate the full length of nerve root in the canal or in the intervertebral foramen, the two important areas of nerve root entrapment.

Neurography—the Latest MRI Technology

With new software in 3 Tesla MRI machine it is now possible to delineate the nerve root throughout the canal and into the foramen and find out if it is compressed and to what extent in the lateral recess. To give one example, two weeks back I had one patient admitted with acute back pain and left sciatica. I had operated on her back 12 years earlier and she was all right. She was a frail 63 years. Old lady fond of adventure and trekking. She went to Kailash Mansarovar and did 14 km horse-riding. She developed back pain and acute left sciatica. Instead of going home to Bihar she came straight from the airport to Mumbai and got admitted to the hospital. Left sciatica clinically was confirmed to be due to left 5th nerve root compression as she had marked weakness in left great toe. X-rays and MRI could not pinpoint the lesion. Neurography showed a piece of bone stuck into the nerve root near the foramen. At micro surgery the piece of bone was from a fracture of the posterior facet which she had developed during horse-riding.

Surgical Management

Internal decompression (IDSS) which the author has popularized is the method of choice in unilateral lumbar canal stenosis. But instead of cutting part of the facet and risking the damage to the facet joint it is better to undercut the facet.[6] This method is also popularized by the author. It was originally described by RB Cloward while he performed PLIF surgery. He used osteotome to undercut the facet. The author uses high speed drill to open the lateral recess. More recently the author has been using the swiveling blade of ultrasound to undercut the bone without any risk of damaging the neural tissue. The advantage of swiveling blade is to undercut the intervertebral foramen keeping the nerve root intact till it emerges out of the foramen. The IDSS or internal decompression technique had been described elsewhere in this book.

Results

Results are good and outcome is satisfactory but one should possess a good microscope, high speed drill and ultrasound blades in the operation theatre.

On the whole the decompression in degenerative lateral recess stenosis by micro techniques is good until the degenerative process causes further compression and stenosis and cause recurrence of symptoms.

REFERENCES

1. Bilimoria PE. Stenosis of one half of lumbar spinal canal. Quoted by Pandya S, Book review. Neurology India 2018;66; 898–901.
2. Cloward RB. The treatment of ruptured intervertebral disc by interbody fusion. Indications, operative treatment, after care. J Neurosurg 1953;10(2);154–68.
3. Crawshaw C, Kean DM, Mulholand RC et.al. The use of NMR in the diagnosis of lateral canal entrapment. Bone and Jt. Surg. 1984;66-B; 711–6.
4. Critchley EMR. Lumbar Canal stenosis. Br. Med J, 1982;284;1588–89.
5. Crock HV. Normal and pathological anatomy of the lumbar spinal nerve root canals. J Bone Joint Surg (Br) 1981;63-B;487–90.
6. Getty CJM, Johnson JR, Kirwan EOG et al. Partial undercutting facetectomy for bony entrapment of the lumbar nerve root. J Bone Joint Surg (Br) 1981;63-B; 330–5.
7. Haughton VM, Syvertsen A, Williams Al. Soft tissue anatomy within the spinal canal as seen by computed tomography. Radiology 1980;134;649–55.
8. Heitoff K. CT scanning of lumbar spine. The procedure of choice in the diagnosis of radicular pain due to spinal nerve root entrapment. Orthopaedic transactions 1984;374–86.

Importance of Maintaining Sagittal Balance of the Spine in Reconstruction

Ahmed Nouby

INTRODUCTION

The sagittal balance of spine helps us to maintain good posture in standing position with minimum effort. The balance is maintained as a result of interaction between different factors such as bone morphology, elasticity in the ligaments (ligament tension), healthy joints and good tone in the muscles supporting the spine.

Radiologically the spine can be considered in good sagittal balance when a vertical line passing down from the centre of C7 vertebra (plumb line) crosses the first sacral end plate within 2.5 cm from its posterosuperior corner. The line then should ideally pass through the centre of femoral head as shown in Fig. 11.1.

If it passes anterior to the femoral head, then anterior imbalance is created in the spine as happens in exaggerated lumbar lordosis.[21,23] If the line passes posterior to the sacral end plate it creates posterior imbalance as happens in flat back in elderly population. Both these imbalances are the main cause of low back pain and needs to be corrected to get relief from back pain.

Understanding Sagittal Balance

Three parameters are important and they are measured on digital lateral X-ray of the spine taken in a specific format.

1. Sacral slope (SS)

It is the angle between a line drawn along the sacral end plate and another line drawn horizontal to the first line.

Normally, it ranges from 36 to 45 degrees with a mean of 400.

Numerous several studies have reported that patients suffering from chronic degenerative low back pain showed a reduction in the normal sacral slope.[2,3,13,1418]

2. Pelvic tilt (PT)

It is an angle between a line drawn from centre of femoral head to the mid-point of sacral end plate and a perpendicular line drawn upwards from the center of the femoral head.

Normally, it ranges from 12 to 18 degrees with a mean of 15 degrees as shown in Fig. 11.3.

The pelvis can rotate around the femoral heads up to a certain limit. The rotation is known as the pelvic tilt (PT). When the pelvis rotates backwards (retroversion), pelvic tilt increases and when the pelvis rotates forward (anteversion), the pelvic tilt decreases.

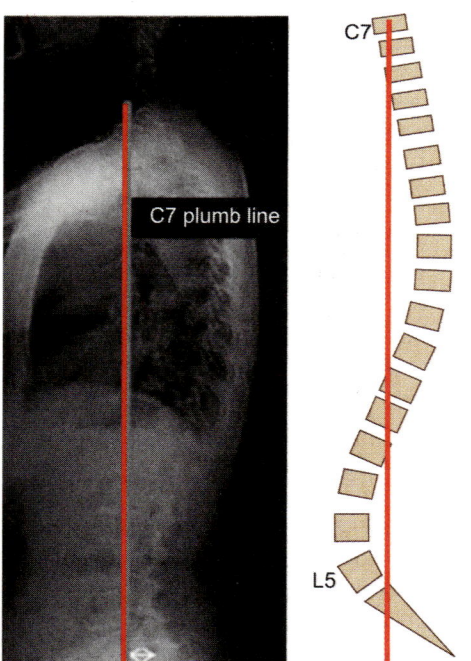

Fig. 11.1: Normal position of the plumb line in a sagittally balanced subject

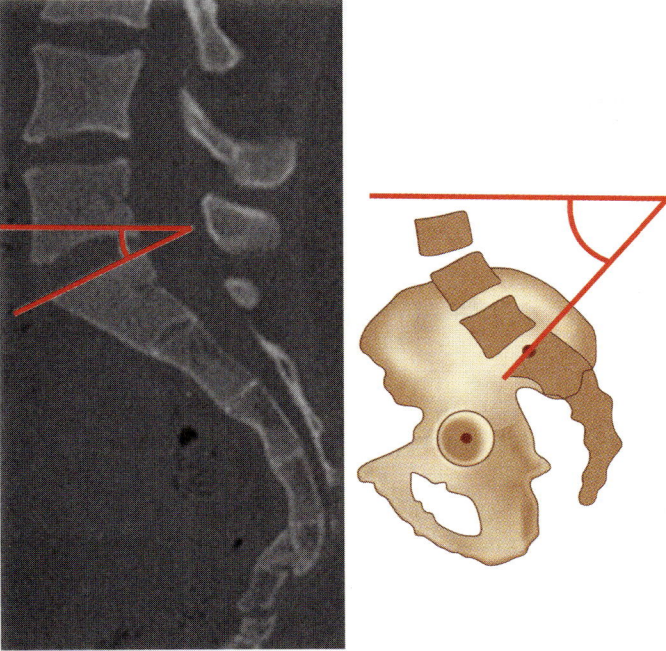

Fig. 11.2: Sacral slope as the angle between a horizontal line and a line drawn along the sacral end plate

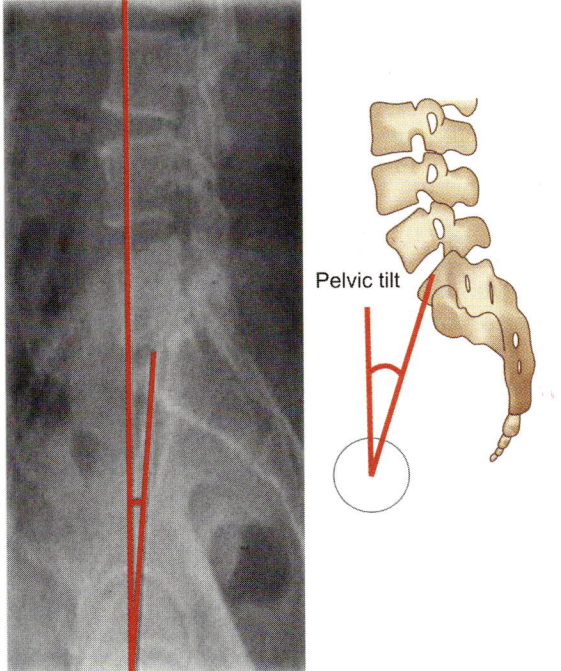

Fig. 11.3: Pelvic tilt as the angle between a vertical line and a line connecting the mid-point of the sacral end plate with the axis of the femoral heads

It has been noticed that in patients with chronic low back pain due to degeneration in the spine, the pelvic tilt increases.[2,3,13,14,18]

Schuller et al[24] has reported a significant increase in pelvic tilt in patients with degenerative spondylolisthesis. They have suggested that the posterior tilt of

the pelvis was a compensatory mechanism to regain the sagittal balance, in a spine with listhesis.

3. Pelvic Incidence (PI)

It is the angle between a line drawn from the center of the femoral head to the midpoint of sacral end plate and a line dropped down perpendicular from this point.

Normally the pelvic incidence ranges from 48 to 55° with a mean of 51 degrees as shown in Fig. 11.4.

As a matter of fact pelvic incidence reading can be obtained by combining sacral slope and pelvic tilt or PI = PT + SS

Pelvic incidence is not influenced by age, posture or tilting of the pelvis.[6]

The pelvis can tilt backwards giving a higher pelvic tilt or forwards giving a lower pelvic tilt so it does not cause significant back pain as there is a much wider range through which adaptation can occur in patients with a high pelvic incidence.

In normal subjects a low pelvic incidence is usually associated with a low lumbar lordosis, whereas a high pelvic incidence is usually associated with a high lumbar lordosis.[29]

Legaye et al [22] reported that a high pelvic incidence indicated a steep sacral slope and exaggerated sagittal curves. Barrey et al. reported that patients with degenerative spondylolisthesis have a higher pelvic incidence—60 degrees than the normal population—52 degrees.

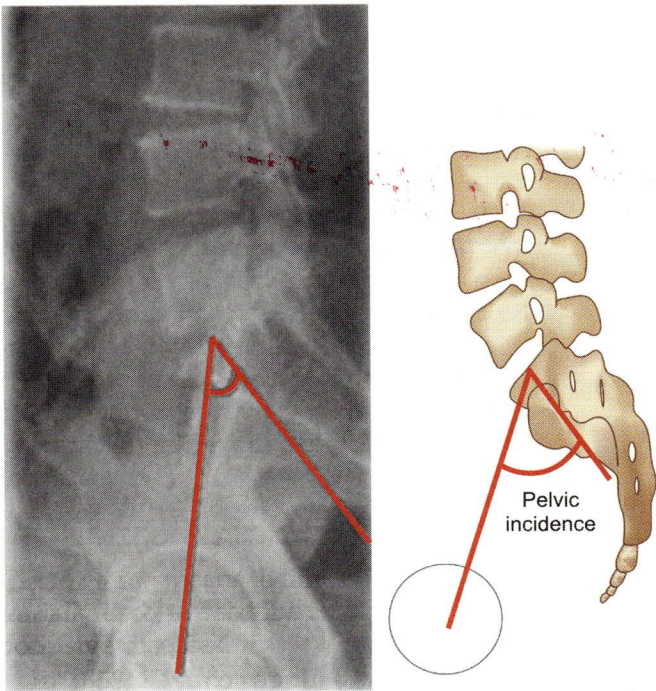

Fig. 11.4: Pelvic incidence as the angle between a line perpendicular to the mid-point of the sacral end plate and a line connecting this midpoint to the axis of the femoral heads

Genesis of Imbalance

Sagittal imbalance causes backpain. Several factors contribute to the imbalance and pain in the back. It can also cause neurological deficit complicating the syndrome. It causes profound decrease in the quality of life which is so important in elderly population. Backpain itself is multifactorial process centered around facet joints. The joints degenerate along with intervertebral disc and cause loss of lumbar lordosis.[27] These changes do occur in the spine as age advances and creates weakness due to atrophy in the extensor muscles of the spine causing progressive kyphosis and sagittal imbalance.[7,17,30] The loss of lumbar lordosis causes increase in the pelvic tilt.[1–3,14]

The degenerative process in the spine is progressive and genetically influenced but the intensity can vary from person to person in spite of the fact that to begin with the pelvic tilt is same in all patients.

Sagittal balance can also be influenced by bad posture, abnormalities of pelvis and lower extremities and abnormalities in the spine itself like degenerative spondylolisthesis or chronic degeneration in the spine.

In such abnormalities which cause kyphosis of the spine, the plumb line falls in front of the hip joint.

Normally a person tries to overcome such abnormality by compensatory mechanisms like vertebral retrolisthesis, pelvic retroversion, knee flexion or thoracic spine compensation curve. The attempt is to maintain balance with effort to see that the plumb line crosses the postero- lateral corner of first sacral end plate. Unfortunately all such compensatory mechanisms are a source of pain making life more miserable to the given patient.[8]

Surgical Management

Surgical treatment for low back pain has always been a controversial topic. Several surgical options have been performed for patients with degenerative lumbar disease. Decompression laminectomy was the most popular treatment of the past. Recurrence of symptoms and high rate of re-exploration compelled surgeons to look for alternative methods.[5] Surgeons then preferred fusion and instrumentation at the time of decompression. Spinal fusion technique has become one of the most common modalities for the management of spinal degenerative diseases. However, spinal fusion has its drawbacks. It interferes with the normal biomechanics of the spine and eliminates mobility.[7,17] Fusion can create flatback syndrome due to loss of lordosis after spinal fusion. The number of surgical procedures of corrective osteotomy for post-fusion. The flatback deformity causes sagittal imbalance.[25]

Importance of Sagittal Balance

In recent years, evaluation of spinal sagittal alignment is becoming increasingly important for investigating and treating different pathologies of the spine with great focus of degenerative spinal diseases. Recently the concept of analysis of sagittal balance is being used as an important step for optimizing the management of lumbar degenerative pathologies, especially when surgery with spinal fusion and instrumentation is planned as this may result in loss of lumbar lordosis (LL). Loss of lumbar lordosis activates compensatory mechanisms like decreased sacral slope (SS), increased risk of adjacent segment degeneration and increased pelvic tilt (PT) and these factors by themselves can be a source of back pain.[12,19,20,30] Recognizing the use of spinopelvic parameters to predict outcomes in such patients has now become important.

Materials and Methods

Present series consists of 80 patients (M = 41, F = 39) with age ranging from 20 to 70 years with different back pathologies who attended the outpatient clinic and in-house patients at the Lilavati Hospital and Research Centre, Mumbai, India between 12th of May and 12th of July 2018. We evaluated the parameters of the sagittal balance, which include the pelvic incidence (PI), pelvic tilt (PT) and sacral slope (SS) in 69 subjects (19 with lumbar canal stenosis, 19 with lumbar disc prolapse, 13 with spondylolisthesis and 18 with mechanical low back pain) who were treated conservatively, in addition to 11 subjects (7 patients with degenerative LCS and LDP, 4 patients with degenerative spondylolisthesis) who were treated surgically, correlating the pre-operative and the postoperative sagittal parameters with the clinical outcome (Tables 11.1 to 11.3).

Table 11.1: Admitted or outpatients	
Total number of patients	80
Outpatients	69
Patients who have surgery	11

Table 11.2: Various pathologies	
Patients with various lower back pathologies	80
Lumbar canal stenosis	26
Lumbar disc prolapse	19
Degenerative spondylolisthesis	17
Mechanical low back pain	18

Table 11.3: Pathology in inpatients	
Patients who had surgery	11
Lumbar canal stenosis	7
Degenerative spondylolisthesis	4

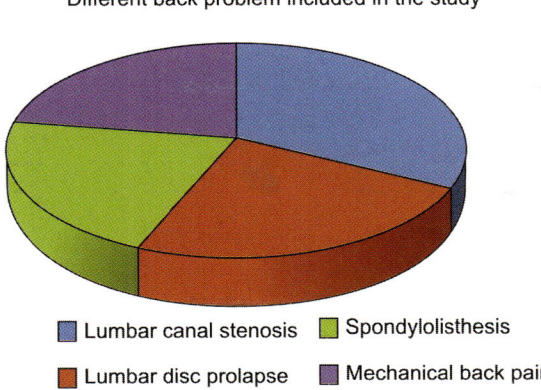

Different back problem included in the study

Fig. 11.5: This study included patients with various back problems: Lumbar canal stenosis (26 patients), lumbar disc prolapse (22 patients), spondylolisthesis (17 patients) and mechanical back pain (15 patients)

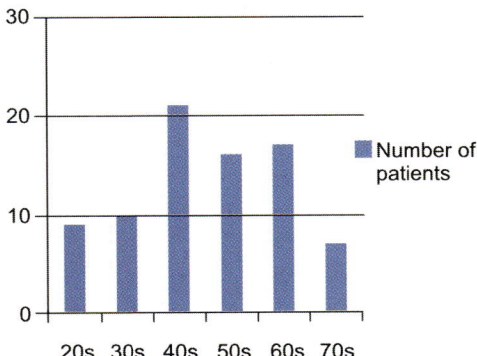

Fig. 11.6: The majority of the patients with varied back problems were in their 40s (21 patients) followed by the 50s and 60s age groups (16 patients each) followed by the 20s and 30s age groups (10 patients each) followed by the 70s age group (7 patients), which proves that back problems are not just age related

Sex

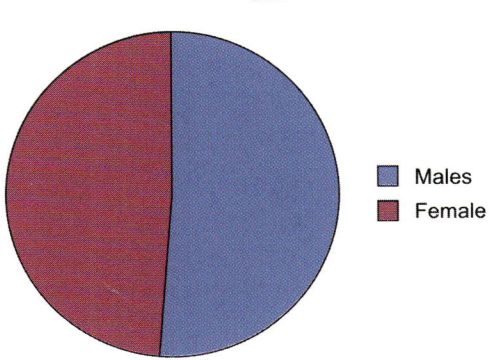

Fig. 11.7: There was no significant difference regarding sex and difference back problems

Inclusion Criteria

- Patients attending the OPD with back problems.
- Patients admitted to the ward for surgery.
- Age 18 to 90 years.
- Patients undergoing conservative or surgical management.

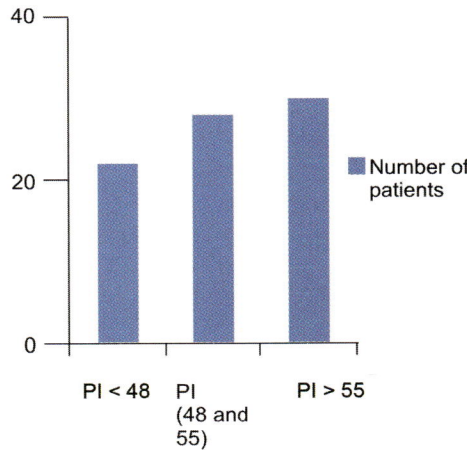

Fig. 11.8: 22 patients had a PI below 48, 28 patients had a pelvic incidence between 48 and 55 and 30 patients had a pelvic incidence above 55, which shows the strong relationship between a high pelvic incidence and various lumbar pathologies

Spondylolisthesis and PI

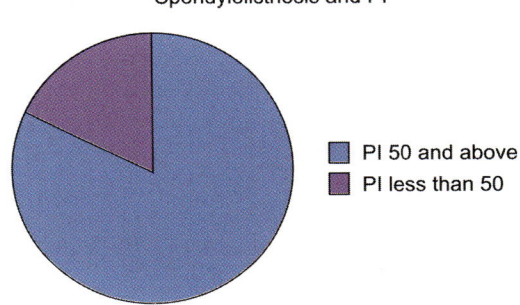

Fig. 11.9: This study included 17 patients with spondylolisthesis: 14 of those patients had a pelvic incidence of 50 and above and only 3 patients had a pelvic incidence below 50, which proves that patients with a high pelvic incidence are at higher risk of developing spondylolisthesis

Exclusion Criteria

- Spinal cord tumor
- Infective pathologies
- Congenital anomalies

Statistical Analysis

Results

This study included 80 patients with different back issues as shown in Fig. 11.5. Even though age is a strong predisposing factor for different back pathologies, it is very important to mention that it is not the only factor and this is illustrated in Fig. 11.6. Our study showed that both males and females are candidates to various back problems with no significant predilection as shown by Fig. 11.7. There is a very strong relationship between a high pelvic incidence and varied back problems specially spondylolisthesis as demonstrated by Figs 11.8 and 11.9. Correction of the pelvic tilt varied from one patient to the other depending on various factors including the type of surgery, the level of motion segment targeted in the surgery and the pelvic incidence of the patient which determines the amount of lumbar lordosis correction needed as outlined in Flowcharts 11.1 to 11.5.

Flowchart 11.1: Patients with decreased SS

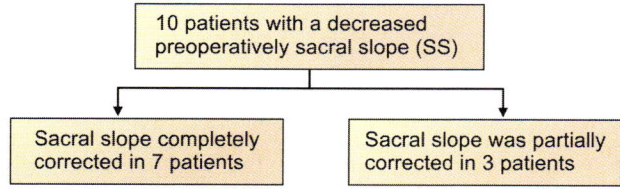

Flowchart 11.2: Patients with high PT

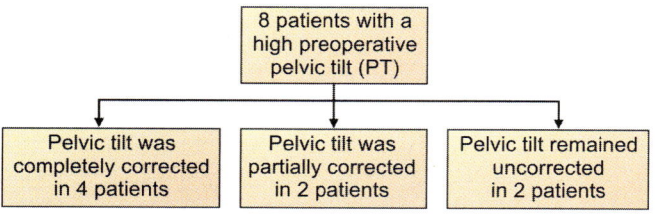

Flowchart 11.3: Patients with high PT and reduced SS

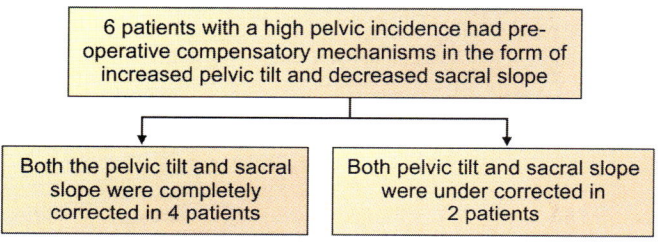

Flowchart 11.4: Patients with PDS device

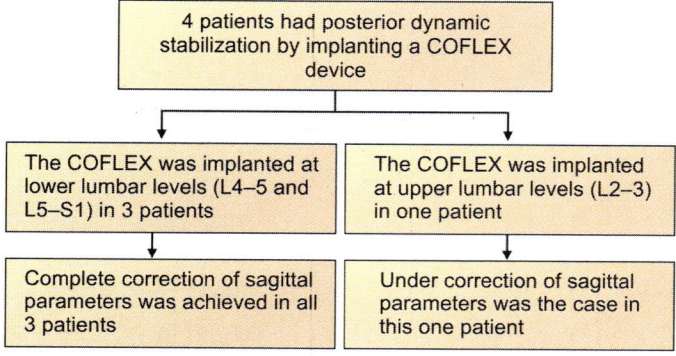

Flowchart 11.5: Patients with spondylolisthesis

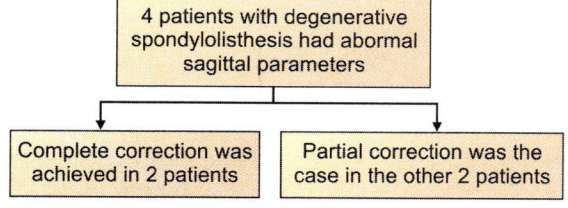

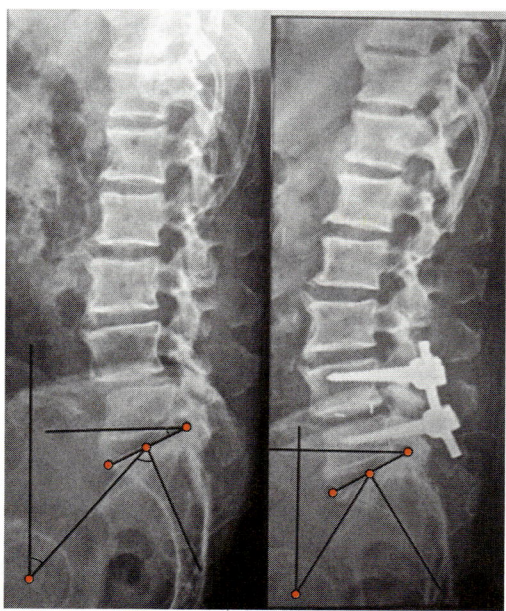

Fig. 11.10: Preoperative and postoperative X-rays of a 70-year-old male patient with grade one degenerative spondylolisthesis who had L4–L5 PLIF surgery showing partial correction of the sagittal parameters postoperatively

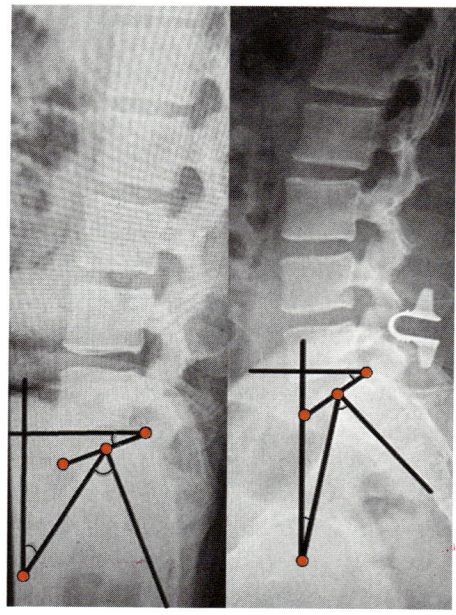

Fig. 11.11: Preoperative and postoperative X-rays of a 40-year-old male with L4–L5 LDP and lateral recess stenosis who had L4–L5 IDSS surgery along with insertion of a COFLEX device at the same level showing complete correction of the sagittal parameters postoperatively

In one patient, e.g. using PDS (posterior dynamic stabilization) with COFLEX done at L4–5 level (Fig. 11.11), the abnormal parameters of the spine were completely corrected, whereas same technique when used at L3–L4 level (Fig. 11.12), the correction of the motion segment had no significant influence on sagittal balance determinants.

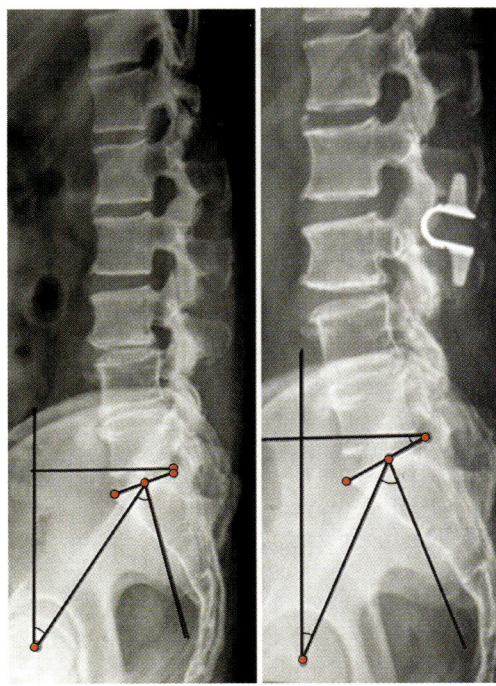

Fig. 11.12: Preoperative and postoperative X-rays of a 63-year-old male patient with recurrent L3–L4 LDP who had discectomy surgery along with insertion of a COFLEX device at the L2–L3 level showing no correction of the sagittal parameters with almost no changes postoperatively

Discussion

Degenerative diseases of the spine such as lumbar canal stenosis and degenerative spondylolisthesis causing low back pain result in disturbances in the normal parameters of sagittal balance. In patients with low back pain due to degenerative spine diseases compared with age-matched controls, Jackson et al. reported that total lumbar lordosis was decreased from 60.9° to 56.3° and sacrum was more vertical with a sacral slope increased from 47.2° to 50.4°.[14] However, C7 plumb line was maintained similar to controls due to compensatory mechanisms (pelvic retroversion and/or increased sacral slope) to compensate the loss of lumbar lordosis. Decline in lumbar lordosis below normal levels in patients with degenerative diseases of the spine and the compensatory decline in the sacral slope and increase in the pelvic tilt was seen in six patients in our study confirming the fact that the spinopelvic parameters can create a state of compensation in these patients.

Lazennec et al compared pelvic parameters in 81 patients of lumbosacral fusion (LDDD n = 44, revision of lumbar fusion n = 13, repeat surgery for disc herniation, n = 12; other n = 12).[20] The subgroup with persistence of pain after fusion surgery were found to have a more vertical sacrum with decreased sacral slope and an increased pelvic tilt suggesting straightening of

the spine and creating imbalance. In fact finding increased pelvic tilt with persistent pain after fusion and was almost twice the normal value. Sacral slope in the standing position was also correlated with the presence of post-fusion pain resulting from a sacrum that was abnormally vertical. These results suggest that failing to restore appropriate lumbar lordosis during surgery is associated with excessive pelvic tilt, which is a cause of chronic pain. In our study, 7 patients had a decreased sacral slope preoperatively returned to normal postoperatively, while 3 were partially corrected and no patient was left uncorrected. The pelvic tilt in 8 patients was increased before surgery and 4 of them returned to normal postoperatively, 2 were partially corrected and 2 remained uncorrected. The clinical outcome in all patients was satisfactory using the VAS score but this is only on short-term basis and since the sagittal imbalance tends to affect the spine on the long-term basis, longer periods of follow-up is required.

Abnormal pre- and/or postoperative sagittal spinopelvic parameters are now widely recognised to affect clinical outcomes in spinal surgery, specifically spinal fusion. Early studies, published 10 to 15 years ago, showed that lumbar fusion in degenerative spine disease can lead to deleterious effects on sagittal spinal balance.[10,15,19,20,28] The retrospective study by Tribus et al[28] assessed radiological parameters in 28 patients undergoing posterior-spinal fusions using the knee-chest position. Spinal fusions were performed at L4–L5 level in seven patients and at L5–S1 level in 13 and L4 to S1 levels in eight. While average lumbar lordosis was unchanged before and after surgery in all the patients, the sacral slope decreased significantly (from 49° to 45°; p = 0.039) in the subgroup of patients undergoing L4–S1 spinal fusion, while it remained unchanged in the other subgroups. This study showed that postoperative sagittal alignment and compensatory mechanisms depended on surgical methods and fusion levels. In our study 1 patient showed reduction in the sacral slope postoperatively while 8 patients showed an increase in the sacral slope but as mentioned earlier, longer follow-up is required to assess the impact of sagittal balance on the spine postoperatively.

Flatback syndrome can result from loss of lordosis after spinal fusion. Spinopelvic parameters, including determination of the optimal amount of lumbar lordosis, must be measured and taken into account before performing lumbar fusion in order to prevent fixed sagittal imbalance.[11] Cho et al. retrospectively analysed 45 patients who underwent long posterior instrumentation and fusion for adult lumbar degenerative scoliosis. Sagittal decompensation occurred in 19 patients (42%).[26] Compared with patients who were sagittally balanced after fusion, a high pelvic incidence was the most significant risk for sagittal decompensation. In our series, 6 patients had a high pelvic incidence with abnormally high pelvic tilt and a significantly low sacral slope (compensatory mechanisms) preoperatively, in 4 of these patients both the pelvic tilt and sacral slope were corrected while 2 patients showed under correction. As a rule high pelvic incidence requires more lumbar lordosis correction.

When rectangular cages were used, global lumbar lordosis and segmental lordosis of the fused segments decreased, and sagittal balance was maintained by compensatory modifications[9] of sacral slope which decreased from 440 to 400. Better results were obtained with wedge-shaped cages, with significant increase in segmental lordosis and lumbar lordosis; sacral tilt increased from 420 to 450. These results indicate the importance of taking into account parameters of sagittal balance to compare methods or devices for surgery of degenerative spinal pathologies. In our series 4 patients had posterior dynamic stabilization with COFLEX implant. One patient who had COFLEX implanted at upper lumbar levels (L2–3) (Fig. 11.13), the sagittal imbalance could not be completely corrected suggesting that level where stabilization is carried out in the spine is important. 3 patients who had COFLEX implanted at lower lumbar levels (L4–5 and L5–S1) (Fig. 11.11), the sagittal parameters were completely corrected post-operatively and this is due to the fact that most of the lumbar lordosis is at lower lumbar levels. This fact is of great importance in patients with high pelvic incidence who require more correction of lumbar lordosis which is easily achieved through the lower lumbar levels rather than the upper levels.

Compared with the normal, asymptomatic population, patients with degenerative spondylolisthesis show higher pelvic tilt and sacral slope values, thus indicating pelvic compensation.[4] The retrospective study by Barrey et al assessed sagittal balance parameters in 85 patients with three different types of LDDD (disc herniation, n = 25; LDDD n = 32; degenerative spondylolisthesis, n = 28) and compared them with controls.[2] LDDD showed significantly higher in patients with degenerative spondylolisthesis (60.00). Nevertheless, sacral slope and lumbar lordosis were decreased in all three degenerative pathologies, an observation that is consistent with the study of Jackson et al. in patients with low back pain and described above.[14] Results for degenerative spondylolisthesis were extended by the same authors in a series of 40 patients.[3] These patients had a higher pelvic incidence, which could be a predisposing factor of degenerative spondylolisthesis. Our study included 11 patients who had surgery (7 patients with degenrative

lumbar canal stenosis and 4 patients with degenerative spondylolisthesis). The pelvic incidence was significantly higher in patients with degenerative spondylolithesis and this can be due to the fact that a high pelvic incidence increases the shear stress at the LSJ which is a very strong predisposing factor for the development of slippage.

The retrospective pilot study by Kim et al. was the first to evaluate the impact of sagittal balance in 18 patients with degenerative spondylolisthesis who underwent fusion surgery.[16] The relationship between sagittal lumbar balance and clinical outcomes was assessed after PLIF for the relief of radicular leg and back pain. Patients were divided into two groups: Those without postoperative improvement of PT value (group A; n = 10) and those with improvement of postoperative pelvic tilt value (group B; n = 8). In group A, improvement of quality of life assessed using the visual analogue scale (VAS) was significantly correlated to postoperative lumbar lordosis (r = 0.829; p = 0.003); similarly, improvement in the Oswestry Disability Index (ODI) score was also positively correlated with postoperative lumbar lordosis (r = 0.700; p = 0.024). In group B, VAS and improvement in ODI were not significantly correlated with postoperative lumbar lordosis or other spinopelvic parameters. In conclusion, this pilot study suggested that patients in whom pelvic tilt improved after fusion achieved good clinical outcomes. These results also show that it is important to quantify sagittal spinopelvic parameters and promote sagittal balance when performing lumbar fusion for degenerative spondylolisthesis. In our study 4 patients with degenerative spondylolithesis and abnormal sagittal parameters underwent fusion surgery, the pelvic tilt was corrected in 2 of these patients and partially corrected in other 2 patients, however, the clinical outcome was satisfactory in all patients immediately postoperatively using the VAS score, but as mentioned before long-term follow-up is required.

Conclusion

Our study and those of others show that if the pelvic incidence angle is more than normal, it needs to be properly corrected with implant surgery to:
1. Achieve sagittal balance
2. Relieve pain and
3. Good outcome

REFERENCES

1. Barrey C. Equilibre sagittal pelvi-rachidienet pathologies lombairesdégénératives. Etude comparative à propos de 100 cas (in French). Thèse de Médecine. Université Claude Bernard, Lyon. 2004.

2. Barrey C, Jund J, Noseda O, Roussouly P. Sagittal balance of the pelvis-spine complex and lumbar degenerative diseases. A comparative study about 85 cases. Eur Spine J. 2007;16:1459–67. doi: 10.1007/s00586-006-0294-6.

3. Barrey C, Jund J, Perrin G, Roussouly P. Spinopelvic alignment of patients with degenerative spondylolisthesis. Neurosurg. 2007; 61:981–6. doi: 10.1227/01.neu.0000303194.02921.30.

4. Chaleat-Valayer E, Mac-Thiong JM, Paquet J, Berthonnaud E, Siani F, Roussouly P. Sagittal spino-pelvic alignment in chronic low back pain. Eur Spine J 20(Suppl 5) 2011;634–40.

5. COST B13 Action. Guidelines for the management of chronic low back pain. www.backpaineurope.org; 2004.

6. Duval-Beaupère G, Schmidt C, Cosson P. A barycentremetric study of the sagittal shape of spine and pelvis: the conditions required for an economic standing position. Ann Biomed Eng. 1992;20:451–462. doi: 10.1007/BF02368136.

7. Gelb DE, Lenke LG, Bridwell KH, Blanke K, MacEnery KW. An analysis of sagittal spinal aligment in 100 asymptomatic middle and older aged volunteers. Spine 1995;20:1351–58.

8. Glassman SD, Berven S, Bridwell K, et al. Correlation of radiographic parameters and clinical symptoms in adult scoliosis. Spine (Phila Pa 1976) 2005;30:682–8. doi: 10.1097/01.brs.0000155425.04536.f7.

9. Godde S, Fritsch E, Dienst M, Kohn D.2003 Influence of cage geometry on sagittal alignment in instrumented posterior lumbar interbody fusion. Spine (Phila Pa 1976).;28:1693–9.

10. Goldstein JA, Macenski MJ, Griffith SL, McAfee PC. 2001 Lumbar sagittal alignment after fusion with a threaded interbody cage. Spine (Phila Pa 1976).; 26: 1137–42.

11. Gottfried ON, Daubs MD, Patel AA, Dailey AT, Brodke DS. Spinopelvic parameters in postfusion flatback deformity patients. Spine J 2009;9:639–647.

12. Izumi Y, Kumano K. Analysis of sagittal lumbar alignment before and after posterior instrumentation: risk factor for adjacent unfused segment. Eur J OrthopSurgTraum. 2001;1:9–13. doi: 10.1007/BF01706654.

13. Jackson RP, Kanemura T, Kawakami N, Hales C. Lumbopelvic lordosis and pelvic balance on repeated standing lateral radiographs of adult volunteers and untreated patients with constant low back pain. Spine 2000;25:575–86. doi: 10.1097/00007632-200003010-00008.

14. Jackson RP, MacManus AC. Radiographic analysis of sagittal plane alignment and balance in standing volunteers and patients with low back pain matched for age, sex and size. Spine 1994;19:1611–8. doi: 10.1097/00007632-199407001-00010.

15. Kawakami M, Tamaki T, Ando M, Yamada H, Hashizume H, Yoshida M.2002 Lumbar sagittal balance influences the clinical outcome after decompression and posterolateral spinal fusion for degenerative lumbar spondylolisthesis. Spine (Phila Pa 1976).;27: 59–64.

16. Kim MK, Lee SH, Kim ES, Eoh W, Chung SS, Lee CS. The impact of sagittal balance on clinical results after posterior interbody fusion for patients with degenerative spondylolisthesis: a pilot study. BMC MusculoskeletDisord 2011;12:69.

17. Kobayashi T, Atsuta Y, Matsuno T, Takeda N. A longitudinal study of congruent sagittal spinal alignment in an adult cohort. Spine 2004;29:671–676. doi: 10.1097/01.BRS.0000115127.51758.A2.

18. Korovessis PG, Dimas A, Iliopoulos P, Lambiris E. Correlative analysis of lateral vertebral radiographic variables and medical outcomes study short-form health survey: a comparative study in asymptomatic volunteers versus patients with low back pain. J Spinal Disord Tech 2002;15:384–90. doi: 10.1097/00024720–200210000-00007.

19. Kumar MN, Baklanov A, Chopin D. Correlation between sagittal plane changes and adjacent segment degeneration following lumbar spine fusion. Eur Spine J 2001;10:314–9. doi: 10.1007/s005860000239.

20. Lazennec JY, Ramare S, Arafati N, Laudet CG, Gorin M, Roger B, Hansen S, Saillant G, Maurs L, Trabelsi R. Sagittal alignment in lumbosacral fusion: relations between radiological parameters and pain. Eur Spine J 2000;9:47–55. doi: 10.1007/s005860050008.

21. Le Huec JC, Leijssen P, Duarte M, Aunoble S. Thoracolumbar imbalance analysis for osteotomy planification using a new method: FBI technique. Eur Spine J. 20(Suppl 5) 2011;S669-S680. doi: 10.1007/s00586-011-1935-y.

22. Legaye J, Duval-Beaupère G, Hecquet J, et al. Pelvic incidence: a fundamental pelvic parameter for three-dimensional regulation of spinal sagittal curves. Eur Spine J 1998;7:99–103. doi: 10.1007/s005860050038.

23. Rose PS, Bridwell KH, Lenke LG, Cronen GA, Mulconrey DS, Buchowski JM, Kim YJ. Role of pelvic incidence, thoracic kyphosis, and patient factors on sagittal plane correction following pedicle subtraction osteotomy. Spine (Phila Pa 1976) 2009;34(8):785–91. doi:10.1097/BRS.0b013e31819d0c86.

24. Schuller S, Charles YP, Steib JP. Sagittal spinopelvic alignment and body mass index in patients with degenerative spondylolisthesis. Eur Spine J 2011;20:713-9.doi: 10.1007/s00586-010-1640-2.

25. Schwab F, Dubey A, Gamez L, El Fegoun AB, Hwang K, Pagala M, et al. Adult scoliosis: prevalence, SF-36, and nutritional parameters in an elderly volunteer population. Spine (Phila Pa 1976) 2005;30:1082–5.

26. Schwab F, Lafage V, Patel A, Farcy JP. Sagittal plane considerations and the pelvis in the adult patient. Spine (Phila Pa 1976) 2009;34: 1828–33.

27. Schwab FJ, Smith VA, Biserni M, Gamez L, Farcy JP, Pagala M. Adult scoliosis: a quantitative radiographic and clinical analysis. Spine 2002;27(4):387–92.

28. Tribus CB, Belanger TA, Zdeblick TA. The effect of operative position and short-segment fusion on maintenance of sagittal alignment of the lumbar spine. Spine (Phila Pa 1976) 1999;24:58–61.

29. Vaz G, Roussouly P, Berthonnaud E, Dimnet J. Sagittal morphology and equilibrium of pelvis and spine. Eur Spine J 2002;1(11):80–7.

30. Vital JM, Gille O, Gangnet N. Equilibre sagittal et applications cliniques (in French) Rev Rhum 2004;71:120–128. doi: 10.1016/j.rhum.2003.09.020.

Management of Lumbar Canal Stenosis Conservative or Surgical

Pragnesh Bhatt, Mohammed Suheel

INTRODUCTION

Lumbar canal stenosis is a common degenerative condition affecting the population and its incidence is only going to increase with aging population. It is the commonest cause for surgery in people older than 65 years. It typically presents with neurogenic claudication with or without back pain. The treatment options range from simple measures like analgesics to complex surgical management. The wide variation in the management is primarily due to the heterogeneity of the condition.

Conservative Management

Patients suffering from the initial symptoms which are not too debilitating could be counselled for activity modification in combination with analgesics. Others include non-steroidal anti-inflammatory drugs, tricyclic compounds and gabapentinoids in appropriate doses.

Physiotherapists most often advocate flexibility exercises (87%), stabilization exercises (86%), strengthening exercises (83%), and joint mobilization (62%).[20] Exercises provide short-term benefit for leg pain compared to no treatment. The other options of physical therapy could be acupuncture, cryotherapy, ultrasound and transcutaneous electrical nerve stimulation (TENS). Though LCS was considered to be a contraindication for spinal manipulation, several studies have recently looked at the effects of flexion-distraction manipulations. A review of chiropractic manipulations found limited benefit and the evidence was of low quality.[19] Similarly, a systematic review in 2013 found "that current evidence for the use of acupuncture in patients with LCS is limited."[8]

Epidural steroid injections have been used by spinal surgeons and/or pain specialists for these patients and outcome has been variable. A most recent meta-analysis found limited short-term and long-term improvement in pain and walking distance.[10] There is some evidence to suggest that interlaminar block is superior to the caudal epidural block although the caudal epidural approach is superior to the transforaminal one.[13] Other modalities include lumbar traction and the use of lumbar corset. More pharmacotherapy includes intramuscular calcitonin, intranasal salmon calcitonin, intravenous lipoprostaglandin E(1), methylcobalamin, prostaglandin E(2), etc. Reduction of significant overweight, activity modification, cessation of smoking and avoiding positions that alleviate pain improves quality of life.

Indications for Conservative Treatment

- The patient is able to tolerate the symptoms and daily functional capacity is adequate.
- The patient does not want to be operated; Worried about assessment of surgery-related risks.

Mechanism of Action of Modalities for Conservative Treatment

The mechanism of action of the various treatments differs. Epidural steroid injections, calcitonin, and NSAIDS aim to reduce nerve root inflammation (Fukusaki 1988; Podichetty 2004). Analgesics, epidural anaesthetic injections, and prostaglandins act to block pain transmission and increase neural blood flow (Fukusaki 1988; Matsudaira 2009). Vitamin B_{12} is thought to increase nerve root blood flow (Waikakul 2000) and neuropathic medications act to block pain transmission. Physical and manual therapies aim to reduce pain and maximize function by improving lumbar spine and lower extremity flexibility, muscular strength, and endurance (Whitman, 2006).

Epidural steroid injection (ESI) provides aggressive-conservative treatment for patients with lumbar spinal stenosis (LSS) who demonstrate limited response to oral medication, physical therapy, and other noninvasive measures. The North American Spine Society (NASS) in its evidence-based guidelines for the diagnosis and treatment of degenerative LSS, suggests that in patients with radiculopathy or neurogenic intermittent claudication from LSS, medium-term pain relief (i.e. 3–36 months) can be achieved with a multiple-injection regimen of radiographically guided transforaminal ESIs or caudal injections. In this regimen, the patient is injected either on demand or when his or her pain exceeds a preset level.[15]

Absolute contraindications to ESIs include systemic infection and pregnancy (because of the teratogenicity of fluoroscopy). Relative contraindications include diabetes mellitus (DM) and congestive heart failure, given the hyperglycemic and fluid retention properties of corticosteroids, respectively. Other relative contraindications include adrenal dysfunction and hypothalamic-pituitary axis suppression. Relative contraindications to ESI include bleeding diathesis and anticoagulation (AC) therapy, because of the increased risk of epidural hematoma. However, the actual incidence of this complication is unknown; estimates in the literature suggest that it occurs in less than 1 in 150,000 outpatient epidural injections.[12]

A multiple injection regimen of radiographically-guided transforaminal epidural steroid injection or caudal injections is suggested to produce medium-term (3–36 months) relief of pain in patients with radiculopathy or neurogenic intermittent claudication (NIC) from lumbar spinal stenosis. Grade of recommendation: C2

Physiotherapy may reduce the need for surgical treatment within one-year follow-up, but it does not seem to improve functional capacity nor to reduce symptoms or use of medications.

The use of a lumbosacral corset is suggested to increase walking distance and decrease pain in patients with lumbar spinal stenosis. There is no evidence that results are sustained once the brace is removed. Grade of recommendation: B2

Determination of Extent and Intensity of Pain

The factors that determine the extent and intensity of the pain in spinal stenosis patients are inflammation and combined pressure or mechanical stimulation at the nerve roots. Howe et al. reported that progression of the inflammatory process induces nerve root sensitization which results in continuing pain signal generation only at mild stimulation. Therefore, inflammation is thought to play an important role in the occurrence of back and lower limb pain in spinal

stenosis patients, and the role of steroids in treatment is not only to inhibit the synthesis or release of proinflammatory substances, but also to reduce the production of arachidonic acid and its metabolites (prostaglandin and leukotriene), which consequently inhibits the inflammatory process and results in the reduction of pain in spinal stenosis patients.

There is low quality evidence that prostaglandins improve walking ability compared with etodolac (NSAID); exercise improves leg pain and function compared with no treatment. Treadmill walking provides similar improvements in pain, function, and walking ability compared with stationary cycling. Direct surgical decompression improves leg pain compared with multimodal nonoperative treatment. There is very low-quality evidence that gabapentin and methylcobalamin improve walking ability compared with placebo and conservative treatment, respectively; calcitonin is no better than placebo or paracetamol; epidural steroid injections improve pain, function, and quality of life, up to two weeks, compared with home exercise or inpatient physical therapy; and indirect surgical nonoperative treatment for lumbar spinal stenosis with neurogenic claudication. Decompression and PDS interspinous spacers improve quality of life and global recovery compared with multimodal nonoperative care.[1,12]

Of patients with mild to moderate lumbar spinal stenosis initially receiving conservative treatment and followed for two to 10 years, approximately 20–40% will ultimately require surgical intervention. Of the patients who do not require surgical intervention, 50–70% will have improvement in their pain.

Surgical Management

Patients with progressively worsening symptoms of neurogenic claudication/radiculopathy with imaging confirmation of stenosis should be offered surgical options. Generally it is undertaken as a planned procedure. In cases of cauda equina compression or rapidly progressive neurological dysfunction surgical option should be offered as an emergency. It is important to rule out associated cervical stenosis since quite often elderly patients have simultaneous degenerative spondylosis in the cervical spine causing cervical cord compression and may need to be addressed as a priority. Elderly patients need thorough preoperative assessment and stabilizing the medical co-morbidities. The contraindication for surgical intervention includes lack of clinicoradiological correlation, significant uncontrolled co-morbidities and unfavorable local skins conditions. The surgical procedure needs to be tailored for individual patients in terms of number of levels to be decompressed and the procedural modifications as required.

Decompressive Laminectomy

Primary aim of surgical management is decompression of neural structures. Laminectomy is a gold standard for central stenosis. We prefer to put patients in prone position on Wilson frame with hips and knees flexed and pressure areas protected. Jacking up of the frame and flexion of the hips results in reduction of lumbar lordosis, thereby opening the inter-laminar space. It is equally important to keep the abdomen free so as to reduce intra-abdominal pressure to avoid venous engorgement and excessive blood loss.

Intraoperative imaging to identify correct level is mandatory. This is all the more important in patients with multi-level degeneration but presenting with symptoms and signs at one or two levels (Fig. 12.1). Use of operating microscope is advisable especially for widening the lateral recesses. When due to anatomic configuration of laminae the surgical approach should be from caudal to cranial in direction. In elderly patients it helps to mobilize the ligamentum flavum first with number 4 dissector before excising it. The exercise will help prevent annoying dural tears.

Lateral recess decompression is performed by partial removal of facets. At least 50% of the facets must be preserved on each side. Location of the lateral edge of pars is important to avoid its inadvertent excision and creating instability. Foraminotomies are best performed from the opposite side.

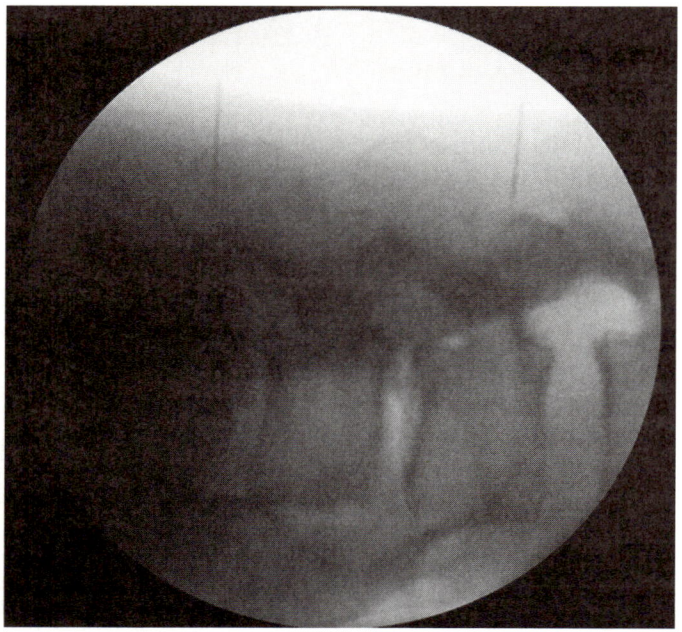

Fig. 12.1: Intraoperative fluoroscopy to confirm the levels

Surgical technique of internal decompression has been described and popularised by PS Ramani.[16]

Laminoplasty

Laminoplasty is not the procedure of choice for a given patient of lumbar canal stenosis and hence will not be described in this book.

Fusion

Indications for fusion include instability (Fig. 12.2), degenerative scoliosis or revisions at the previously operated levels with excessive bone removal. Various studies have shown that patients do better in these situations with instrumented fusion.[21]

Interspinous Stabilization Techniques

Numerous stabilization devices have been introduced recently in the management of lumbar spinal stenosis. The main types of devices include inter-spinous spacers (X-stop, DIAM) and interlaminar spacers (Coflex). The aim of these is to decompress neural structures indirectly by increasing the distance between adjacent posterior elements (lamina and spinous processes).

This mechanical principle is most likely to work in soft disco-ligamentous stenosis and unlikely to work in bony stenosis.[2] The contraindications for their use include severe osteoporosis, degenerative spondylolisthesis higher than grade 1, isthmic spondylolisthesis, scoliotic curve greater than 25 degrees, ankylosis of the stenotic segment, and severe neural impairment.[9]

Commentary

Cochrane review in 2005 showed that there is no statistically significant difference in outcomes following decompression plus fusion or decompression alone.[6] On the other hand, a previously published paper from 1993 concluded that patients with instrumented fusion as compared to non-instrumented fusion had a significantly higher fusion rates, less progressive listhesis and greater improvement in walking.[3]

Interbody fusions of various types ALIF, PLIF and TLIF have shown better fusion rates, however, that adds to surgical time, blood loss and complications.

The rate of surgery for LCS increased almost eight fold between 1979 and 1992. The rate then plateaued apart from those operations that include lumbar fusion.[4] Needless to say that the rates vary widely, more so in terms of fusions, with geographic areas. This can only be explained on the basis of lack of consensus.

Incidence of common complications vary widely depending on the surgical procedure and include CSF leak, mechanical instability, nerve root damage, incidental durotomy, etc. Such complications should

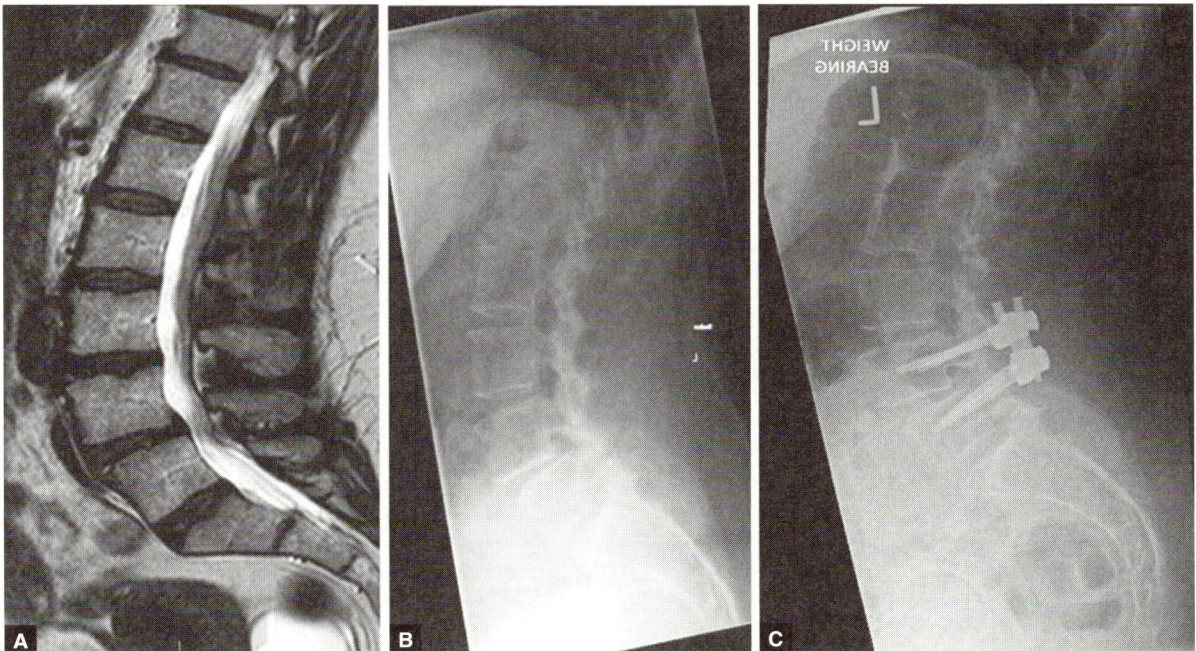

Fig. 12.2A to C: (A) T2W sagittal MRI; (B) Preoperative lateral X-ray; (C) Postoperative lateral X-ray showing L4/5 stenosis with listhesis managed with pedicle screw fixation and autologous bone graft fusion

be identified and managed immediately. Opened dura should be sutured to achieve watertight closure with fine sutures under the microscope. Use of autologous fat graft or dural substitute with synthetic glue might be useful.

If bleeding has been a major challenge, use of subfacial suction drain could be considered especially following multilevel decompressions and those involving fusion procedures.

Interspinous devices have been used either as stand-alone implants or to augment conventional decompression procedures.[14,18] Moojen et al, compared results of decompression to interspinous process devices at 1 year in a randomised controlled trial. No difference was seen in overall outcome in the 2 groups but re-operation rates at the end of first year reached 29% for interspinous process device compared to 8% with conventional decompression.[14] Additional implantation of interspinous device after decompression does not improve the clinical outcomes compared to decompression alone.[17]

Interlaminar stabilization devices are indicated for use in one or two level lumbar stenosis. They are intended to be implanted midline between adjacent lamina of 1 or 2 contiguous lumbar motion segments after decompression of the affected levels.

Davis et al randomized patients with moderate symptoms of lumbar spinal stenosis with or without grade 1 degenerative spondylolisthesis to undergo either decompression with fusion (107 patients) or decompression with interlaminar device (coflex) implantation (215 patients). At 2-year follow-up, they reported comparable clinical outcomes and reoperation rates (10.7% among patients who received interspinous process devices and 7.5% among those who underwent fusion).[5] Surgical treatment with interspinous/interlaminar stabilization techniques is an effective treatment option in selected cases, but the risk of needing early revision surgery is substantially higher compared to conventional decompression procedures.

To Be or Not to Be

Regardless of initial treatment be it conservative or surgical, all patients improved over a period of 2 years follow-up. However, those undergoing surgical decompression reported greater improvement in terms of pain and disability. However, the relative benefits of initial treatment gradually diminished over time but outcomes of surgery and particularly fusion surgery remained favorable.

It has been argued that surgical treatment improves the walking ability.[11] It has also been argued that the improvement observed in nonoperative group could be due to psychological effect of having got better without a surgery. The variation also may reflect the fact that the symptoms in degenerative lumbar canal stenosis fluctuate from time to time and the advice sought during an acute phase may not remain valid during the period or remission. No patient should be considered for surgery if he is feeling better with alternate treatment.[7,11]

Decompression surgery has a definite beneficial effect on backpain and sciatic pain. But notable recoveries have also been observed in the nonoperative treatment group.

Thus patients with degenerative lumbar canal stenosis should first be subjected to conservative treatment and surgical option should only be offered with caution only after conservative treatment has not produced expected benefit. One should follow this philosophy until we have consensus guidelines available, based on randomised and controlled prospective trials based on long-term follow-up of such patients.

REFERENCES

1. Ammendolia C, Stuber KJ, Rok E, et al. Nonoperative treatment for lumbar spinal stenosis with neurogenic claudication (Review). cochrane library. 2013;30(8).
2. Beyer F , Yagdiran F, Neu P. Percutaneous interspinous spacer versus open decompression: a 2-year follow-up of clinical outcome and quality of life. Eur Spine J 2013;22: 2015–21.
3. Bridewell KH, Sedgewick TA, O'Brien Mf, et al. The role of fusion and instrumentation in the treatment of degenerative spondylolisthesis with spinal stenosis. J Spinal Disord 1993;6(6):461–72.
4. Ciol MA, Deyo RA, Howell E, et al. An assessment of surgery for spinal stenosis: time trends, geographic variations, complications, and reoperations. J. Am Geriatr Soc 1996;44: 285–90.
5. Davis R, Errico T, Bae H. Decompression and Coflexinterlaminar stabilization compared with decompression and instrumented spinal fusion for spinal stenosis and low-grade degenerative spondylolisthesis. Two-year results from the prospective, randomized, multicenter, Food and Drug Administration Investigational Device Exemption Trial. Spine 2013;38:1529–39.
6. Gibson JN, Waddell G. Surgery for degenerative lumbar spondylosis: updated Cochrane Rev. Spine 2005;30(20): 2312–20.
7. Hadianfard MJ, Aminlari A, Daneshian A, et al. Effect of acupuncture on pain and quality of life in patients with lumbar spinal stenosis: A case study; J Acupunct Meridian Stud 2016;9(4); 178–82.
8. Kim KH, Kim T-H, Lee BR, et al Acupuncture for lumbar spinal stenosis: A systematic revieiw and meta-analysis. Comlement Ther Med 2013;21:535–56.
9. Kuchta J, Sobottke R, Eysel P. Two-year results of interspinous spacer (X-Stop) implantation in 175 patients with neurologic intermittent claudication due to lumbar spinal stenosis. Eur Spine J 2009;18:823–9.
10. Liu K, Liu P, Liu R, et al. Steroid for epidural injection in spinal stenosis: a systematic review and meta-analysis. Drug Des DevTher 2015;9: 707–16.
11. Malmivaara A, Slatis P, Heliovaara M et.al. Surgical or non operative treatment for lumbar spinal stenosis? A randomized controlled trial; Spine; 2007;1:32; 1–8.
12. Manchikanti L, Falco FJ, Benyamin RM, et al. Assessment of bleeding risk of interventional techniques; a best evidence based synthesis of practice patterns and perioperative management of anticoagulant and antithrombotic therapy. Pain physician 2013;16(2): SE261–318.
13. Manchikanti L, Singh V, Pampati V, et al. Comparison of the efficacy of caudal, interlaminar, and transforaminal epidural injections in managing lumbar disc herniation: is one method superior to the other? Korean J pain 2015;28:11–21.
14. Moojen W, Arts M, Jacobs W.Interspinous process device versus standard conventional surgical decompression for lumbar spinal stenosis: randomized controlled trial. BMJ 2013;347:f6415.
15. NASS evidence based clinical guidelines committee. Diagnosis and treatment of degenerative lumbar spinal stenosis. Revised 2011.
16. Ramani PS, Maheshwari S. Surgical technique of internal decompression for spinal stenosis (IDSS). J Spinal Surg 2011;2(4):556–69.
17. Richter A, Halm H, Hauck M. Two-year follow-up after decompressive surgery with and without implantation of an interspinous device for lumbar spinal stenosis: a prospective controlled study. J Spinal Disord Tech 2014;27:336–41.
18. Strömqvist BH, Berg S, Gerdhem P et al.X-Stop versus decompressive surgery for lumbar neurogenic intermittent claudication. Randomized controlled trial with 2-year follow-up. Spine 201338(17): 1436–42.
19. Stuber K, Sajko S, Kristmanson K. Chiropractic treatment of lumbar spinal stenosis: a review of the literature. J Chiropr Med 2009;8: 77–85.
20. Tomkins CC, Dimoff KH, Forman HS, et al. Physical therapy treatment options for lumbar spinal stenosis. J Back Musculoskelet Rehabil 2010;23: 31–7.
21. Weinstein JN, Lurie JD, Tosteson TD, et al. Surgical versus non-surgical treatment for lumbar spinal stenosis. N Engl J Med 2007;356(22):2257–70.

Lumbar Canal Stenosis: Interventional Pain Management

Jitendra Jain

INTRODUCTION

Lumbar canal stenosis is more symptomatic in elderly people. Pain is always most disturbing and demoralising to the patient with spine issues. The fear of getting disabled and bedridden can cause unnecessary stress and depression in some of these patients. The whole purpose of this chapter to help alleviate pain symptom of the patient provided there are no RED (neurodeficit or infection or inflammation or malignancy) or YELLOW (psychological issues) flags[1] present in the patient. Even if red or yellow flags are present pain control should also be instituted along with other surgical or medical management for lumbar canal stenosis as pain is slowly getting recognized as fifth vital sign.[2,4]

Main purpose of pain management is to improve spinal rehabilitation both physical and mental in patients of lumbar canal stenosis. Nerve block is a misnomer. Interventional pain procedure does not necessarily interrupt pain signal but mostly causes anti-inflammation with steroid unless radio-frequency ablation or neurolysis is planned for patient.

Pain Management Philosophy

Stepwise approach to lumbar canal stenosis pain is to start from least interventional techniques to complicated surgical or interventional procedures as shown in Fig. 13.1.[3]

Step 1 is pain management which includes interventional pain procedure like epidural, transforaminal and caudal epidural steroid blocks.

Key to successful completion of canal stenosis treatment would be breaking the pain cycle and improving physical and mental rehabilitation to prevent recurrence of symptoms in patient.

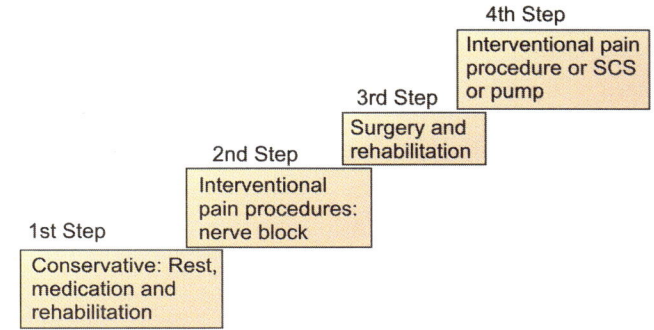

Fig. 13.1: Stepwise approach to lumbar canal stenosis (same can be applied to other spine related pain issues)

Why do Interventional Pain Procedures[5]

Interventional pain procedures are the next possible option if there are no RED or YELLOW flags present in the patient. An interventional pain procedure might be able to decrease perineural inflammation, edema or peridiscal swelling or facet joint inflammation. One of the advantages of doing interventional pain procedure is to do target delivery of therapeutic agents like steroid, local anesthetic or radiofrequency directly to affected area of spine. Trigger point injection may help to break the trigger area and decrease pain. Reasons for considering interventional pain procedure or nerve block are as follows:

- Uncontrollable pain
- Pain limiting patients day-to-day activity
- Poor sleep due to pain
- Failure of pharmacotherapy
- Undesirable side effects to pharmacotherapy
- Immediate pain relief for breaking pain cycle and starting early rehabilitation
- Patient not willing for surgery in absence of RED or YELLOW flags

- Patients who wants to buy time before deciding for spine surgery
- Patients who are not fit for spine surgery like older patients with co-morbidities
- Patients who had spine surgery and still has pain issues

Lumbar canal stenosis could just be a simple nerve root pain or compounded by facet joint pain. Depending on the patients symptom area specific pain management interventional procedure can be offered. Different kinds of nerve blocks or interventional pain procedures are used for different purposes. Nerve block could be a misnomer especially if steroid is injected where it is mainly anti-inflammatory action rather than nerve signal interruption results in pain relief. The potential targets for pain control could be:

- Nerve root by interlaminar or transforaminal or caudal route utilizing epidural space
- Facet joint by facet joint block or radiofrequency ablation
- Myofascial areas by trigger point injection
- Lumbar sympathetic chain for neuropathic leg pain
- Epidural space for utilizing dorsal spine column for spinal cord stimulators
- Intrathecal space for implantable intrathecal pumps

Mechanism of Pain Relief by Interventional Pain Procedures

Mechanism of pain relief with various interventional pain procedures is depending on the procedure and technique used for pain control (Table 13.1). Of the procedures described below most common one is steroid procedure and trigger point injection.

Purpose of improving patients pain control would improve patients moral, physical endurance, body mechanics along with improving body's pain protective techniques. It will also help to decrease his requirements for medicines will improve patients own positive coping skills along with improved emotional control. These will eventually facilitate patient's recovery and rehabilitation to increase the patient's activity level at home and to facilitate a return to work. Multiple factors contributing to degenerative spine problem as shown in Fig. 13.2.

Interventional Pain Procedures

Commonly done interventional pain procedures are:
- Interlaminar epidural steroid block
- Transforaminal epidural steroid block
- Caudal epidural steroid block
- Facet joint steroid block and median branch radiofrequency ablation

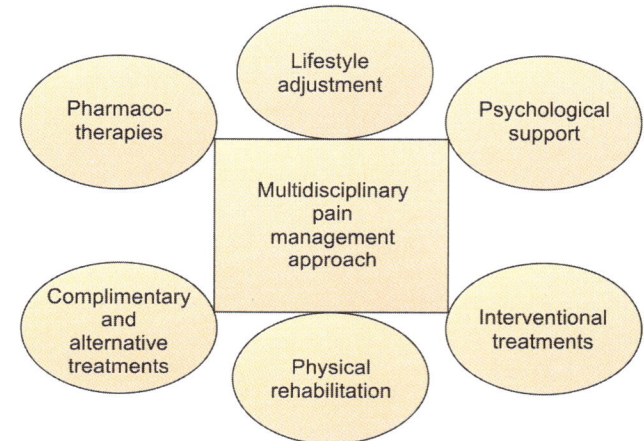

Fig. 13.2: Multidisciplinary approach[7] to lumbar canal stenosis pain management

Table 13.1: Mechanism of pain relief in various procedures[6]		
Procedure	Target area	Mechanism of relief
Steroid procedure	Nerve root (in epidural space by interlaminar, transforaminal or caudal space), facet joint and disc	Anti-inflammatory action on nerve root and intervertebral disc
Radiofrequency ablation	Ablation of facet joint median branch of nerve or sympathetic chain	Desensitization of facet joint (sympatholysis) for neuropathic pain relief in lower limb
Trigger point injection	Myofascial trigger or tender muscles (paravertebral, gluteal or leg muscles)	Breaks the pain cycle by breaking trigger points and relaxing tight muscles
Neurolysis	Sympathetic chain in lumbar area	Sympathetic chain neural destruction.
Spinal cord stimulator	Epidural space for stimulating the dorsal spinal column of spinal cord, and in some cases specific nerve roots	Diverting the pain signals and replacing with tingling by electrical means
Implantable intrathecal pump	Intrathecal space	Direct delivery of pain killers like morphine into intrathecal space

- Trigger point injections
- Resistant case might need spinal cord stimulator and implantable intrathecal pump.

General pattern of doing these procedures involves following salient features:

- Most of these procedures are done on day care basis, under local anesthesia.
- These procedures are percutaneous procedures, non-surgical minimally invasive procedures.
- It is to be done using imaging modalities like C-arm (fluroscopy) or ultrasound or CT guided procedure so as to be more accurate and safe.

Interlaminar Epidural Steroid Block[8]

It was one of the most commonly done interventional pain procedures before transforaminal epidural steroid became more relevant (Fig. 13.3).

Technique: It is done in the same way like introducing needle in the epidural space for the purpose of instillation of drugs. Preferably it should be done under fluoroscopy guided so that it is targeted directly at the affected level. It can be done in sitting or prone position, prone preferable under fluoroscopy (Fig. 13.4). Once local anesthesia is given epidural Tuohy's needle is commonly (18 G or 16 G in adult) used to reach epidural space. LOR (loss of resistance) is commonly used to detect epidural space. After confirming contrast spread in desired space 40 mg Triamcinolone or 6 mg Betamethasone or 8 mg Dexamethasone with or without local anesthetic with a volume of about 8 to 10 ml diluted in normal saline. Postprocedure observation is done in day care for allergy and hemodynamic stability.

Advantages

- Simple to perform

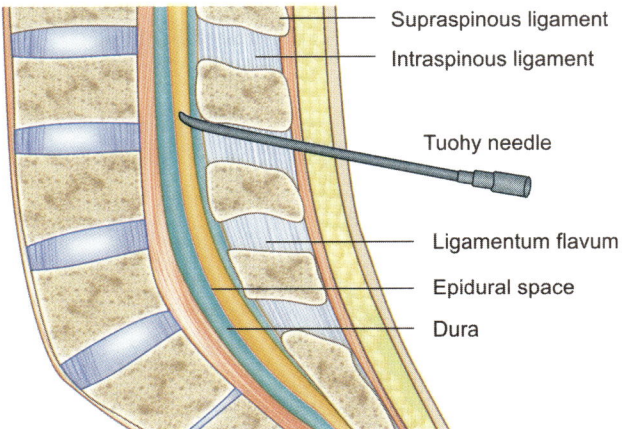

Fig. 13.3: Interlaminar Epidural procedure for lumbar canal stenosis

Supraspinous ligament

Intraspinous ligament

Tuohy needle

Ligamentum flavum

Epidural space

Dura

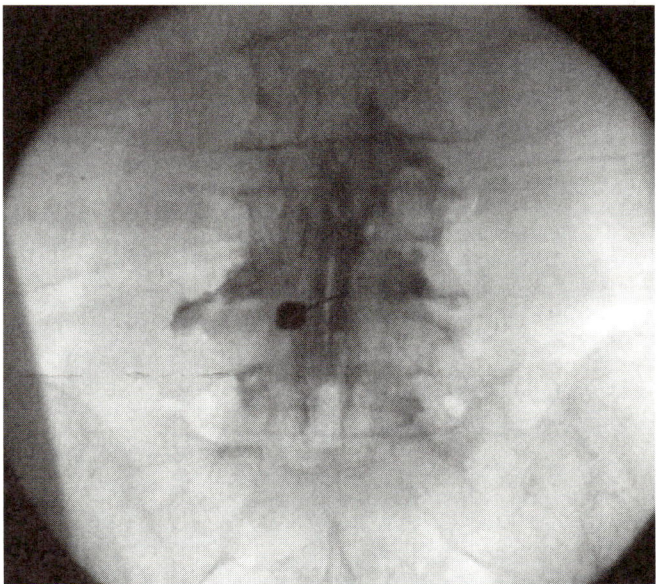

Fig. 13.4: Interlaminar epidural steroid in L4–5 interspinous space under C-arm and non-ionic contrast (Iopamide) guidance

- Both sides and multiple levels can be covered with single needle prick
- A big volume can be injected to be effective
- In most patients the relief is maintained for 3–6 months
- The epidural block can be repeated if pain recurs

Disadvantages

- In case of tight/severe canal stenosis steroid might not reach the lateral or anterior epidural space
- Volume required to reach therapeutic space or nerve might be more causing hypotension or nerve root pressure causing weakness of lower limb especially if local anesthetic is used
- Epidural space bleeding due to epidural vessel puncture can cause neurological deficit in lower limb
- Epidural infection although rare is a possibility
- Dural puncture with steroid intrathecally can cause arachnoiditis especially if patient has tight central canal stenosis.

Lumbar Transforaminal Epidural Steroid[9,10]

It is one of the most commonly done procedure to get relief from sciatic pain in patients with degenerative lumbar canal stenosis. In this technique, the intervertebral foramen space is used to reach the affected stenotic nerve root (Fig. 13.5).

Transforaminal epidural is done to inject a mixture of steroids and local anesthetic in lateral and anterior epidural space through oblique approach under fluoroscopy guidance. It is done in prone position under

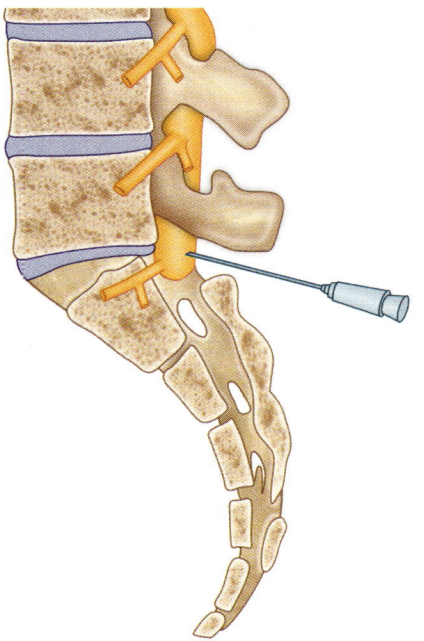

Fig. 13.5: Lumbar transforaminal epidural steroid procedure at L5–S1 level

fluoroscopy (Fig. 13.6). It is usually done under local anesthesia. Spinal needle 22 G is used. Gun barrel approach is commonly used in interventional pain procedure. It means that the needle is parallel to the X-ray beams of the fluoroscopy. For transforaminal procedure usually the respective end plate of the vertebral body is squared and oblique direction to 15 degrees is done. Once satisfied with the C-arm placement local anesthesia is first given to decrease procedure pain and to mark the entry point for the spinal needle at a depth of about 3–5 cm. As shown in the X-ray picture below needle is usually in the upper half and center of the intervertebral foramen. Contrast dye with iopamide about 1 ml is injected to reconfirm

needle in the transforaminal space (covering nerve root and epidural space both) and also making sure that there is no vascular or intrathecal spread. 40 mg Triamcenalone or 6 mg Betamethasone or 8 mg Dexamethasone with or without local anesthetic with a volume of about 2 ml diluted in normal saline is then injected. Postprocedure observation is done in day care for allergy and hemodynamic stability.

Advantages

- Simple and easy to perform
- Safer procedure in comparison to epidural steroid injection for one or two levels
- Small volume of 1–5 to 2 ml is sufficient to perform this procedure
- Anterior and lateral epidural space can be covered by transforaminal approach
- Gives longer pain relief as compared to epidural or caudal steroid injection
- For tight spinal stenosis it is a much better procedure in comparison to other procedures
- It can be easily repeated if pain recurs

Disadvantages

- For multiple and bilateral spinal canal pain symptom issues it might be uncomfortable for patients as multiple needle pricks will be involved.
- In patients with huge facet joints and past history of bony fusion surgeries there might be technical issues to reach intervertebral foraminal space.
- Epidural space bleeding due to epidural vessel puncture can cause neurodeficit in lower limb.
- Epidural infection although rare but is a possibility.
- Dural puncture with steroid intrathecally can cause arachnoiditis.

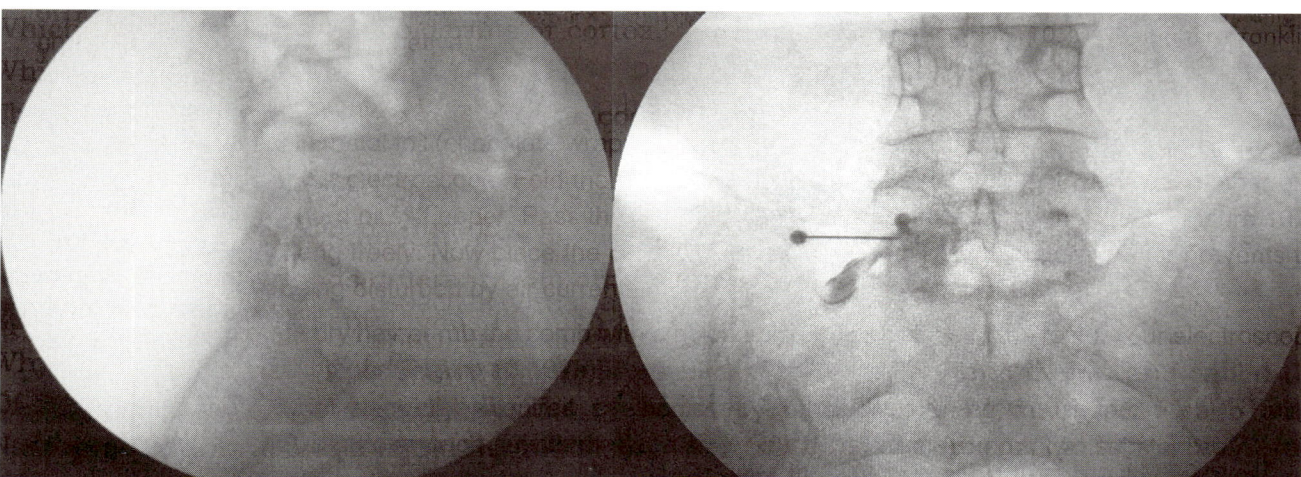

Fig. 13.6: Lumbar transforaminal epidural steroid under C-arm guidance (lateral and AP)

Caudal Epidural Steroid Procedure

It was one of the most commonly used interventional pain procedures before transforaminal epidural steroid became more popular (Fig. 13.7). It is still widely practiced, commonly done blindly as most anesthetists would give for postoperative analgesia.

Technique: Caudal epidural steroid procedure is done under local anesthesia, position of the patient might be lateral if done blindly and prone if done under C-arm guidance. Blind caudal is done by feeling Sacral hiatus in between the sacral cornu in lower part of sacral spine. Local anesthesia with 2% lignocaine is given. Needle is

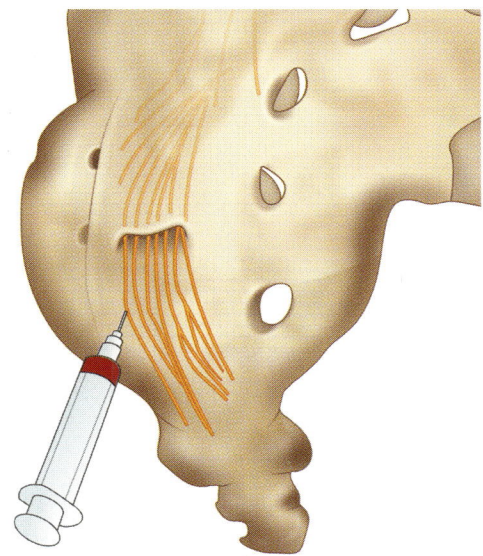

Fig. 13.7: Caudal epidural diagram for caudal epidural steroid procedure in lumbar canal stenosis patient

introduced in the center of sacral hiatus, feeling a "pop" when sacrococcygeal ligament is pierced. The needle angle is changed to keep it parallel to sacram as needle goes 2–3 cm further inside. Once negative for blood or CSF the desired 10–15 ml solution of 40 mg Triamcenalone with or without local anesthetic is injected. Under fluoroscopy similar technique (Fig. 13.8) is followed but the needle is directed to the affected side (left side of sacral hiatus if left leg is involved). Contrast is injected to confirm needle position. Typically in center a Christmas tree appearance is hallmark of a successful caudal epidural block. Postprocedure observation is done in day care for allergy and hemodynamic stability.

Caudal epidural adhesiolysis[11, 12] (Fig. 13.9): It is a modification of caudal epidural procedure. It is mainly done for the patients who have post-laminectomy radiculopathy. In this Tuohy's needle is used to enter caudal space, then a stiff catheter directed to the affected side (right side if right leg or L4–5, L5–S1 on right side is involved). The purpose is push the catheter in the anterior epidural space to break the smaller fibrosis and to deflect the scar tissue if possible so that therapeutic steroid can work on the affected nerve roots and higher volume and mechanical catheter can break the fibrosis and try to soften the scar tissue with hyaluronidase (1500 units).

Advantages

- Simple to perform
- Both sides and multiple levels can be covered with single needle prick especially if lower L4–5–S1 levels involved.

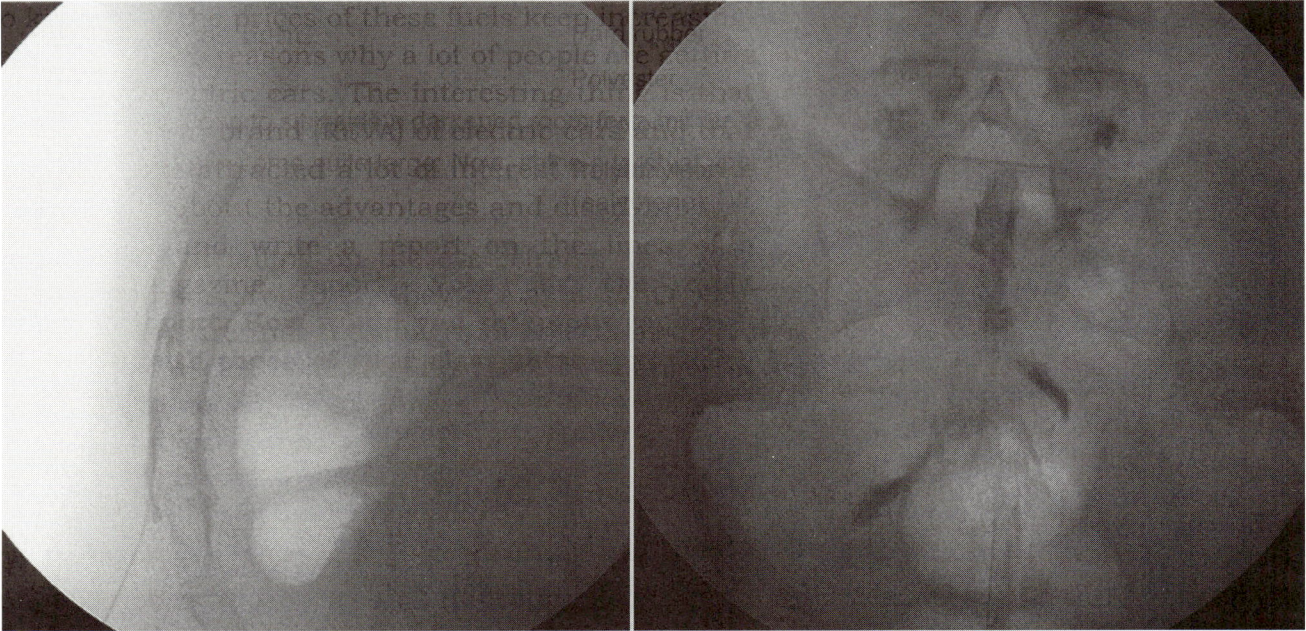

Fig. 13.8: Caudal epidural steroid under C-arm guidance

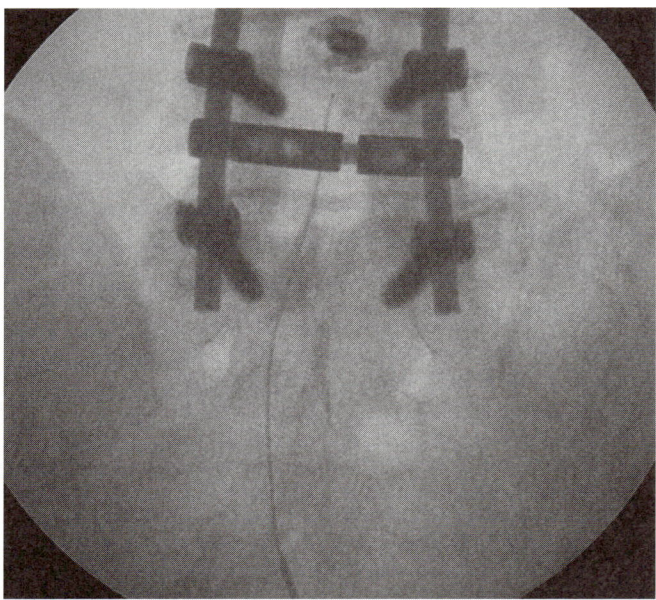

Fig. 13.9: Caudal epidural neuroplasty or adhesiolysis

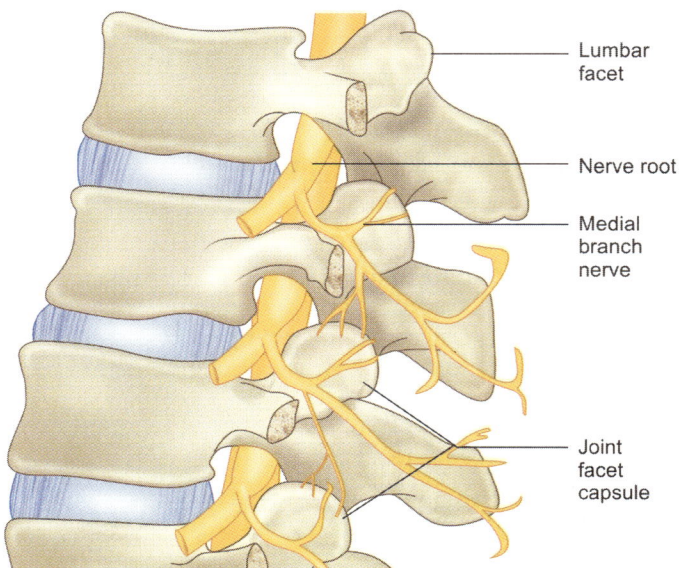

Fig. 13.10: Lumbar medial branch around facet joint

- A big volume can be injected to be effective epidural block
- It can give relief for 3–6 months in most patients
- It can be performed blind but under fluoroscopy it is more accurate and more effective
- Anterior epidural space is more accessible with caudal in comparison to interlaminar epidural procedure
- It can be easily repeated if pain recurs

Disadvantages

- In case of tight/severe canal stenosis steroid might not reach to lateral or anterior epidural space especially if it is postsurgery
- Volume required to reach therapeutic space or nerve might be more causing hypotension or nerve root pressure causing weakness of lower limb especially if local anesthetic is used
- Caudal space bleeding due to epidural vessel puncture is a possibility
- Caudal epidural infection although rare but is a possibility
- Dural puncture is possible if needle is pushed too much inside the caudal epidural space with steroid intrathecally can cause arachnoiditis

Lumbar Facet Radiofrequency Ablation

It is mainly done for the patients with back pain, lumbar paravertebral pain with or without radicular or neurogenic claudication pain. Initial form of this was facet joint steroid procedure (Fig. 13.11) which has slowly being replaced by facet joint medial branch nerve

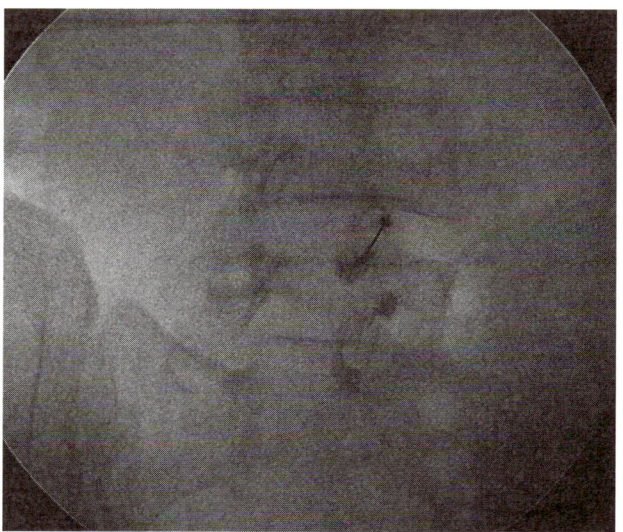

Fig. 13.11: Lumbar facet joint procedure

radiofrequency ablation. Medial branch (Fig. 13.10) is division of dorsal root around the base of superior articular facet nerve supplying the facet joint and multifidis muscle. If the medial branch block is positive with local anesthesia (2% Lignocaine or 0.5% Bupivacaine), then patient can undergo lumbar facet medial branch radiofrequency ablation.

Technique: It is done under fluoroscopy guidance. Entry of the needle is such that the radiofrequency needle is parallel to the medial branch at the junction of transverse process and superior articular facet (Fig. 13.12). Once confirmed by C-arm, sensory and motor stimulation of medial branch radiofrequency ablation is performed usually at 80° centigrade for 75 seconds and

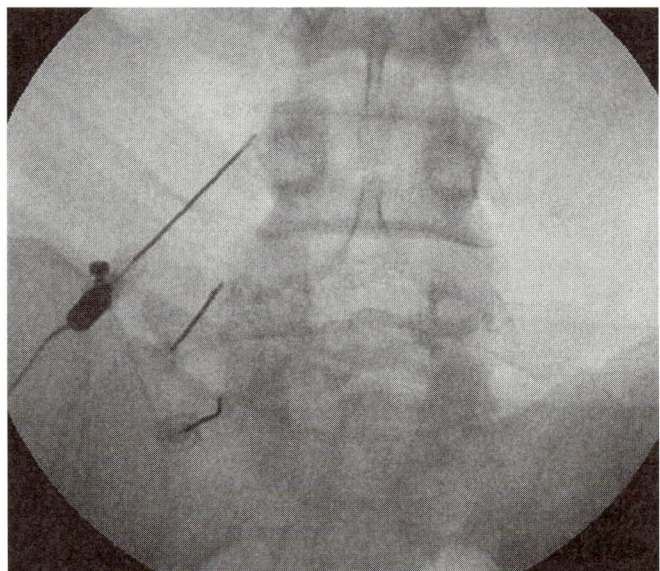

Fig. 13.12: Lumbar facet radiofrequency ablation

two lesion at each joint is performed so as to increase the size of medial branch lesion. If one has to ablate L4–5 facet joint then one level above and one level below is also covered.

Advantages

- Simple procedure to relieve back pain
- Can be done under local anesthesia
- Relief of pain is for usually a year or more
- Procedure can be repeated if pain recurs
- Usually immediate pain relief and initiate early rehabilitation in patients

Disadvantages

- Needs radiofrequency generator to do ablation
- Cannot be done without fluoroscopy
- Rarely can cause discomfort of back for a few weeks postprocedure
- Too much sedation or general anesthesia should be avoided for this procedure or else sometimes nerve root ablation can cause weakness of lower limb.

Trigger Point Injection[13]

Trigger points are the muscles knots which on pressure of those muscles will cause referred pain in the area away from tender muscle. Commonly seen in the chronic spine pain areas leading to lumbar paraverte-bral or gluteal or lower limb muscle trigger points (Fig. 13.12). If conservative option are not working, then a simple trigger point injection with local anesthetic like 2% lignocaine can decrease the pain significantly. Patient should be counselled before that there might be repeat trigger point procedures and physical and

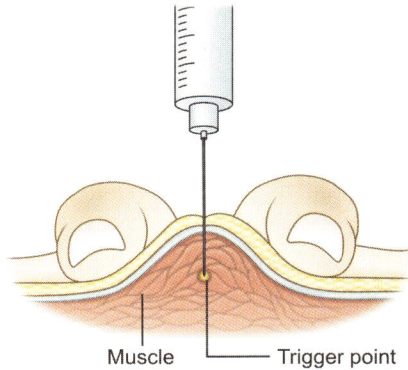

Fig. 13.13: Trigger point injection

mental rehabilitation needs to be combined to have a long-term pain relief of patient's symptoms.

It is simple OPD-based procedure. There is no need of operation theatre or C-arm. Nowadays, ultrasound is used to do trigger point injection. But it should be done only if facility for resuscitation is available in nearby area as local anesthetic like Lignocaine and Bupivacaine with or without steroid is used for it. Area of trigger is marked and injected with local anesthetic. Usually 2–3 ml Lignocaine is good enough for pain relief and breaking the tight band and pain cycle. This could be followed by ice compression of local area 2–3 times a day for next one week with stretch of trigger muscle.

Rarely infection or bleeding inside the muscle can be an issue but is can be managed if one is alert and does it cleanly.

Spinal cord stimulator[14] and implantable intrathecal pump[15] are generally not used in patients with lumbar canal stenosis and will not be discussed in this chapter.

Evidence for Interventional Pain Procedures[7,9,14,15]

Summary of the evidence and recommendations are given in Table 3.2.

Table 13.2: Evidence for interventional pain procedures	
Procedure	*Evidence level*
Interlaminar epidural steroid block	Fair in short term (less than 6 months)
Transforaminal epidural steroid block	Good in short and fair in long term (6 to 12 months)
Caudal epidural steroid block	Fair in short term (less than 6 months)
Facet joint radiofrequency ablation	Good in short to long term for back pain not radicular complain
Trigger point injection	Fair to poor in short term
Spinal cord stimulator	Good in long term
Implantable intrathecal pump	Good in long term

Lumbar canal stenosis can be complicated if treatment fails and if the patient selection for treatment is inappropriate. Step ladder approach is the safest way to avoid confusion and unnecessary complications in patients treatment. From the evidence it is clear that transforaminal epidural steroid procedure is simplest kind of treatment option to improve pain of the patient. Advanced procedure like spinal cord stimulator and intrathecal pump can be thought if the patient is resistant to most treatment options described in the step ladder approach to control pain of lumbar canal stenosis patient.

REFERENCES

1. Sizer PS Jr1, Brismée JM, Cook C: Pain Practice: Medical screening for red flags in the diagnosis and management of musculoskeletal spine pain;2007 Mar;7(1):53–71.

2. Walid MS1, Donahue SN, Darmohray DM, Hyer LA Jr, Robinson JS Jr. Pain Practice: The fifth vital sign—what does it mean; 2008 Nov-Dec;8(6):417–22.

3. Jitendra Jain: Handbook of Pain management;2017: (6)96–122.

4. American pain society: Pain: Current understanding of assessment, managements and treatments: Pain as fifth vital sign;1996:20–29.

5. Smith H, Youn Y, Guay RC, Laufer A, Pilitsis JG. The Role of Invasive Pain Management Modalities in the Treatment of Chronic Pain;2016: Med Clin North Am.: Jan;100(1):103–15.

6. Manchikanti L, Falco FJ, Singh V, Benyamin RM, Racz GB, Helm S 2nd, Caraway DL, Calodney AK, Snook LT, Smith HS, Gupta S, Ward SP, Grider JS, Hirsch JA. An update of comprehensive evidence-based guidelines for interventional techniques in chronic spinal pain. Part I: introduction and general considerations;2013: Pain Physician. 2013 Apr;16(2 Suppl):S1–48.

7. IASP: Pain clinic guidelines: Recommendation for pain treatment services: John Loeser et al;2009.

8. Park CH1, Lee SH. Correlation between severity of lumbar spinal stenosis and lumbar epidural steroid injection;2014: Pain Med.: Apr;15(4):556–61.

9. Manchikanti L, Buenaventura RM, Manchikanti KN, Ruan X, Gupta S, Smith HS, Christo PJ, Ward SP. Effectiveness of therapeutic lumbar transforaminal epidural steroid injections in managing lumbar spinal pain;2012: Pain Physician.: May-Jun;15(3):E199–245.

10. Davis N, Hourigan P, Clarke A. Transforaminal epidural steroid injection in lumbar spinal stenosis: an observational study with two-year follow-up;2017: Br J Neurosurg.; Apr;31(2):205–8.

11. Parr AT, Manchikanti L, Hameed H, Conn A, Manchikanti KN, Benyamin RM, Diwan S, Singh V, Abdi S. Caudal epidural injections in the management of chronic low back pain: a systematic appraisal of the literature;2012: Pain Physician.; May-Jun;15(3):E159–98.

12. Jamison DE, Hsu E, Cohen SP. Epidural adhesiolysis: an evidence-based review;2014: J Neurosurg Sci.: Jun;58(2):65–76.

13. Gerwin RD. Myofascial Trigger Point Pain Syndromes;2016: Semin Neurol.; Oct;36(5):469–73. Epub 2016 Sep 23.

14. Walsh KM, Machado AG, Krishnaney AA. Spinal cord stimulation: a review of the safety literature and proposal for perioperative evaluation and management; 2015: Spine J; Aug 1;15(8):1864–9.

15. Rainov NG, Heidecke V. Management of chronic back and leg pain by intrathecal drug delivery;2007: Acta Neurochir Suppl; 97(Pt 1):49–56.

Role of Laminectomy in Lumbar Canal Stenosis

JKBC Parthiban

INTRODUCTION

Ever since lumbar canal stenosis was recognised, lumbar laminectomy has established itself as the standard surgical procedure for its management and has never been ignored by surgeons. Lumbar canal stenosis by its terminology indicates that the canal being narrowed and its contents are in constant compression and finally produces symptoms and later signs that warrant attention beyond which a man cannot function freely due to severe reduction in quality of life. The commonest cause of canal stenosis is due to degenerative changes that occur during ageing and strain of lumbar disc (degenerative disc disease, its bulge, osteophytes), facets and its joints (arthropathy, hypertrophy), buckling of ligamentum flavum (so called thickened ligament), associated fusion or lysthesis, all leading to narrow canal, compression of nerve roots and blood vessels in particular the veins that drain through the root canals and foramen. The stagnant venous blood and the congestion at and above the stenosis cause claudication pain along with root pains in legs, in isolation or in combination, unilateral or bilateral, later leading to even neurological deficits in worst cases. Lumbar canal stenosis can be central, lateral and foraminal by anatomical definition and cause appropriate neurovascular compressions and produce symptoms accordingly. Facetal arthropathy, segmental instability and paraspinal spasm secondary to abnormal positioning can cause low backache.

Rationale

Laminectomy of lumbar canal achieves decompression of nerve roots and improves venous flow and hence decongest the dural space and nerve roots. Though symptoms due to lumbar canal stenosis get better with postural adjustments like stooping forward and flexing the lumbar spine at early stages of the disease, they may not work for long time and patients at some point of time like to seek for better treatment to improve quality of life. Sciatica in association with back pain become unresponsive to medical management at some point of time. Moreover, medical managements and rehab programmes do not meet the patient satisfaction. Many of them walk less, wheel chaired and some bedridden. Lumbar canal decompression in the form of laminectomy, lateral canal deroofing and for aminotomy provide excellent relief of pain and prevent progression of neurological deficit, thus preventing patients from leading poor quality of life particularly in elderly population. Early surgical decompression, hence sounds sensible in the management of symptomatic lumbar canal stenosis.

Techniques

Techniques to address lumbar canal stenosis depends on radiology and clinical status. Often patients who seek surgical management have a significant canal stenosis and may be associated with instability or lysthesis. Lumbar laminectomy *per se* involves excision of spinous process and lamina as lateral as possible without disturbing facet joints and pars. Bony excision alone may not achieve decompression until the buckled ligamentum flavum is removed meticulously. Often due to long duration of compression the dura will be thin and compression impressions will be seen on dura. Simple laminectomy is suffice for central canal stenosis. However, when the lateral canal is also seen stenosed, then undercutting of facet joint complex, lateral lamina, neural foramen, thick ligamentum flavum is mandatory. While this being done the dural sleeve and nerve root guide the surgeons towards exit of neural foramen. Point worth mentioning here is the meticulous way the lateral most fibres of ligamentum flavum being excised. Dura is thin and hence can tear which may need suturing. Finally a good laminectomy should provide good decompression of dura and nerve roots from midline to far lateral and up to neural foramen exit (Figs 14.1A to J and 14.2A to D).

In the event of instability appreciated on table, preoperatively detected by radiology or expected to occur in postoperative period, then it is preferred to stabilise the segments with pedicle screw fixation and add trans-

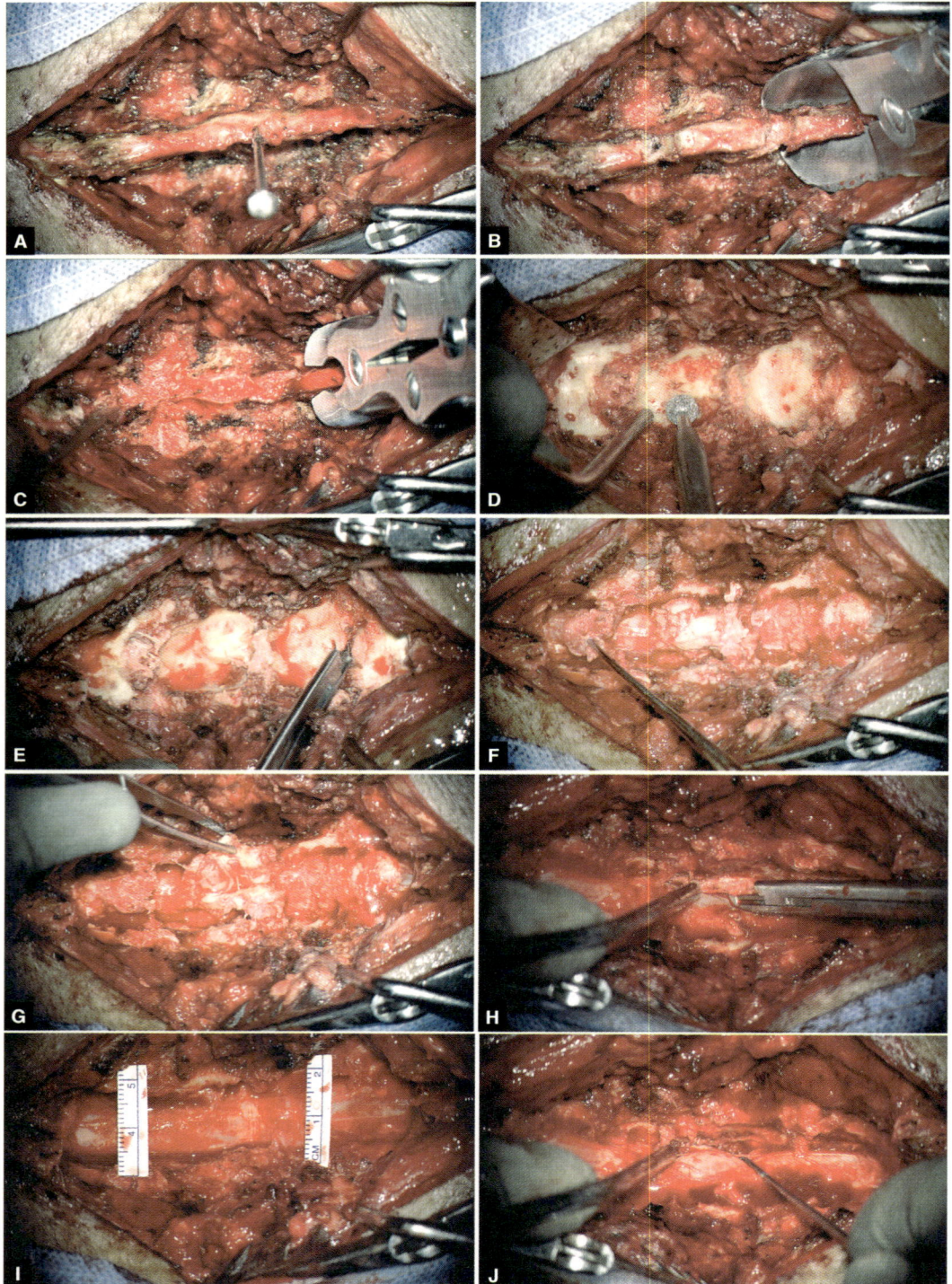

Fig. 14.1A to J: (A) Paraspinal muscles are dissected away from spinolaminar surface; (B) After excising interspinous ligament spinous process base is cut; (C) Spinous base and lamina nibbled; (D) Lamina is drilled to inner table; (E) Lamina excised; (F) Dura and the buckled ligamentum flavum at multiple levels; (G) Ligamentum flavum excision at midline; (H) Ligamentum flavum excised at lateral canal to deroof and decompress nerve root; (I) Free nerve root in lateral canal towards foramen; (J) Completed laminectomy

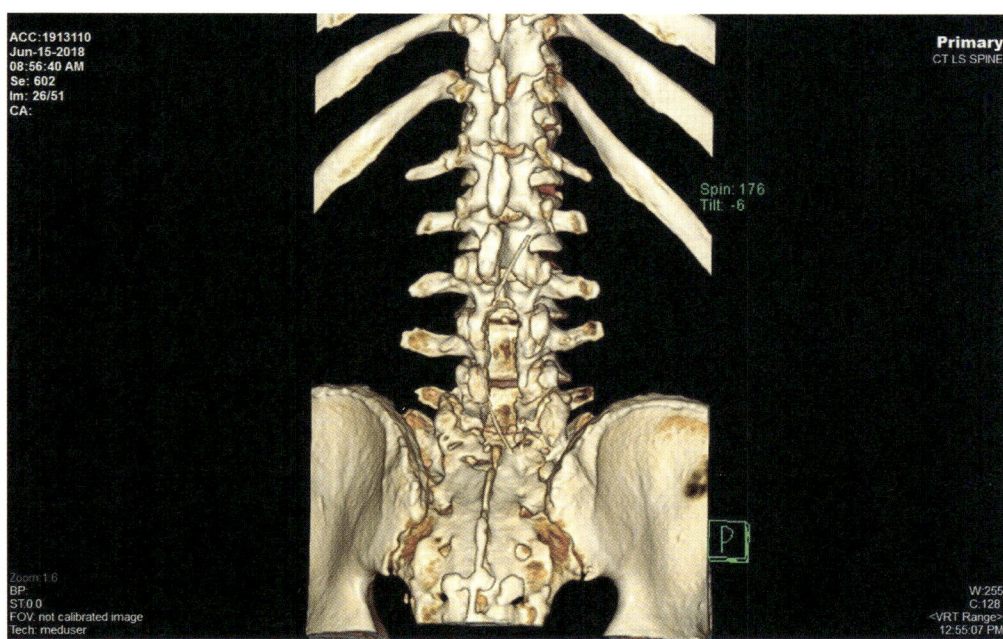

Fig. 14.2A: Postoperative 3D posterior view of laminectomy

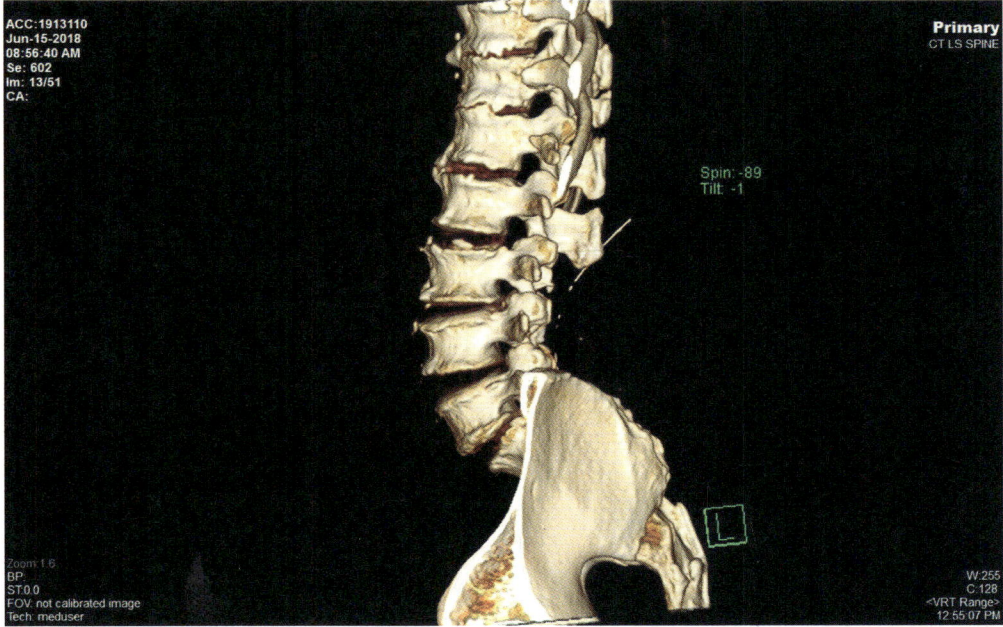

Fig. 14.2B: Postoperative 3D lateral view of laminectomy

foraminal interbody fusion or posterolateral fusion along with.

Though most of the time laminectomy is done by excising spinolaminar bone along with interspinous ligaments through a midline approach and paraspinal muscle dissection, to preserve posterior anatomical complex and replacing the tension band in young patients we practice subspinous laminectomy. In this technique the paraspinal muscles are separated from spinolaminar surface, interspinous ligament is cut at the lowest level of interest, base spinous processes are cut over midlamina and the full segment along with desired spinous processes and ligament is reflected up for further laminectomy and later to be replaced and sutured back anatomically. This technique provides good repositioning of paraspinal muscles and keeps the tension band anatomically connected when healing occur.

Postoperatively patients are mobilised with lumbosacral corset or thoracolumbar sacral orthosis for 6 weeks and advised to avoid abnormal flexion and overstraining.

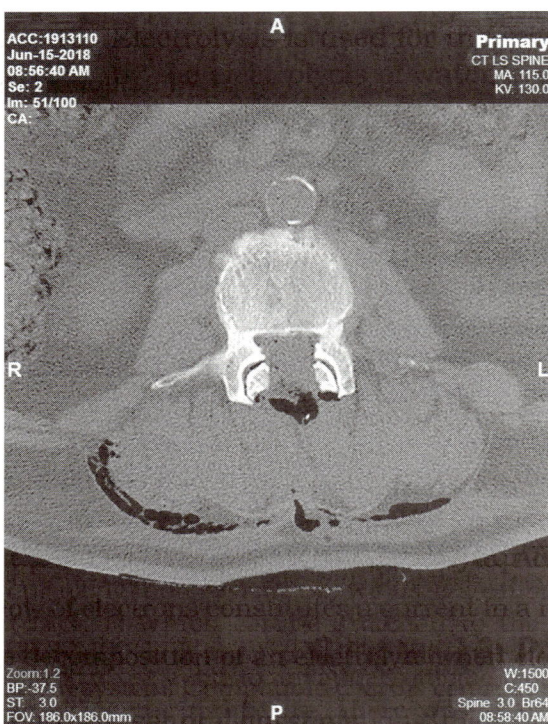

Fig. 14.2C: Postoperative axial CT cut showing the extent of laminectomy

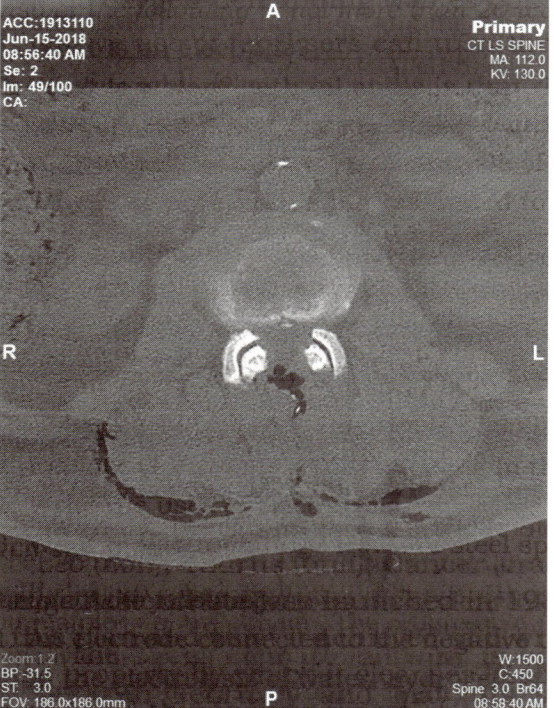

Fig. 14.2D: Postoperative axial CT cut showing undercutting of facets

Results

Careful and rigid selection of cases and perfect execution of surgery finally decides best outcome in individual patient. In majority of patients where claudication pain was the main presenting symptom laminectomy alone gives excellent relief of pain that can be appreciated in the immediate postoperative period. Many patients feel free and relieved of pain on bed in supine position and could walk for more distance in the immediate postoperative period. The distance and comfort increases by days and majority of them get into better quality of life. We observed in a few patients experiencing a tingling mild electric like feeling in lower limbs on the day of surgery in postoperative period, particularly who had long history and associated with diabetes. These sensations subside over a period of time. Patients with preoperative sensory disturbances, in particular with motor weakness do not improve quickly though pain comes down and they could walk better. Numbness and weakness like foot drop do not improve well. Postoperative medical management with Gabapentin and vitamins need to be continued for long period of time along with rehab programmes. Generally when pain disappears posture, gait and quality of life improves. The stooped posture disappears, distance covered without break prolongs and hence improved mobility. Laminectomy is one of the most rewarding and gratifying treatments for patients suffering from claudication pain due to lumbar canal stenosis. Low backache in lumbar canal stenosis generally get relieved with laminectomy alone if not associated with hypertrophic bulky facet joints.

Overall literature shows a success rate of around 88% in the first few months that drops by few percentages in six months. Patients with central canal stenosis have better result than with lateral canal stenosis alone. A small percent of patients either stay unchanged in their symptomatology or even worsen particularly when stenosis was significant with long duration history and neurological deficits. Motor weakness in the form of foot drop, severe wasting of leg muscles and bladder bowel deficits do not improve well. Though the results of laminectomy is always compared with other newer techniques, the author feels unlimitedly case selection and surgical execution decides the outcome.

Complications

The most important complication that is preventable with meticulous surgical technique is dural tear and the resultant cerebrospinal fluid leak. Since the dura is thin, dural tear tends to occur while excising ligamentum flavum particularly at lateral canal and at L5/S1 region where the dorsal dural is seen surfacing close due to lumbosacral curve. Dural tear if detected should be sutured with microsurgical technique and if

2

not possible at lateral canal and foramen, then it is better to use muscle fat patches to seal the rent. Use of sealants on top is advisable if available. A good closure of paraspinal muscle, facia and skin will avoid CSF leak in the postoperative period. It is also advisable to mobilise the patients at earliest to prevent CSF leak.

REFERENCES

1. Javid, Manucher & J. Hadar, Eldad. (1998). Long-term follow-up review of patients who underwent laminectomy for lumbar steno- sis: A prospective study. Journal of neurosurgery. 89. 1–7. 10.3171/ jns.1998.89.1.0001.

2. Munting E, Roder C, Sobottke R, et al. Patient outcomes after lami- notomy, hemilaminectomy, laminectomy and laminectomy with instrumented fusion for spinal canal stenosis or degenerative spondylolisthesis. Eur Spine J 2013;22:S653–84.

3. Phan K, Mobbs RJ. Minimally invasive versus open laminectomy for lumbar stenosis: a systematic review and meta-analysis. Spine (Phila Pa 1976) 2016;41:E91–E100.

4. Tuite GF, Stem JD, Doran SE, Papadopoulos SM, McGillicuddy JE, Oyedijo DI, et al: Outcome after laminectomy for lumbar spinal stenosis. Part I: clinical correlations. J Neurosurg 1994;81: 699–706.

Role of IDSS in Surgical Management of Lumbar Canal Stenosis

Sumeet Pawar, PS Ramani

INTRODUCTION

Lumbar canal stenosis remains the most frequent indication for surgery in elderly patients.[3]

Pain in lumbar canal stenosis occurs due to compression on neural and vascular elements in the lumbar spine due to nonavailability of space as a result of narrowing of the canal.

While both conservative and surgical treatments are suggested, the effect of conservative therapy is very limited and hence surgical intervention is recommended.

The challenge facing surgical management of lumbar spinal stenosis is to be able to decompress the cauda equina and the nerve roots while preserving the integrity of the spine. A frequently used surgical technique for lumbar spinal stenosis is laminectomy.[1,2,17] Laminectomy involves an extensive removal of tissues of the posterior elements of the spine. This results in a high risk of postoperative instability.[16] Moreover, the extensive removal of posterior elements results in extensive scar formation that can also be a cause of persistent postoperative pain due to scar tension.[5] There are still a few conditions in which laminectomy plays an important role which is discussed in details in other chapter in the book.

The drawbacks of laminectomy has necessitated the development of minimal invasive spinal surgery (MISS) which involves minimal dissection of tissue and minimal bone removal.[9,10,13,14] Benefits of MISS are as follows:

- Better cosmetic results from smaller skin incisions (sometimes as small as 2 cm)
- Less blood loss from surgery
- Reduced risk of muscle damage
- Reduced risk of infection and postoperative pain
- Faster recovery from surgery and less rehabilitation required

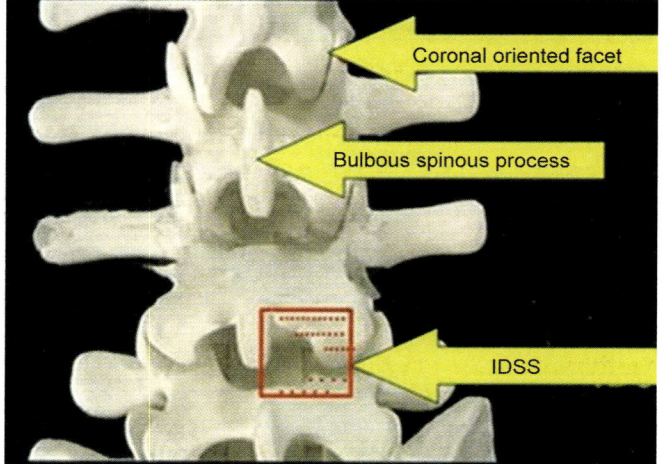

Fig. 15.1: Concept of IDSS

- Diminished reliance on pain medications after surgery

Internal decompression of spinal stenosis (IDSS)[8,15] involves limited resection of superior and inferior laminae along with ligamentum flavum while preserving the supra- and interspinous ligament and the spinous process and facet joints at the level involved, producing a fenestration that allows the decompression of the cauda equina and nerve roots using an undercutting technique, with limited loss of tissues of the posterior elements, while preserving the integrity of the facet joints (Fig. 15.1).

SURGICAL TECHNIQUE

The procedure is done under general anesthesia in prone position with a midline incision.

Patient Positioning

A radiolucent table is used. The patient is placed in prone position over the bolsters and the table may be flexed slightly to decrease the lordosis of the spine and open up the interlaminar space. Care is taken that the abdomen is free to avoid increase in abdominal pressure and thereby increased venous oozing during surgery. Adequate cushioning is given at all pressure points and eyes.

Incision and Exposure

After painting and draping, midline incision is taken. For single level surgery, not more than 3 cm is required. In a 4 cm incision, 2 levels can be done easily by maneuvering the retractors. Subperiosteal muscle resection is done to expose the posterior elements of the spine using monopolar cutting cautery. The lateral extent of the dissection is the facets. Care should be taken not to damage the facet capsule as it can lead to further secondary degeneration. Muscle retractors are then placed.

IDSS

The IDSS consists of removal of inferior margin of upper lamina and superior margin of lower lamina. This creates a window for the decompression of the neural elements. This laminotomy can be done using high-speed drill as well. The partial medial facetectomy is then done till the lateral margin of the canal is approached which is marked by the pedicle. After the window is created, careful and meticulous foramino-tomy is done. This is the most essential step of the surgery as the degeneration which cause hypertrophy of the facets impinges on the nerve root. Without adequate foraminotomy, patient cannot get complete relief of symptoms. The end result is assessed on table using Ramani's nerve root probe.

Similar decompression is done on the opposite side and any other level involved.

Closure

After achieving hemostasis, minivac drain is placed, the surgical site is then infiltrated with 0.25% or 0.5% Bupivicaine and wound is closed in layers. Sutures are removed 7–10 days postoperatively.

Photographs

We did a study to evaluate the changes in visual Analogue Scale (VAS), Oswestry disability index (ODI) and overall satisfaction in patients operated for lumbar canal stenosis by IDSS.

Objective

To evaluate the clinical outcome in patients operated with IDSS in lumbar canal stenosis at 3 years follow up.

Material and Methods

This is a hospital-based prospective study. The Institutional Ethical Committee approved it. The study population consisted of patients with a history of low back pain with or without pain radiating down to lower limbs and who were operated with internal decom-pression of spinal stenosis during 1st March 2011 to

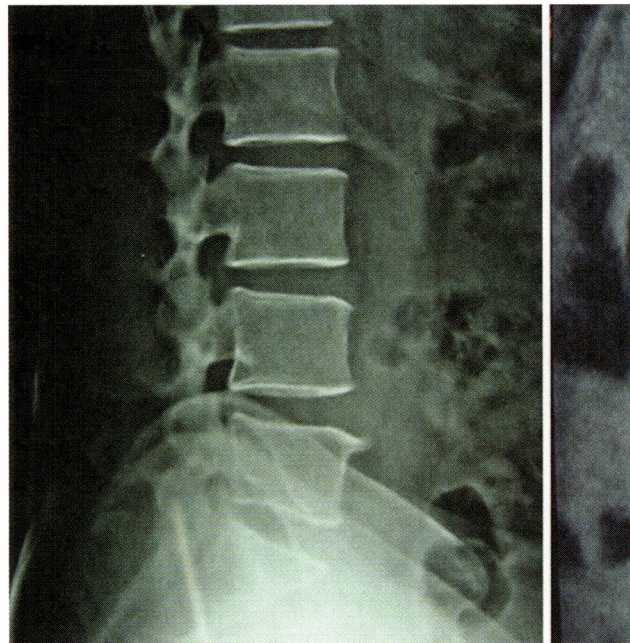
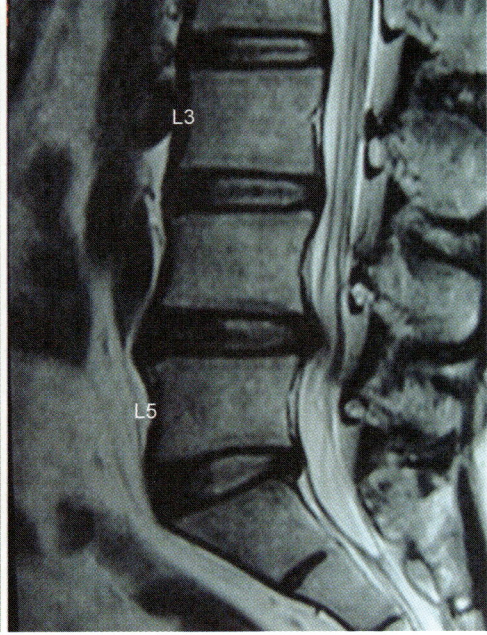

Fig. 15.2: Representative X-ray lateral and MRI sagittal view of the lumbar spine demonstrating degenerative changes with canal stenosis at L4–L5

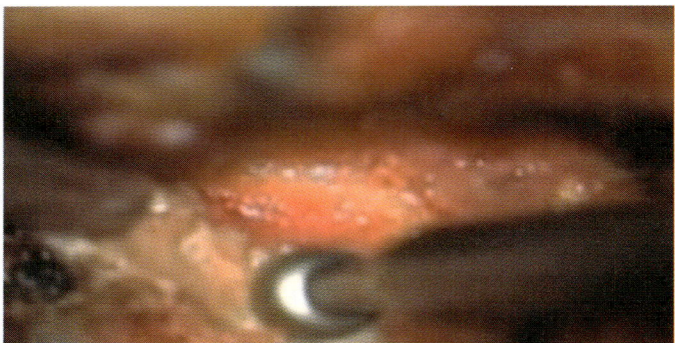

Fig. 15.3: High-speed drill being used to thin the lamina

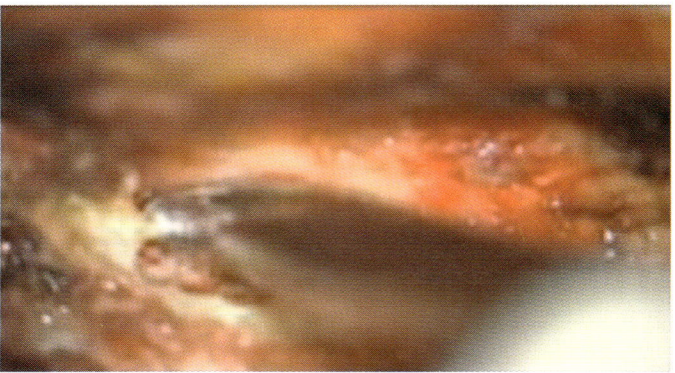

Fig. 15.4: Kerrison bone rongeur being used to remove the thinned out upper lamina

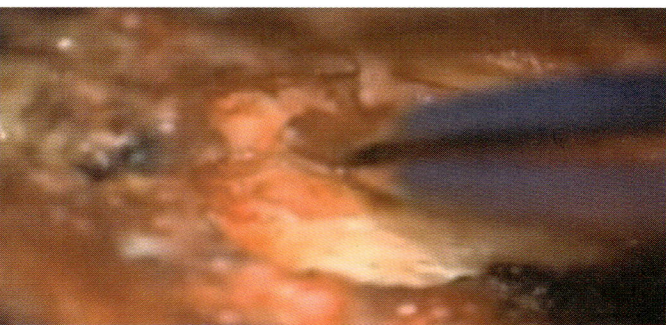

Fig. 15.5: Bipolar coagulation can be used to control the epidural venous oozing which starts soon after decompression of the lateral recess

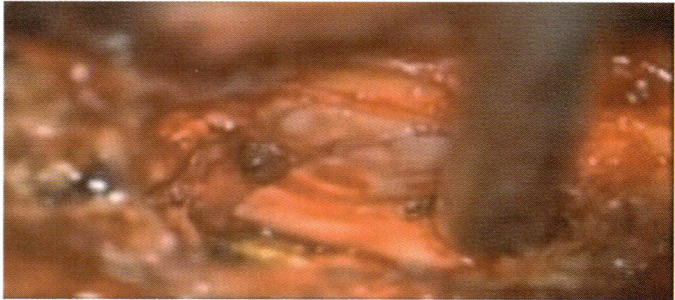

Fig. 15.6: The final state of neural elements. The nerve can be seen going freely into the foramen

29th February 2012. Detailed history of patients with low back pain and low back pain with radiation to

lower limb(s) was taken using Oswestry disability index (ODI) and visual analogue scale (VAS). The study was carried out in Lilavati Hospital and Research Centre, Mumbai.

Design of study: Hospital based prospective study.

Sample size: Throughout the duration of our study, we studied 50 consecutive patients who were operated by IDSS during 1st March 2011 and 29th February 2012 and they were followed up for a period of 3 years.

Inclusion Criteria

1. Age group: 18 years and above.
2. Persistent low back pain with or without radiation to lower limbs associated with neurogenic claudication.
3. Positive imaging findings on X-ray and/or MRI attributable to the symptoms.
4. Failed trial of conservative management for 3 months
5. Degenerative spondylolisthesis up to grade I identified on digital dynamic X-ray, MRI of lumbosacral spine.
6. Degenerative disc disease with retrolisthesis with disc prolapse at single or more levels on MRI of lumbosacral spine.

Exclusion Criteria

1. Age group: <18 years of age (pediatric patients).
2. >grade I spondylolisthesis on digital dynamic X-ray, MRI of lumbosacral spine.
3. Severe osteoporosis.
4. Fractures.
5. Scoliotic deformity at that level.
6. Infection.
7. Morbid obesity.
8. Previous surgery.
9. Post-trauma patients.

Results

Our study was conducted at Lilavati Hospital and Research Centre, Mumbai between March 2011 and February 2015. 50 indoor patients were evaluated using Oswestry disability index and visual analogue scale preoperatively along with routine general and neurological examination. This was a prospective study where the patients were operated by internal decompression of spinal stenosis (IDSS).

Statistical Analysis

After data collection, data entry was done in Excel.

Data analysis is done with the help of SPSS software version 15 and Sigmaplot version 11.

Table 15.1: Comparison among study group for ODI score

ODI score	N	Mean	Std. Dev	Median	IQR	Friedman RM analysis		Minimum	Maximum
ODI pre OP.	50	44.93	7.73	44.00	13.11	Chi-square	P value	31.11	62.22
ODI post 10 days	50	33.37	6.32	32.00	7.64	133.82	<0.001	22.22	57.77
ODI post 3 months	48	18.68	4.72	18.00	4.34	Difference is significant		11.11	35.55
ODI PO 6 months	47	10.58	3.95	8.88	5.33			4.00	26.00
ODI at 1 year	47	10.28	3.35	8.4				6.22	22.00
ODI at 2 years	47	11.46	3.88	8.9				7.87	24
ODI at 3 years	47	11.82	4.12	9.6				8.11	27

Note: Normality test (Saphiro Whilks) failed, thus Friedman repeated measures analysis of variance on ranks test applied.

Table 15.2: All pairwise multiple comparison procedures (Tukey test)

Comparison	P<0.05	Difference is
ODI pre OP. vs ODI PO 3 years		
ODI pre OP. vs ODI PO 2 years		
ODI pre OP. vs ODI PO 1 year		
ODI pre OP. vs ODI PO 6 months		
ODI pre OP. vs ODI PO 3 months		
ODI pre OP. vs ODI PO 10 days		
ODI PO 10 days vs ODI PO 3 years		
ODI PO 10 days vs ODI PO 2 years		
ODI PO 10 days vs ODI PO 1 year		
ODI PO 10 days vs ODI PO 6 months		
ODI PO 10 days vs ODI PO 3 months	Yes	Significant
ODI PO 3 months vs ODI PO 3 years		
ODI PO 3 months vs ODI PO 2 years		
ODI PO 3 months vs ODI PO 1 year		
ODI PO 3 months vs ODI PO 6 months		
ODI PO 6 months vs ODI PO 3 years		
ODI PO 6 months vs ODI PO 2 years		
ODI PO 6 months vs ODI PO 1 year		
ODI PO 1 year vs ODI PO 3 years		
ODI PO 1 year vs ODI PO 2 years		
ODI PO 2 years vs ODI PO 3 years		

Quantitative data is presented with the help of mean, standard deviation, median and IQR, pre- and post-operative comparison among study group is done with the help of Friedman RM Analysis as per results of normality test, multiple pairwise comparison among group is done with Tukey test.

Qualitative data is presented with the help of frequency and percentage table, association among study group is assessed with the help of Chi-Square test.

P value less than 0.05 is taken as significant level.

Normality test (Saphiro Whilks) failed, thus Friedman repeated measures analysis of variance on ranks test was applied for analysis of Oswestry Disability Index and Visual Analogue Scale at different time intervals.

There was statistically significant difference in ODI postoperatively at 10 days, 3 months, 6 months, 1 year, 2 years and 3 years (P <0.001) as compared to before the operation.

All Pairwise Multiple Comparison Procedures (Tukey test) showed statistically significant difference (P <0.05) in ODI preoperative versus postoperative at 10 days, 3 months, 6 months, 1 year, 2 years and 3 years. Also statistical significant difference (P <0.05) 10 days postoperatively versus 3 and 6 months, 1 year, 2 years and 3 years. And statistical significant difference (P < 0.05) 3 months postoperatively versus 6 months, 1 year,

Table 15.3: Comparison among study group for VAS score

VAS score	N	Mean	Std. Dev	Median	IQR	Friedman RM analysis		Minimum	Maximum
VAS pre OP	50	4.86	1.12	5.00	1.13	Chi-square	P value	2.00	7.00
VAS post OP 10 days	50	5.87	1.31	6.20	2.45	121.02	<0.001	3.00	8.30
VAS post OP 3 mths	48	2.87	0.92	3.00	1.10	Difference is significant		1.50	6.00
VAS post OP 6 mths	47	1.22	0.78	1.10	0.40			0.30	5.10
VAS post OP 1 year	47	1.18	0.89	1.10				0.40	4.90
VAS post OP 2 years	47	1.38	0.87	1.40				0.30	5.20
VAS post OP 3 years	47	1.47	0.93	1.60				0.40	5.70

Note: Normality test (Saphiro Whilks) failed, thus Friedman repeated measures analysis of variance on ranks test applied.

Table 15.4: All pairwise multiple comparison procedures (Tukey test)

Comparison	P<0.05	Difference is
VAS pre OP. vs ODI PO 3 years		
VAS pre OP. vs ODI PO 2 years		
VAS pre OP. vs ODI PO 1 year		
VAS pre OP. vs ODI PO 6 months		
VAS pre OP. vs ODI PO 3 months		
VAS pre OP. vs ODI PO 10 days		
VAS PO 10 days vs ODI PO 3 years		
VAS PO 10 days vs ODI PO 2 years		
VAS PO 10 days vs ODI PO 1 year		
VAS PO 10 days vs ODI PO 6 months		
VAS PO 10 days vs ODI PO 3 months	Yes	Significant
VAS PO 3 months vs ODI PO 3 years		
VAS PO 3 months vs ODI PO 2 years		
VAS PO 3 months vs ODI PO 1 year		
VAS PO 3 months vs ODI PO 6 months		
VAS PO 6 months vs ODI PO 3 years		
VAS PO 6 months vs ODI PO 2 years		
VAS PO 6 months vs ODI PO 1 year		
VAS PO 1 year vs ODI PO 3 years		
VAS PO 1 year vs ODI PO 2 years		
VAS PO 2 years vs ODI PO 3 years		

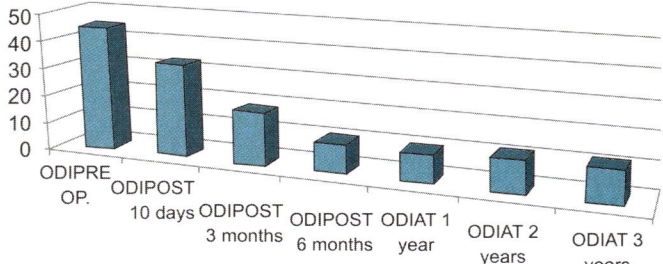

Graph 15.1: Comparison of ODI score among study group

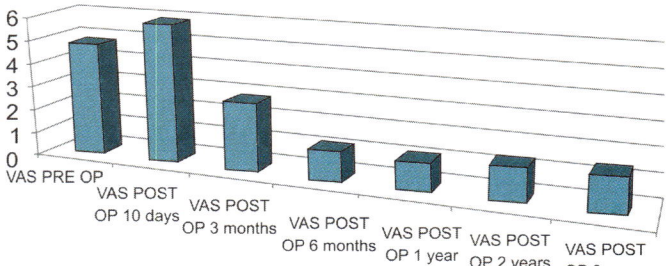

Graph 15.2: Comparison of VAS score among study group

2 years and 3 years postoperatively. There was statistical significant difference (P <0.05) 6 months postoperatively versus 1 year, 2 years and 3 years postoperatively, statistical significant difference (P <0.05) 1 year postoperatively versus 2 years and 3 years post operatively and statistical significant difference (P<0.05) 2 years postoperatively versus 3 years postoperatively.

The mean ODI for the study group preoperatively was 44.93% ± 7.73 and postoperatively at 10 days, 3 months, 6 months, 1 year, 2 years and 3 years were 33.37% ± 6.32, 18.68% ± 4.72, 10.58 % ± 3.95, 10.28% + 3.35, 11.46% + 3.88 and 11.82% + 4.12 respectively. The ODI decreased by 34.35 percentage points, an improvement by 77.44% at 6 months as compared to preoperatively.

All pairwise multiple comparison procedures (Tukey test) showed statistically significant difference (P <0.05) in VAS preoperative versus postoperative at 10 days, 3 months, 6 months, 1 year, 2 years and 3 years. Also statistical significant difference (P <0.05) 10 days postoperatively versus 3 and 6 months, 1 year, 2 years and 3 years. And statistical significant difference (P <0.05) 3 months postoperatively versus 6 months, 1 year, 2 years and 3 years postoperatively. There was statistical significant difference (P <0.05) 6 months

postoperatively versus 1 year, 2 years and 3 years postoperatively, statistical significant difference (P <0.05) 1 year postoperatively versus 2 years and 3 years postoperatively and statistical significant difference (P<0.05) 2 years postoperatively versus 3 years postoperatively.

The mean VAS score was 4.86 ± 1.12 points before the surgery and 5.86 ± 1.31, 2.86 ± 0.92, 1.22 ± 0.78, 1.18 + 0.89, 1.38 + 0.87, 1.47 + 0. 93 at the 10 days, 3 months, 6 months, 1 year, 2 years and 3 years respectively. The VAS score decreased by 3.64 points, an improvement by 74.89% at 6 months compared to preoperatively.

Complications

Two patients suffered intraoperative dural nick which was managed by muscle patch and Tisseal solution. They did not show any deterioration postoperatively or any deviation in their improvement pattern.

DISCUSSION

The primary aim of this study was to evaluate the clinical outcome of patients at 3 years follow-up postoperatively.

The main advantage of IDSS is sparing of supraspinous and intraspinous ligaments along with the spinous process while adequately decompressing the neural elements. This surgery achieves the perfect balance between extensive laminectomy which may lead to instability and inadequate decompression which does not give patient relief from his symptoms.

Lin PM in his technical note on internal decompression of spinal stenosis had noted that use of the wide decompressive procedure for neural compression in cases of lumbar canal stenosis without regard for the integrity of facets led to instability and the chronic pain syndrome. His technique achieves the necessary internal decompression of the multiple levels of spinal stenosis without interruption of the integrity of the motion segment. The spinous processes and the supraspinous ligaments and the lateral half of the facet, with its firm fibrous capsules, were scrupulously preserved. The disc is not removed unless it is overtly extruded.[9]

Ramani PS popularized the technique of IDSS in India and in its neighboring countries. He described the technique which involved minimal disruption of bony elements preserving the motion segment and thereby the stability of the spine. This technique involved decompression by inferior and superior marginal laminotomy, minimal medial facetectomy and foraminotomy with an angle bone punch. Various methods were applied to achieve this result such as angled Kerrison bone punched, high speed drills and supersonic bone cutters. The bone decompression was considered adequate after the nerve root could be seen free without any compression of bone, ligament or disc.[13,14]

Jalil et al in their clinical outcome study were able to demonstrate that using the interspinous approach for lumbar spinal stenosis showed a favorable maintenance of improvement in symptoms. Radiological data showed that this approach did not alter the stability of the spine. Their clinical long-term outcome was evaluated retrospectively using self-rating questionnaires: the Oswestry disability index, visual analogue scale (0–10), walking capacity (1–5), progress in walking capacity and global activity, and level of satisfaction in 106 patients. The risk of postoperative instability was evaluated on the basis of dynamic radiographs of the lumbar spine.[9]

Similar method described by Iwatsuki et al in 2007 where they used unilateral approach to decompress the bilateral nerve roots using Casper's retractors under microscope and found satisfactory relief in neurogenic claudication outcome score (NCOS). 2 patients described the procedure to be "fairly successful" and "not very successful".[8]

In a 2008 study by Sasai et al, surgical outcome of 48 patients has been reported over a 24 months follow-up. The surgical outcome was evaluated using the neurogenic claudication outcome score (NCOS) and the Oswestry disability index (ODI). Additionally, the back pain score within the NCOS was also compared. This is the only study which described the midterm follow up (>2 years) of the surgical outcome.[15]

Furthermore, a study by Musluman describes his series of patients with lumbar degenerative spondylolisthesis. Operations were performed in 84 selected patients with lumbar DS. The selection criteria included lower back pain with or without sciatica, neurogenic claudication that had not improved after at least 6 months of conservative treatment, and a radiological diagnosis of Grade I DS and lumbar stenosis. Decompression was performed at 3 levels in 15.5%, 2 levels in 54.8%, and 1 level in 29.7% of the patients with 1 level of spondylolisthesis. All patients were followed up for at least 24 months. For clinical evaluations, a visual analog scale, Oswestry disability index (ODI), and neurogenic claudication outcome score (NCOS) were used. Good or excellent results were obtained in 80% patients with one patient requiring secondary fusion.[11]

Since the method of surgery and approach varies greatly amongst the studies done on IDSS, there is no unified opinion on the satisfactory outcome in patients with lumbar canal stenosis and hence the need to study the clinical outcome in patients with lumbar canal stenosis who were operated by minimal invasive IDSS.

The short-term results of IDSS have been assessed and found to be satisfactory. In this study we found that the midterm results at 3 years have been satisfactory and there has been no case of iatrogenic instability in our series.

We compare our results with similar study done by Sangwan et al[18] published in 2014 and another by Hrabálek et al[6] in 2013 and Huodek et al[7] in 2012.

a. ODI

The mean ODI for the study group preoperatively was 44.93% ± 7.73 and postoperatively at 10 days, 3 months and 6 months were 33.37% ± 6.32, 18.68% ± 4.72 and 10.58 % ± 3.95 respectively. It was close to a study done by Houdek et al[7] with an average ODI of 47.2% preoperatively and 17.48% at 6 months postoperatively while in our study the average ODI was 10. 58% at 6 months postoperatively which suggests better improvement as compared to above mention study. In a study done by Zhou et al the average ODI was 10.6 ± 2.1 postoperatively at 6 months.[4]

ODI (%) (average)	Our study	Houdek et al	Hrabálek et al
Preoperative	44.93% ± 7.73	47.20%	58.4%
Postoperative (at 6 months)	10.58% ± 3.95	17.48%	23.9%

b. VAS Score

The mean VAS score was 4.86 ± 1.12 points before the surgery and 5.86 ± 1.31, 2.86 ± 0.92 and 1.22 ± 0.78 at the 10 days, 3 months and 6 months respectively. In a study done by Houdek et al[7] with an average VAS score of 6.62 preoperatively and 2.96 points at 6 months post-operatively. In another study by Hrabalek et al for juxtfacet cyst by the same method, average VAS score was 6.7 points preoperatively and 3.5 points post-operatively. In a study done by Zhou et al the average VAS score was 1.5± 0.7 postoperatively at 6 months.[4]

VAS score (average)	Our study	Houdek et al	Hrabálek et al	Zhou et al
Preoperative	4.86 ± 1.12	6.62	6.7	7.8 ± 2.1
Postoperative	1.22 ± 0.78	2.96	3.5	1.5 ± 0.7

Sangwan et al demonstrated improvement clinically using claudication distance and Japanese Orthopedic Association score. They found statistically significant improvement in JOA scores and claudication distance postoperatively for average follow-up of 32 months (range 24–41 months).

Conclusion

IDSS for lateral recess stenosis was performed with micro techniques using micro lumbar approach and is also minimally invasive. The postoperative morbidity is the least and quick mobilization within hours of the surgery and quick discharge from the hospital gives added confidence to the patient.

The results were statistically significant at 3 years follow-up. There was no incidence of re-exploration or worsening.

REFERENCES

1. Airaksinen O, Herno A, Turunen V, et al. Surgical outcome of 438 patients treated surgically for lumbar spinal stenosis. Spine 1997;22:2278–82.
2. Benz RJ, Garfin SR. Current technique of decompression of lumbar spine. ClinOrthopRelat Res 2001;384:75–81.
3. Deyo RA. Treatment of lumbar spinal stenosis: a balancing act. Spine J 2010;10(7):625–7.
4. Dong Zhou, Lu Ming Nong, Rui Du, Gong Ming Gao, Yu Qing Jiang, Nan Wei Xu: Effects of interspinous spacers on lumbar degenerative disease. 10.3892/etm 2013;894; 952–6.
5. Herno A, Airaksinen O, Saari T, et al. The predictive value of preoperative myelography in lumbar spinal stenosis. Spine 1994;19:1335–8.
6. Hrabálek L, Wanek T, Adamus M: Percutaneous dynamic interspinous stabilisation for the treatment of juxtafacet cysts of the lumbar spine: prospective study. ActaChirOrthopTraumatolCech 2013;79(2):144–9.
7. Hrabálek L, Wanek T, Macha J, Vaverka M, Langová K, Kalita O, Krahulík D, Novák V, Houdek M: Percutaneous interspinous dynamic stabilization (in-space) in patients with degenerative disease of the lumbosacral spine, a prospective study 2012;91(6):311–6.
8. Iwatsuki K, Yoshimine T, Aoki M. Bilateral interlaminar fenestration and unroofing for the decompression of nerve roots by using a unilateral approach in lumbar canal stenosis. Surg Neurol 2007;68(5):487–92.
9. Jalil Y, Carvalho C, Becker R: Long-term clinical and radiological postoperative outcomes after an interspinous microdecompression of degenerative lumbar spinal stenosis. Spine 2014;39(5): 368–73.
10. Lin PM. Internal decompression for multiple levels of lumbar spinal stenosis: a technical note. Neurosurgery 1982;Oct;11(4):546–9.
11. Müslüman AM, Cansever T, Yılmaz A, Çavusoglu H, Yüce I, Aydın Y. Midterm outcome after a microsurgical unilateral approach for bilateral decompression of lumbar degenerative spondylolisthesis. J Neurosurg Spine. 16(1):68-76; 2012.
12. North American Spine Society. Evidence Based Clinical Guidelines for Multidisciplinary Spine Care: Diagnosis and Treatment of Degenerative Lumbar Spinal Stenosis. In. Burr Ridge, IL.: North American Spine Society; 2007.
13. Ramani PS, Maheshwari S. Surgical technique of internal decompression for spinal stenosis (IDSS). J Spinal Surg 2011;2(4):566–9.
14. Ramani PS, Singh A, Cahyadi A, Babhulkar SS, Pawar SG: Use of technological advance in surgical management of Internal Decompression for Spinal Stenosis (IDSS) in lumbar canal stenosis J. Spinal Surg 2012;4(3):992–5.
15. Sasai K, Umeda M, Maruyama T, Wakabayashi E, Iida H.: Microsurgical bilateral decompression via a unilateral approach for lumbar spinal canal stenosis including degenerative spondylolisthesis. J Neurosurg Spine 2008;9(6):554–9.
16. Schultz KP. Risk of instability following decompression surgery for lumbar spinal stenosis. Z OrthopIhre Grenzgeb 1995;133:236–41.
17. Silvers HR, Lewis PJ, Asch HL. Decompressive lumbar laminectomy for spinal stenosis. J Neurosurg 1993;78:695–701.
18. Sukhbir Singh Sangwan, Rakesh Garg, ParitoshGogna, Zile Singh Kundu, Vinay Gupta, Pradeep Kamboj Limited Laminectomy and Restorative Spinoplasty in Spinal Canal Stenosis. Asian Spine J. 2014;8(4):462–8.

Instability in Lumbar Canal Stenosis

Shradha Maheshwari

INTRODUCTION

Instability of the spine as a whole is a complex subject with many controversies in its diagnosis and management. With more advances in the understanding of biomechanics of spine, there is now some consensus as regards to the diagnosis and treatment of the spinal instability. However, multiple factors along with biomechanics are involved in rendering the spine unstable.

Degenerative process in the joint is a disease that primarily involves the articular cartilage. Degeneration is the leading cause of chronic disability all over the world and usually presents with joint pain, tenderness, stiffness, locking, and effusion.[1] Muscle atrophy, joint instability and deformity may develop in advanced cases.

Degenerative spondylolisthesis (DS) is an acquired anterior vertebral displacement without a disruption of the pars interarticularis. It results from degenerative changes of aging occuring in the intervertebral discs, facet joints, osteophytes formation on vertebral edges and ligament hypertrophy and then buckling.[8,13]

Pathophysiology

At any level, the functional spinal unit consists of three joints; the intervertebral disc and two facet joints. These three joints along with the various ligaments are anatomically linked to maintain the mechanical balance of the spine. Hence any stress or trauma to one joint will automatically reflect on the other two joints depending on the changes it brings in the biomechanics of the spine. The natural history of degeneration in the spine follows three phases; inflammation, instability and re-stabilization in deformity.[27]

Degeneration can start in any one of the joints (disc or facets), but eventually involves all three joints. It is well known fact that with normal aging, the intervertebral disc starts degenerating as the nucleus pulposus loses water causing reduction in disc height. The facets, which are diarthrodial joints, begin degenerating by developing synovitis.[28] The joint cartilage then becomes thin and the facet capsule becomes loose. Since this loosening allows for greater spinal motion albeit abnormal, the degeneration of the intervertebral disc is accelerated. The natural history of the disease, at this stage, tries to restabilise the unstable motion segment by forming osteophytes around the facet joints and traction spurs along the vertebral bodies. The process help to stabilise the spine but it also complicates the process by producing lateral recess stenosis and lumbar canal stenosis. Degeneration of the intervertebral disc (nucleus) and the facets joints causes hypermobility in the motion segment thus giving rise to instability. All the same, it is not often that these abnormal movements are sufficient to constitute gross mechanical instability. With change in the weight bearing axis due to hypermobility, degenerative spondylolisthesis starts to develop. When the laxity predominates in the intervertebral disc, retro-listhesis occurs and it can be well demonstrated in sagittal extension view of the spine.

The degenerative changes are more common in the motion segments which are subjected to stress of load bearing area with greater mobility and pressure. L4/5 region is the most commonly affected followed by L3/4, L2/3 and then L5/S1.[6] Although degeneration affects various levels in this order of frequency, different stages of arthritis can be observed simultaneously in one segment of the spine.[11]

Clinical Presentation

While patients with disc prolapse present with classical symptoms of radiculopathy, patients with instability generally have slow and progressive course of symptoms. Back pain is usually the first symptom, which is initially aggravated on exertion and relieved with rest but eventually becomes chronic and persistent in nature. They classically complain of morning stiffness and find it difficult to get out of bed. The distribution of pain in the lower extremities is dependent on the area of stenosis. Pain in the legs is usually bilateral. It improves with trunk flexion, sitting, stooping or lying down and aggravates with prolonged standing or lumbar extension. As the condition becomes more advanced, sitting or lying down is less helpful in relieving the pain. Symptoms of neurogenic claudication is generally seen in these patients. Rest pain or a neurogenic bladder can develop in advanced cases.[24]

On examination, physical findings are inconsistent and the localising signs are often absent. The back is usually stiff with obliterated lordosis and spinal movements are painful. Straight leg raising and femoral nerve stretching tests are usually negative.[17] The neurological examination is not contributory but some abnormality may be detected, if the patient is forced to walk beyond the limit of pain. The gait and posture after walking may reveal a positive "stoop test". In this test, on brisk walking, the patients tends to assume stooped posture to relieve the symptoms of claudication.[5]

Investigations

Plain X-rays

Plain X- rays of the spine are important as preliminary investigation to make the diagnosis of instability. Evaluation of patients with low back pain typically includes anterior–posterior (AP) and lateral radiographs of the lumbar spine. X-rays are helpful in evaluating alignment, loss of disc height and osteophyte formation (Fig. 16.1). A key component to radiographic evaluation

is obtaining flexion/extension dynamic X-rays. Translation of more than 5 mm, or rotation of more than 10 to 15° in the dynamic view, indicates instability. A reversal of the normal trapezoidal intervertebral space geometry with widening posteriorly and narrowing anteriorly may also indicate instability (Fig. 16.2).[10]

Magnetic Resonance Imaging

Magnetic resonance imaging (MRI) is a noninvasive and suitable method for assessment of soft tissue structures. MRI best demonstrates compressive changes of the thecal sac due to disc disease, ligamentous compression, facetal hypertrophy, listhesis and other neural pathology. Because of its ability to differentiate tissues and assess the status of the intervertebral disc, central and lateral recess stenosis are easily demonstrated on MRI. Midline T2 sagittal images may be useful in diagnosing central stenosis by noting sagittal narrowing of the intervertebral canal. Sagittal T1- weighted images

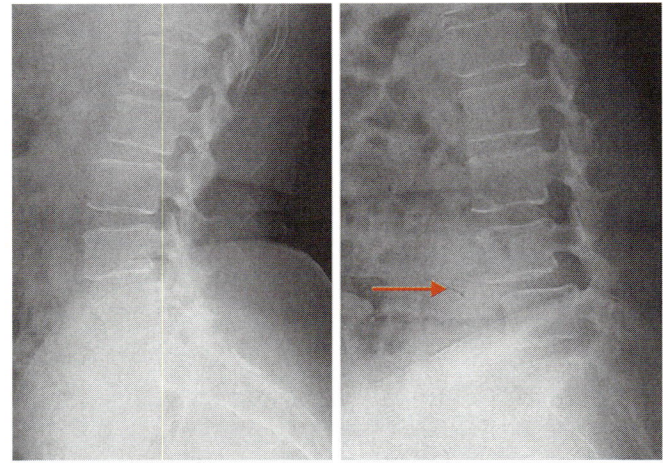

Fig. 16.2: Dynamic X-rays showing early instability with opening of the joint

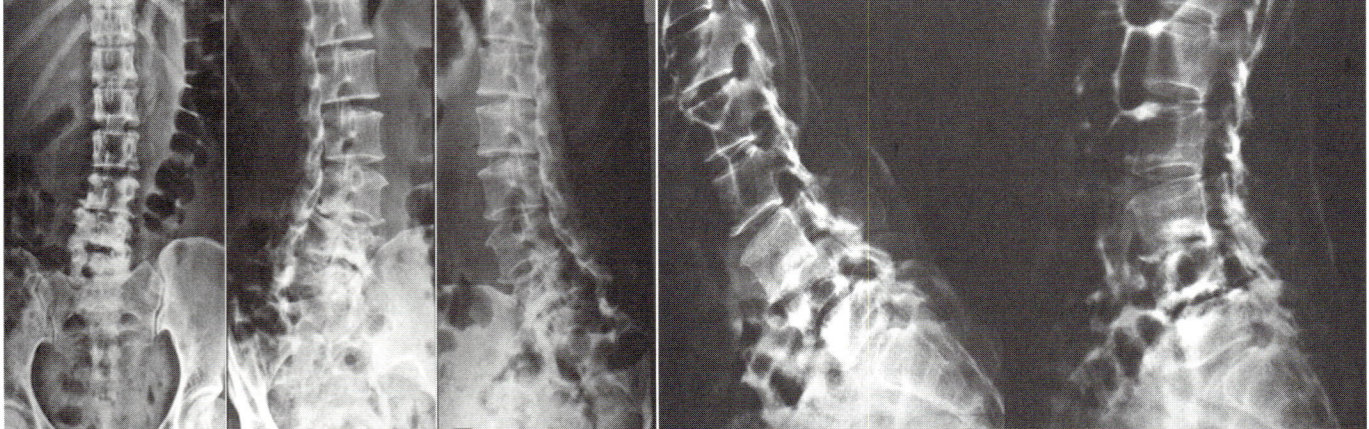

Fig. 16.1: Standard AP, oblique and lateral X-rays views showing degenerative instability with early degenerative scoliosis

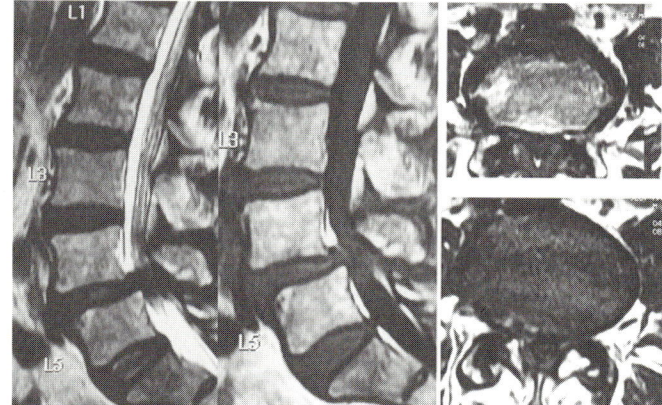

Fig. 16.3: MRI showing severe degenerative stenosis with instability at L4/5 level

are evaluated with particular attention focused on the foramen. An absence of normal fat around the root indicates foraminal stenosis (Fig. 16.3).[4] Lumbar instability associated with lumbar canal stenosis can also be documented on MRI.[22] It is as accurate as CT and myelography in diagnosing spinal stenosis, while being more sensitive at identifying disc degeneration.[25]

CT Scan and CT Myelography

CT scan and CT myelography are the best suited for patients with dynamic stenosis, postoperative leg pain, severe scoliosis or spondylolisthesis, metallic implants, any contraindications to MRI and lower extremity symptoms in the absence of suitable findings on MRI (Fig. 16.4).[3] This combined study gives an excellent picture of the central and lateral canal and defines any extradural cause of compression. However, direct measurement of the bony canal on CT images often gives an inaccurate assessment of the degree of stenosis.[12]

Treatment

Non-operative Treatment

Non-operative modalities include activity restriction, non-steroid anti-inflammatory drugs (NSAIDs) and physical therapy. They remain the first-line therapy for patients with degenerative spondylolisthesis without any obvious neurological deficit. In one study of 145 patients with non-operative management, 76% patients without neurological deficits remained asymptomatic at 10 years follow up.[19] However, 83% patients that did have neurological deficit experienced progression of symptoms over 10 years. Progression of spondylolisthesis was not correlated with progression of symptoms.

The degree of listhesis, disk space narrowing, and hypermobility at the affected motion segment may be the predictors which help in deciding if the patient will respond to conservative treatment.[13] In patients with mobile or low-grade spondylolisthesis, without neurological deficits, a trial of non-operative therapy is certainly indicated and generally associated with good clinical outcomes.

Surgical Treatment

In patients with debilitating lumbar degenerative spondylolisthesis and stenosis, surgery compared to nonsurgical treatment can provide substantial improvement in pain and function. Although, a few would argue that the fusion of the diseased segment appears to offer the best and most durable results, treatment of this disease is best tailored to the individual. The following risk factors must be taken into consideration while deciding the surgical modality

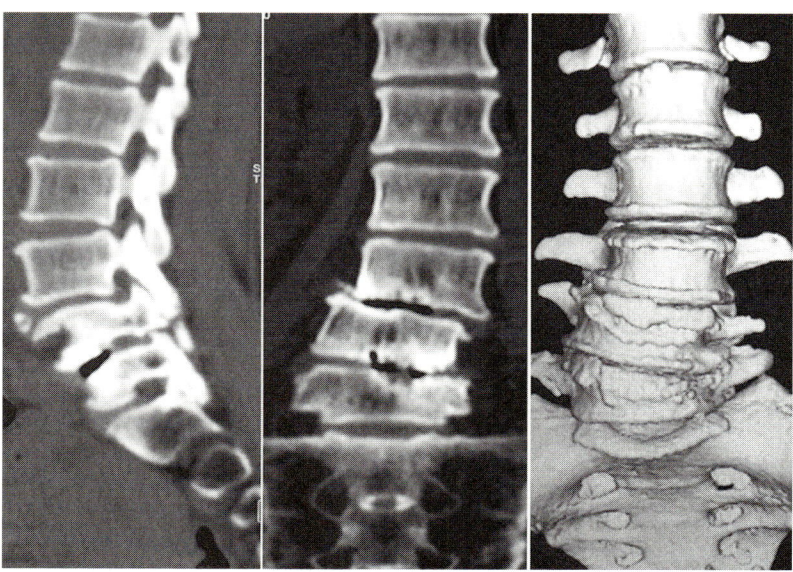

Fig. 16.4: CT spine showing severe degeneration with osteophyte formation and scoliosis

of treatment: Anteroposterior hypermobility, angular hypermobility and large disc height.

Decompression Alone

In degenerative spondylolisthesis, which is generally associated with stenosis, decompression of the spinal canal is of utmost importance. Even a strong construct for fusion without decompression may fail to provide symptomatic relief in these patients. The North American Spine Society's (NASS) guidelines state that surgical decompression may be considered for patients with low-grade degenerative spondylolisthesis and symptomatic spinal stenosis that is refractory to conservative therapy. For single-level degenerative spondylolisthesis that is symptomatic, low-grade, with only central stenosis (no foraminal stenosis), decompression provides equivalent outcomes compared to decompression with fusion.[18]

Dynamic Stabilisation/Non-fusion Techniques

The concept of dynamic stabilization of the lumbar spine for treatment of degenerative instability has been introduced almost two decades ago. Internal decompression of spinal stenosis (IDSS) and posterior dynamic stabilization (PDS) form a bridge between decompression laminectomy alone and rigid fusion. It combines beneficial effects of decompression and stabilization in an attempt to prevent bad effects of relentless degeneration.[7] Various interspinous process spacers (like X-stop, device for intervertebral assisted motion (DIAM), interspinous posterior device (IPD), coflex, etc.) or pedicle-based systems (like PercuDyn, or dynesys) have been introduced in this category (Fig. 16.5).

Advantages of these non-fusion implants include retention and protection of the intervertebral disc, sparing of the soft tissues and bony structures of the

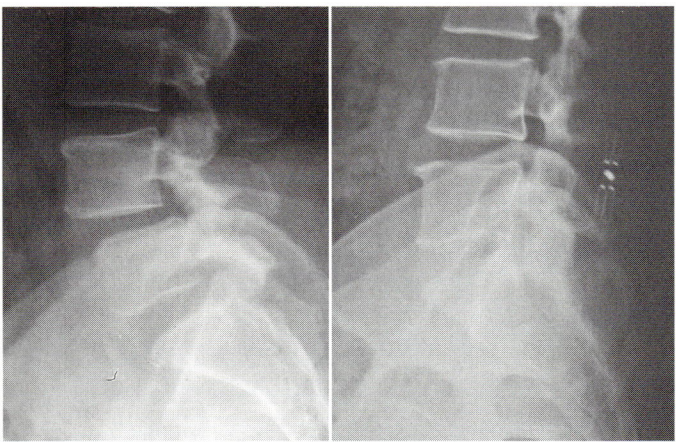

Fig. 16.5: Pre- and postoperative X-rays of grade I degenerative listhesis treated with IDSS and dynamic stabilization using in-space

posterior spine, application of minimally invasive technique, lesser operative time and preservation of the motion (dynamic stabilization).[20] These devices fairly distract the intervertebral space, reduce stress on the affected segment by providing load transfer of the spinal segment without fusion and may therefore reduce the probability of adjacent segment disease. Reinmuller et al recently analyzed the longitudinal reoperation rate due to adjacent segment disease and screw loosening and overall reoperation in patients who underwent dynamic stabilization and rigid stabilization. They found that reoperation rates after dynamic stabilization of the lumbar spine are comparable to rigid fixations.[21]

Posterior Spinal Fusion

The existing body of evidence supports spinal fusion surgery for patients with symptomatic degenerative spondylolisthesis that has failed a course of conservative treatment. Whenever, it is necessary to correct the underlying spinal deformities such as degenerative scoliosis or degenerative kyphosis associated with spinal stenosis, instrumented fusion is recommended. Multiple studies have demonstrated improved long-term outcomes of fusions compared with decompression surgery alone.

Although there has been tremendous improvement in the design and structure of pedicle screw systems, one must gain appropriate training and learning before attempting these procedures. The clinicians should not forget that in every spinal procedure for achieving spinal fusion, the fusion stage is the most important stage in the whole procedure. If the fusion fails, the whole construct is doomed to fail. Spinal fusion is usually achieved by applying autogenous or allogenous bone graft over the decorticated bone surfaces. Instrumentation is used to improve and supplement the fusion rate and to correct the underlying deformity.[16]

Interbody Fusion

Although there are no absolute indications for interbody fusion in degenerative stenosis and listhesis, the most accepted indications include intractable lumbar discogenic pain, spondylolisthesis, revision surgeries for recurrent disc herniation and symptomatic pseudoarthrosis.[15,23,26] Complete excision of the intervertebral disc tissues and interbody fusion can significantly improve the discogenic pain. The interbody cage not only restores the normal intervertebral lumbar lordosis, but also increases the likelihood of achieving an appropriate fusion in the weight bearing area of the vertebral body.[14] During the postoperative healing process until solid fusion is achieved, there will be much less stress on the pedicular screws that have already been augmented with interbody cages thus decreasing the occurrence of implant failure.[9]

Minimally Invasive Techniques

Minimally invasive techniques (MIS) are increasingly being utilized for both decompression and fusion surgeries with more and more studies showing equivalent outcomes and lower postoperative morbidity for patients. Minimally invasive techniques (MIS) for spine surgery reduce surgical morbidity and maintain posterior midline structures such as the multifidus muscle, which play a role in spine stability.[2] As this new field grows, investigation of MIS techniques for treatment of degenerative spondylolisthesis has also been increasingly studied. However, the most current NASS guidelines state that there is conflicting evidence regarding whether MIS techniques or traditional spinal fusion leads to better outcomes.

Conclusions

One must judiciously evaluate the patients with degenerative disc disease for evidence of associated instability. Current evidence supports surgical treatment of degenerative spondylolisthesis. Posterolateral spinal fusion remains the treatment of choice for this disease. Solid bony fusion should be the goal for treatment of these cases. The use of decompressions without fusion and dynamic stabilization may be efficacious in select cases. However, additional high-quality evidence is awaited, especially in newer areas of practice such as minimally invasive techniques and sagittal balance correction.

REFERENCES

1. Arden NK, Leyland KM. Osteoarthritis year 2013 in review: clinical Osteoarthritis Cartilage 2013;21:1409–13.
2. Asgarzadie F, Khoo LT. Minimally invasive operative management for lumbar spinal stenosis: overview of early and long-term outcomes. Orthop Clin North Am. 2007;38:387–99.
3. Bolender NF, Schonstrom NS, Spengler DM. Role of computed tomography and myelography in the diagnosis of central spinal stenosis. J Bone Joint Surg Am. 1985;67:240–6.
4. Crawshaw C, Kean DM, Mulholland RC, et al. The use of nuclear magnetic resonance in the diagnosis of lateral canal entrapment. J Bone Joint Surg Br. 1984;66:711–5.
5. Dyck P. The stoop-test in lumbar entrapment radiculopathy. Spine (Phila Pa 1976) 1979;4:89-92.Kim CW, Siemionow K, Anderson DG, Phillips FM. The current state of minimally invasive spine surgery. J Bone Joint Surg Am. 2011;93:582–96.
6. Epstein NE. Decompression in the surgical management of degenerative spondylolisthesis: Advantages of conservative approach in 290 patients. J. Spinal Disord. 1998;11:116–122.
7. Hobart J, Gilkes C, Adams W, Germon T. Interspinous spacers for lumbar foraminal stenosis: formal trials are justified. Eur Spine J 2013; 22 Suppl 1:S47–53.
8. Jacobsen S, Sonne-Holm S, Rovsing H, Monrad H, Gebuhr P. Degenerative lumbar spondylolisthesis: an epidemiological perspective: the Copenhagen Osteoarthritis Study. Spine (Phila Pa 1976). 2007;32(1):120–125.
9. Kim CW, Siemionow K, Anderson DG, Phillips FM. The current state of minimally invasive spine surgery. J Bone Joint Surg Am 2011;93:582–96.
10. Lee SY, Kim TH, Oh JK, Lee SJ, Park MS. Lumbar Stenosis: A Recent Update by Review of Literature. Asian Spine J 2015;9(5):818–828.
11. Leone A, Guglielmi G, Cassar-Pullicino VN, Bonomo L. Lumbar intervertebral instability: a review. Radiology 2007;245:62–77.
12. Matsunaga S, Ijiri K, Hayashi K. Nonsurgically managed patients with degenerative spondylolisthesis: a 10- to 18-year follow-up study. J Neurosurg. 2000;93(2 Suppl):194–19.
13. Matz PG, Meagher RJ, Lamer T, Tontz WL, Jr, Annaswamy TM, Cassidy RC, et al. Guideline summary review: an evidence-based clinical guideline for the diagnosis and treatment of degenerative lumbar spondylolisthesis. Spine J. 2016;16(3):439–448.
14. Meng C, Tang K, Ou Y, et al. Effectiveness of posterior pedicle screw system combined with interbody fusion in treating lumbar spondylolisthesis. Zhongguo Xiu Fu Chong Jian Wai Ke Za Zhi. 2010;24:904–7.
15. Mobbs RJ, Loganathan A, Yeung V, Rao PJ. Indications for anterior lumbar interbody fusion. Orthop Surg. 2013;5:153–63.
16. Nasca RJ. Newer lumbar interbody fusion techniques. J Surg Orthop Adv 2013;22:113–7.
17. Natelson SE. The injudicious laminectomy. Spine (Phila Pa 1976). 1986;11:966–9.
18. Pawar SG, Dhar A, Prasad A, Munjal S, Ramani PS. Internal decompression for spinal stenosis (IDSS) for decompression and use of interlaminar dynamic device (CoflexTM) for stabilization in the surgical management of degenerative lumbar canal stenosis with or without mild segmental instability: our initial results. Neurol Res. Apr; 2017;39(4):305–10.
19. Pearson AM, Lurie JD, Blood EA, Frymoyer JW, Braeutigam H, An H, et al. Spine patient outcomes research trial: radiographic predictors of clinical outcomes after operative or nonoperative treatment of degenerative spondylolisthesis. Spine (Phila Pa 1976) 2008;33(25):2759–66.
20. Rienmüller AC, Krieg SM, Schmidt FA, Meyer EL, Meyer B. Reoperation rates and risk factors for revision 4 years after dynamic stabilization of the lumbar spine. Spine J. 2018;7. pii: S1529-9430(18)30250-X.
21. Resnick DK, Choudhri TF, Dailey AT, et al. Guidelines for the performance of fusion procedures for degenerative disease of the lumbar spine. Part 9: fusion in patients with stenosis and spondylolisthesis. J Neurosurg Spine 2005;2:679–85.
22. Schnebel B, Kingston S, Watkins R, Dillin W. Comparison of MRI to contrast CT in the diagnosis of spinal stenosis. Spine (Phila Pa 1976) 1989;14:332–7.
23. Shen FH, Samartzis D, Khanna AJ, Anderson DG. Minimally invasive techniques for lumbar interbody fusions. Orthop Clin North Am 2007;38:373–86.
24. Smith AY, Woodside JR. Urodynamic evaluation of patients with spinal stenosis. Urology 1988;32:474–7.
25. Uden A, Johnsson KE, Jonsson K, Pettersson H. Myelography in the elderly and the diagnosis of spinal stenosis. Spine (Phila Pa 1976) 1985;10:171–4.
26. Xiao YX, Chen QX, Li FC. Unilateral transforaminal lumbar interbody fusion: a review of the technique, indications and graft materials. J Int Med Res 2009;37:908–17.
27. Yong-Hing K. Pathophysiology and rationale for treatment in lumbar spondylosis and instability. Chir Organi Mov 1994;79:3–10.
28. Yong-Hing K, Kirkaldy-Willis WH. The pathophysiology of degenerative disease of the lumbar spine. Orthop Clin North Am 1983;14:491–504.

Role of Fusion in Lumbar Canal Stenosis

PS Ramani

INTRODUCTION

Instability in the spine is the main cause for fusion in patients with lumbar canal stenosis both adults and elderly (above the age of 65 years) undergoing surgical intervention for symptoms like neurogenic claudication, chronic low back pain and the quality of life.[18,28,34,36]

The choice of an appropriate surgical intervention is indeed difficult and includes complications and expected outcome.[2,19,23,28]

While surgical intervention definitely produces relief from symptoms and improves quality of life including mobility, one has to be cautious to use implants for stability in presence of osteoporosis.[20] All the same, the perioperative complications rate is comparable and not adverse.[27] Even Deyo and his colleagues studying the medical database of 30,000 patients undergoing surgical intervention were of similar opinion. They also notices that role of fusion in these patients with instability was 18.4% and scoliosis 5.1%.[9]

When necessary surgical intervention has to be undertaken keeping in mind that in patients with obesity and diabetes the outcome may not be as satisfactory.

Indications

1. At times, the intervertebral disc degeneration is unilateral causing settlement of the disc space unilaterally causing lateral kyphosis in the lumbar spine. Only appropriate method of reconstructing the spine with fusion will help correct such deformities.[34]
2. Lumbar scoliosis is seen in patients with stenosis[11]
3. Degenerative spondylolisthesis creates instability necessitating fusion.[1,6,7,8,10,14,15,24,25,32,33] There are two

characteristics of degenerative spondylolisthesis. (a) Usually, it is not more than grade I, and (b) all the time it occurs at the level of L4/L5 (Figs 17.1, 17.2, and 17.4).

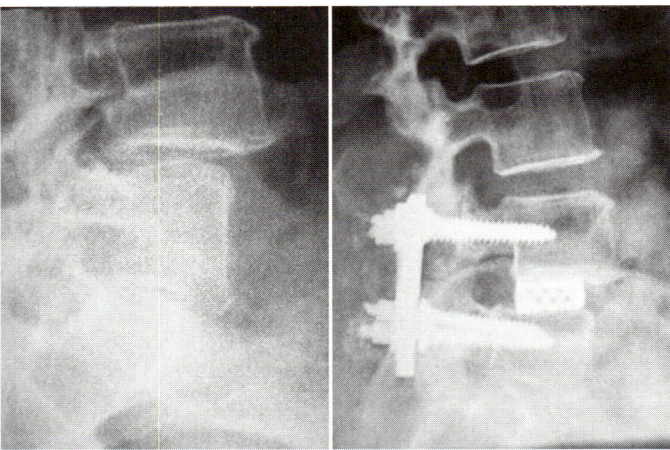

Fig. 17.1: Degenerative spondylolisthesis corrected with interbody fusion and 2-level pedicle screws

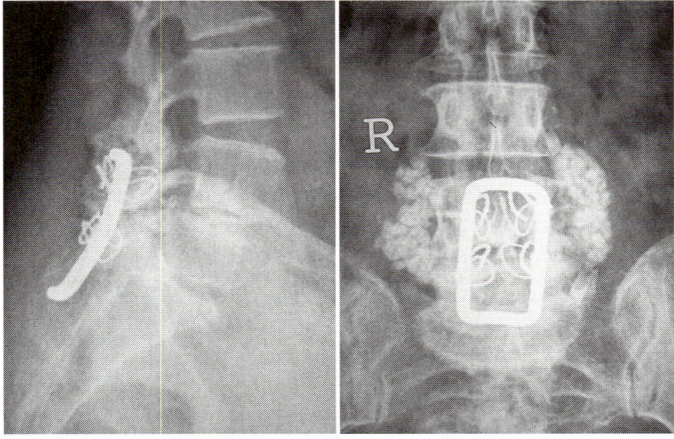

Fig. 17.2: Degenerative spondylolisthesis corrected with Hartshil ring stabilization and posterolateral fusion in the past

4. In elderly people with significant degenerative changes, it is common to see retrolisthesis specially at the level of L3/L4 (Fig. 17.3).

5. Several times we see abnormal anterior opening of the disc space on sagittal and digital X-ray films in extension. It reverts back to normal in flexion. The sign is an indicator of presence of instability requiring fusion.

6. Chronic axial backpain lasting for several years is due to degeneration in the lumbar spine. Such patients are not happy with decompression as there is no significant compression on neural tissue. The pain which is at times most excruciating and/or severe is essentially due to microabnormal motion in the degenerated spine. Multilevel fusion in such patients helps to relieve nagging back pain (Fig. 17.5).

Genesis of Chronicity in Low Back Pain; Instability in Degenerated Spine

The slightest degeneration in the lumbar intervertebral disc produces stress on the respective facet joint of the motion segment.

Even in absence of prolapse, disc degeneration along is an important cause of chronic low back pain. As

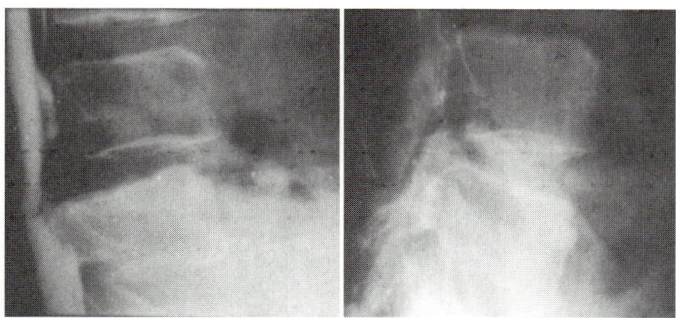

Fig. 17.3: Degenerative retrolisthesis. Corrected with interbody fusion using autologous bone graft from iliac crest

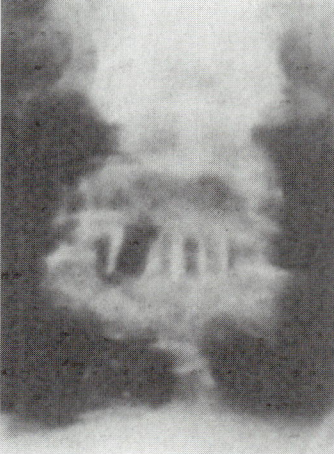

Fig. 17.4: Degenerative spondylolisthesis treated with a combination of auto- and allo-bone grafts (from the iliac crest and bone bank) in the past

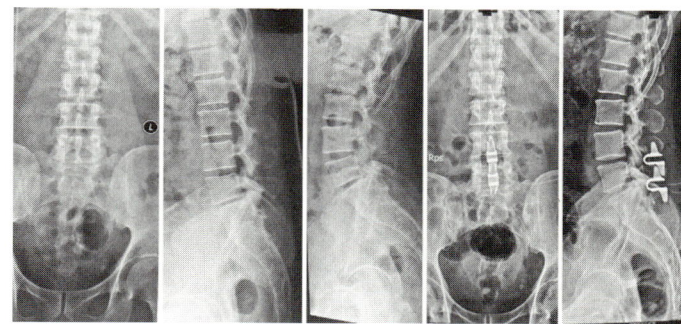

Fig. 17.5: Lateral recess stenosis treated with bilateral IDSS, bilateral foraminotomy and posterior dynamic stabilization at 2 levels with inter-laminar device CoFlex

degeneration progresses the facet joint becomes thick and hypertrophied in an attempt to bear the brunt of the degenerative ongoing process.[16,17]

The facet joint then subluxates and there is abnormal movement in the joint. The superior facet moves upwards and downwards during flexion and extension movements of the spine. The process causes recurrent or intermittent entrapment of the nerve roots.

Clinically, patient's symptoms of back pain and particularly axial pain becomes more severe and more frequent. At times the pain becomes unbearable. He complains of morning stiffness and difficulty in getting out of bed. Imaging shows radiological abnormalities including instability, evidence of additional mechanical stress on the joints and chronic low back pain becomes a permanent feature.

Similarly once the slippage becomes 25% or more, chronic low back pain becomes a permanent feature.

Abnormal lateral translation of vertebrae produces chronic low back pain. This is the time when patient seeks medical advice for management.

Fixed Deformity in the Lumbar Spine

Majority of the patients fall in this group.[16] Severe degenerative changes in the intervertebral disc and the posterior facet joints results in ankylosis of the spine and instability gives way to fixed deformity, reduced movements and fixed entrapment of nerve roots. Relief with conservative measures is not satisfactory. Decompression alone has unsatisfactory long term outcome in these patients.

Two Nerve Roots are at Risk

At any one given motion segment, two nerve roots are at risk of getting entrapped. The exiting nerve root gets entrapped due to upward migration of superior facet, the tip of which impinges into the nerve root and pushes it against the inferior border of the pedicle (foraminal stenosis). The traversing nerve root is compressed by the overgrowth of facet joint surfaces and is trapped in the vertebral canal by the medial edge of rotated and hypertrophied posterior facet. The curling in of the ligamentum flavum into the lateral recess by the hypertrophied facet adds further to the compression of traversing nerve root.

A Classical Example

A classical example is a 60 years old lady who consulted me recently for severe chronic low back pain, neurogenic claudication of 12 years duration. For the last three months she was bed ridden and could not help herself with any activities of the daily living. Clinically, she had now developed weakness in right tibialis anterior and right extensor halluces longus muscles with wasting in right quadriceps. Her both ankle jerks and right knee jerk were absent. The spine was stiff and bent to right side. Movements were grossly restricted.

X-rays of the spine showed scoliosis with lateral bend in the lumbar spine due to unilateral settlement of L3/4 disc space on the right side. There was significant degeneration in the spine and MRI showed indentation in the thecal sac at 4th and 3rd disc levels due to hypertrophied facet joints (Figs 17.6 to 17.9).

Decompression of the thecal sac and the nerve roots followed by right L3/4 interbody fusion and four level pedicle screws with posterolateral fusion resulted in relief of pain. Straightening the spine and her resuming normal activities once again.

Discussion

When the lumbar disc is degenerated, there is settlement of the disc space and the narrowing of the disc space is followed by the sequential changes in the motion segment as described in the text. Posterior spur formation in the respective vertebral bodies. Facet overriding with spur formation in the facets, internal invagination of ligamentum flavum causes disruption in the functions of the given motion segment and it has definite influence on adjacent motion segment leading to its adjacent segment degeneration or adjacent segment disease[13] and adding to the already severe symptomatology of the patient.[3] The progressive nature of spinal stenosis is multifactorial with significant contribution from facet joints.[3,29] Any operative procedure does not arrest the progression of disease which is multifactorial.

Most of the patients of lumbar canal stenosis opting for surgical intervention are elderly (above the age of 65) usually associated with co-morbidities like obesity, diabetes, osteoporosis, etc.[12] and are likely to have operative complications. But they need decompression

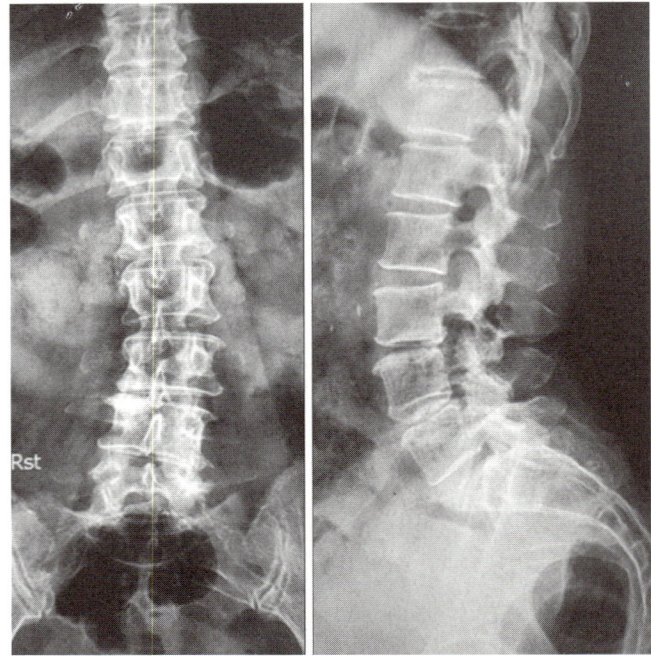

Fig. 17.6: Degenerative lateral scoliosis at L3–L4 due to unilateral settlement of the disc space

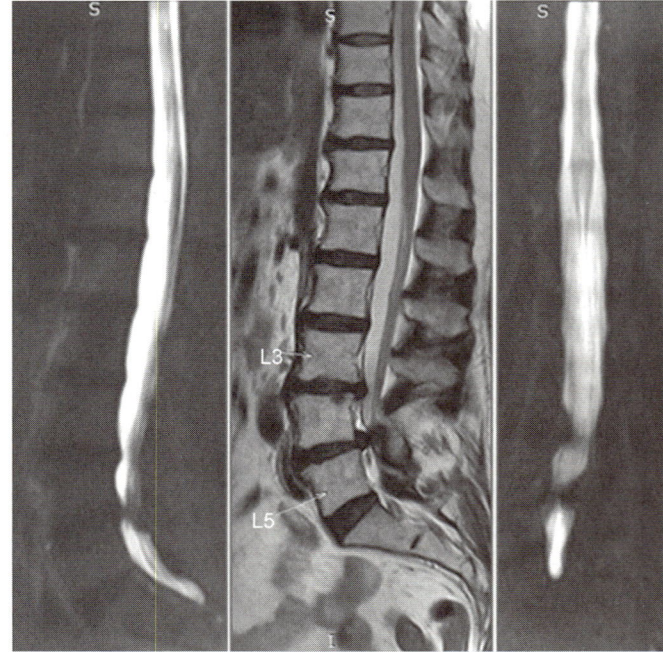

Fig. 17.7: MR myelogram and MRI sagittal coronal view showing degenerative lateral recess stenosis at multiple levels

to get relief from nerve pain but also needs fusion when associated with instability or other conditions as described earlier.

The whole pathological process has to be reverted to give lasting relief to the patient from pain and morbidity.

Fifty years ago decompression alone was the standard treatment for relieving pain and neurogenic

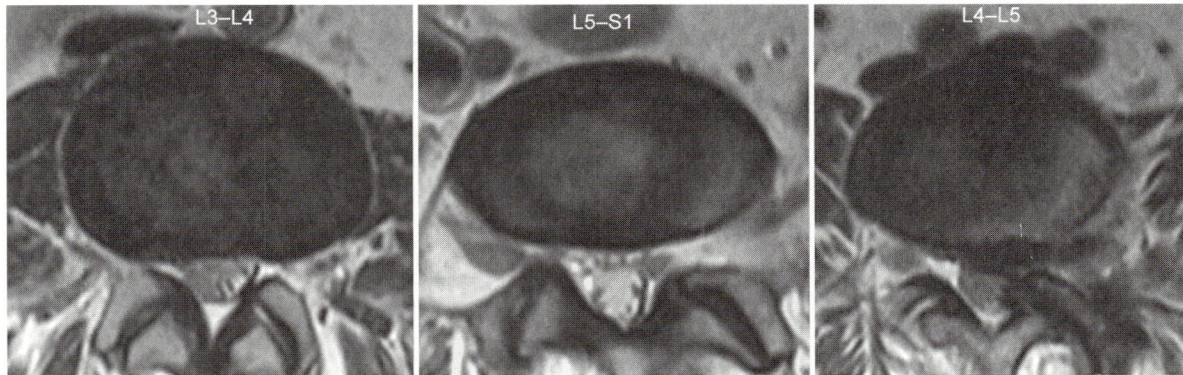

Fig. 17.8: Axial cuts showing lateral recess stenosis at multiple levels with significant diffuse disc prolapse at L4–L5

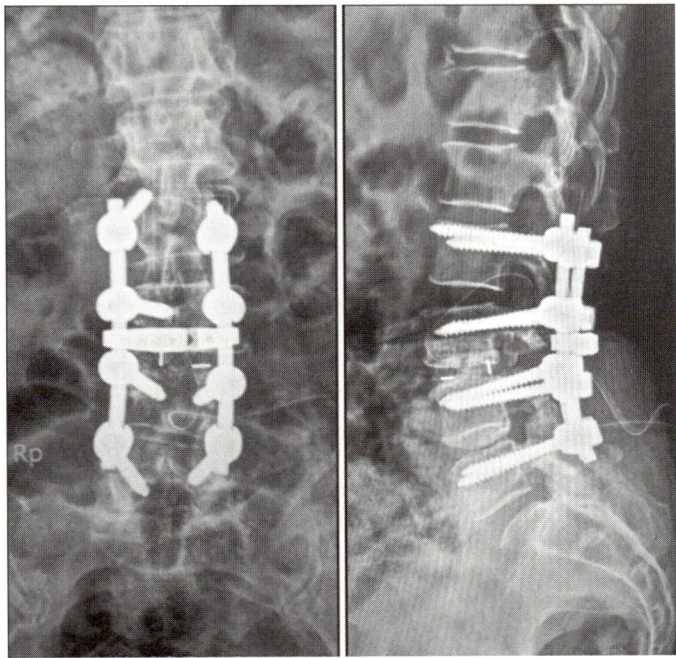

Fig. 17.9: Patient discussed in Figs 17.6 to 17.8 was surgically managed with multiple pedicle screws along with interbody fusion and cross-link to correct lateral scoliosis

claudication along with sciatic pain in patients suffering from lumbar canal stenosis.[5,19,30,31] We now know that it addresses the presenting symptoms of the patient but does not arrest the progression of the disease. Now we also know that neither decompression alone or decompression with fusion is the effective treatment.[29] The progressive nature of spinal stenosis is multifactorial.

Fusion rates have increased significantly in recent times and it has rained concerns regarding overuse of implants.[11]

In one series of decompression alone the readmission rates were 8 to 10% every year for revision or convention to fusion.[21] The Spine Patient Outcome Research Trial (SPORT) reported re-operation rates ranging from 8% at 2 years to 13% at 4 years following decompression.[27,35]

Internal decompression as described by this author and described in details in another chapter along with posterior interlaminar stabilization offers a satisfactory solution in patients with moderate spinal stenosis including up to grade I instability in this complex and nagging issue of lumbar canal stenosis.[22,26]

Conclusions

Lumbar canal stenosis is a chronic degenerative process. It causes nagging low back pain followed by morning stiffness and later neurogenic claudication. If not treated in time the process becomes chronic and eventually, the patients finds it difficult even to help himself or herself for activities of daily living. Good internal decompression along with fusion offers a viable solution to give long term lasting relief in such patients.

Management

This being the first visit of patient to the doctor, he may not agree for surgery. Conservative treatment should be tried.

Bed rest helps to relieve pain. Use of lumbosacral belt is definitely indicated to prevent abnormal movements and physiotherapist has a tremendous role to play by way of hear treatment, muscle mobilization exercises and gait training.

Role for Surgery, Role for Fusion

Unstable spine in instability phase is to be treated with fusion (posterior lumbar interbody fusion) involving the use of interbody cages, pedicle screws and rods and sometimes posterolateral fusion.

The percentage of patients in this phase of instability opting for interbody fusion is relatively less.

If the pain is chronic and becoming progressively worse then he should be considered for fusion even in the absence of instability.

Neurogenic claudication in elderly patients with or without sciatic pain can be considered for fusion for better long term outcome.

Similarly patients with chronic low back pain who are now unable to pursue activities of daily living due to pain should have fusion.

In such patients 92% relief from pain can be obtained on long term follow up.

If the pain is moderate and the instability is relatively less in magnitude, posterior dynamic stabilization along with bilateral internal decompression for spinal stenosis (IDSS) is useful. At least two levels should be stabilized for better relief from pain.

REFERENCES

1. Alexander E. Significance of small lumbar canal. Cauda equina compression syndrome due to spondylosis. J Neurosurg. 1969;31; 513–19.
2. Bae HW, Rajaee SS, Kanim LE. Nationwide trends in the surgical management of lumbar spinal stenosis. Spine (Phila Pa 1976) 2013;38(11): 916–26.
3. Baliga S, Treon K, John N, et al. Low Back Pain: Current surgical approaches: Asian Spine Journal 2015;9(4),645–657.
4. Berven SH, Deviren V, Mitchell B, et al. Operative management of degenerative scoliosis: an evidence-based approach to surgical strategies based on clinical and radiographic outcomes. Neurosurg Clin N Am 2007;18(2):261–72.
5. Bouras T, Sttanjalis G. Loufardaki M, et al. Predictors of long-term outcome in an elderly group after laminectomy for lumbar stenosis. J Neurosurg Spine 2010;13(3):329–34.
6. Ciric I, Michael AM. The lateral recess syndrome. Neurosurgery (ed). Wilkins, Rengachary 2279–82.
7. Clark K. Significance of small lumbar canal. Cauda equina compression syndrome due to spondylosis. J. Neurosurg 1969;31:495–98.
8. Cloward RB. Spinal Stenosis. Treatment by posterior lumbar interbody fusion. Spine 1987;1;457–516.
9. Deyo RA, Mirza SK, Martin BI, et al. Trends in major medical complications associated with surgery for lumbar spinal stenosis in older adults JAMA 2010;303 (13);1259–65.
10. Epstein JA, Epstein N. Lumbar spondylosis and spinal stenosis. Neurosurgery (ed.) Wilkins and Rengachary; 2272–78.
11. Forsth P. Olafsson G, Carlsson T, et al. A randomized controlled trial of fusion surgery for lumbar canal stenosis. N Eng J Med. 2016; 374:1413–1424.
12. Gepstein R, Shabat S, Arinzon ZH, et al. Does obesity affect the results of lumbar decompressive spinal surgery in the elderly? Clin Orthop Relat Res 2004;426:138–44.
13. Gillet P. The fate of the adjacent motion segments after lumbar fusion. J Spinal Disord Tech 2003;16:338–45.
14. Herkowitz HN, Kurz LJ. Degenerative lumbar spondylolisthesis with spinal stenosis; J Bone Jt Surg 1991;73; 802–08.
15. Hope E, Tsou PM. Postdecompression lumbar instability; Clin Orthop 1988;143–51.
16. Johnsson KE, Rosen I, Uden A. The natural course of lumbar spinal stenosis. Clin Ortop 1992;279:82–6.
17. Junghans J. Schmorl G. The human spine in health and disease. Published Grune and Stratton NY 1977;(2nd ed) 35–7.
18. Kaptan H, Kasimcan O, Cakiroglu K, et al. Lumbar spinal stenosis in elderly patients. Ann N Y Acad Sci. 2007;1100:173–78.
19. Katz JN, Lipson SJ, Chang LC, et al. Seven to ten year outcome of decompressive surgery for degenerative lumbar spinal stenosis. Spine (Phila Pa 1976). 1996;21(1):92–98.
20. Lee BH, Moon SH, Kim HJ, et al. Osteoporotic profile in elderly patient with symptomatic lumbar canal stenosis: Indian J. Orthop2012;46(3):279–84.
21. Modhia U, Takemoto S, Braid Forbes MJ, et al. Readmission rates after decompression surgery in patients with lumbar canal stenosis among Medicare beneficiaries. Spine 2013;38:591–596.
22. Pawar SG, Dhar A, Ramani PS, et al. Internal decompression for spinal stenosis (IDSS) for decompression and use of interlaminar dynamic device (Coflex TM) for stabilization in the surgical management of degenerative lumbar canal stenosis with or without mild segmenta insability; Our initial results. Neurological Research; 2017;1–6.
23. Rajaee SS, Kanim LE, Bae HW. National trends in revision spinal fusion in the USA: patient characteristics and complications. Bone Joint J. 2014;96-B(6):807–16.
24. Ramain PS. Introduction; Posterior lumbar interbody fusion. PS Ramani (Ed.) 1989;1–10.
25. Ramani PS, Sharma A. Brief history of Spinal Surgery. 1994;13–6.
26. Richter A, Schutz C, Hauck M, Halm H. Does an interspinous device (Coflex) improve the outcome of decompressive surgery in lumbar spinal stenosis? One-year follow up of a prospective case control study of 60 patients. Eur Spine J 2010;19:283–9.
27. Rihn JA, Hilibrand AS, Zhou W, et al. Effectiveness of surgery for lumbar stenosis and degenerative spondylolisthesis in the octogenerial population. Analysis of SPORT (Spine Patient Outcome Research Trial) data: J Bone Joint Surg Am 2015;97:177–85.
28. Sanderson PL. Wood PL. Surgery for lumbar spinal stenosis in old people. J Bone Joint Surg Br. 1993;75(3):393–97.
29. Schmidt S, Franke J, Rauschmann M, et al. Prospective, randomized, multicenter study with 2-year follo-up to compare the performance of decompression with and without interlaminar stabilization. J Neurosurg Spine 2018;28(4):406–415.
30. Shabat S, Arinzon Z, Folman Y, et al. Long-term outcome of decompressive surgery for lumbar spinal stenosis in octogenarians. Eur Spine J 2008;17(2):193–98.
31. Shamji MF, Mroz T, Hsu W, et al. Management of degenerative lumbar canal stenosis in the elderly. Neurosurgery 2015;77;568–74.
32. Verbiest H. A radicular syndrome from developmental narrowing of the lumbar verterbral canal. J Bone Joint Surg 1954;36;230–37.
33. Verbiest H. Further experience on the pathological influence of a developmental narrowing of the lumbar vertebral canal. J Bone Joint Surg 1955;37;576–81.
34. Wang MY. Improvement of sagittal balance and lumbar lordosis following less invasive adult spinal deformity surgery with expandable cages and percutaneous instrumentation. J Neurosurg Spine 2013; 18(1):4–12.
35. Weinstein JN, Tosteson TD, Lurie JD, et al. Surgical versus non surgical therapy for lumbar canal stenosis. N Eng J Med 2008;358:794–810.
36. Weinstein JN, Tosteson TD, Lurie JD, et al. Surgical versus nonoperative treatment for lumbar spinal stenosis, four-year results of the Spine Patient Outcomes Research Trial. Spine (Phila Pa 1976). 2010;35(14): 1329–38.

Posterior Dynamic Stabilization (PDS) of Spine

PS Ramani

INTRODUCTION

The concept of dynamic stabilization of spine is more than 20 years old. It as introduced as a follow-up technique to minimally invasive internal decompression of lumbar spine in lumbar spinal stenosis (IDSS). The role, if IDSS has been popularized by the author (Dr PS Ramani) as a minimally invasive technique (MISS) in the surgical treatment of lumbar canal stenosis. It is described in a separate chapter. Both these attempts (IDSS and PDS) are aimed at preserving posterior motion segment of the spine so that patient even after surgery is mobile and active as before the surgery.

These techniques form a bridge between decompression laminectomy alone and decompression with rigid fusion. Much to the dismay of surgeons both the techniques (decompression and fusion) were associated with high rate of recurrence of symptoms and reoperation in some over a long term follow up of these patients.[3] Various interspinous process spacers (like X-stop, device for intervertebral assisted motion (DIAM) (Fig. 18.1) interspinous posterior device (IPD), Coflex, etc.) or pedicle-based systems (like PercuDyn, or Dynesys) have been introduced in this category. Co-flex is an interlaminar spacer which besides opening canal stenosis also opens foraminal stenosis. Some formal trials justify this view.[4] There are various inter- spinous and inter-laminar spacers in the market.

Author's Experience

The author having tried DIAM (Fig. 18.1) at first in few cases (22 cases) then was happy to use in-space (Fig. 18.2) for a long time in 78 patients.

But then settled to use Coflex interlaminar device for along time now (more than 400 patients) (Fig. 18.4) as it is easy to use and medial range follow up results are available and it is FDA approved product. In the

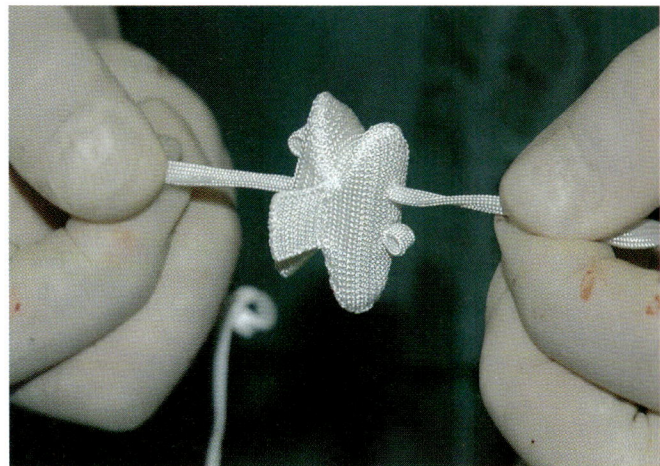

Fig. 18.1: PDS device DIAM

opinion of North American Spine Society (NASS) PDS with Coflex gives durable pain relief, achieves stability and mobility (Figs 18.2, 18.5 and 18.6) and has good follow-up outcome in patients with moderate and severe lumbar canal stenosis. Grade I evidence is now available for the use of Coflex after IDSS as recommended by the author in the surgical management of lumbar canal stenosis.[8,11] Prospective randomized multicenter study with 2 years follow up to compare the performance of decompression with and without interlaminar stabilization.

Device

Coflex (paradigm spine, Germany) is interlaminar posterior dynamic stabilization device approved by FDA and made from titanium alloy. The device has been extensively tried in the world.

It was invented by French orthopaedic surgeon Jacques Samani in 1994 and he called it Interspinous U. Subsequently, it has been modified to its present

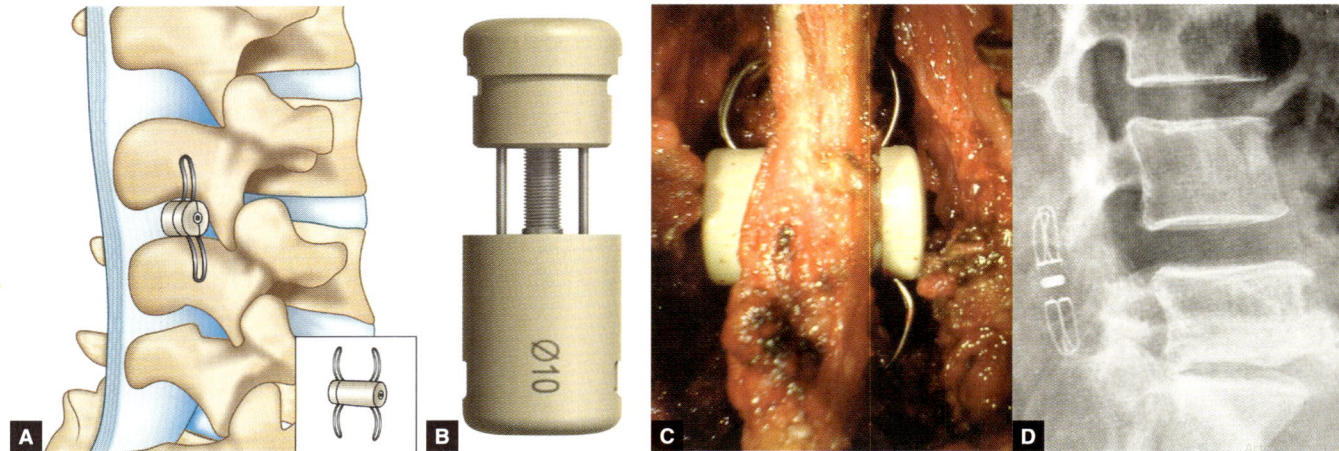

Fig. 18.2A to D: In-space interspinous PDS device

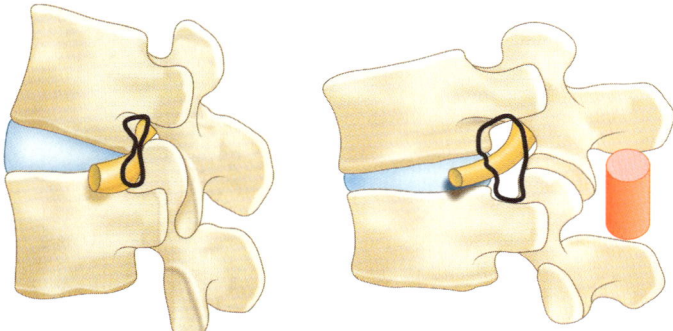

Fig. 18.3: PDS device restores foraminal height

interlaminar form and varies in sizes from 8, 10, 12, 14 and 16 mm with two wings on upper and lower ends. After decompression of neural elements with IDSS, the device is place in the interlaminar space and its wings are crimped over the adjacent spinous processes.

Several biomechanical studies have been performed and the device has been shown to limit extension, increase foraminal height, maintain disc height, offload the facet joints and perhaps decreases the incidence of adjacent segment degeneration.

Operative Technique

After general anesthesia the patient is placed on two bolsters in prone position.

A small midline incision is taken between two spinous processes.

Paraspinal muscles are separated subperiosteally.

Supraspinous ligament is preserved.

IDSS is performed.[7,9] Foraminotomy is done.

The supraspinous ligament is separated from the two spinous processes and held apart.

The interspinous ligament is excised.

The space is fashioned with high speed drill to accommodate the device.

The space is measured with spacers. The device should be fitting snuggly. Neither loose not too tight.

The appropriate device is mounted on holder or carrier and gently hammered into the space.

The undersurface is checked to be free and not compressing on the dura.

The wings are compressed on the spinous process with a crimper.

The supraspinous ligament is then replaced to its natural place and while taking a stich to approximate the muscles the supraspinous ligament in involved in the stitch.

The wound is closed without a drain. The steps are shown in Fig. 18.7.

Advantages

The advantages of PDS are several and as follows:
1. It takes off the burden and reduces intradiscal pressure. Thus it protects the disc from further degeneration.
2. It helps to preserve the posterior motion segment so important for maintained normal mobility of spine in the lumbar region.
3. The operative procedure is a minimally invasive technique creating less morbidity in the patient.
4. Less operating time.
5. Hardly any blood loss
6. Distracts the intervertebral space and opens up the foramina to decompress the nerve roots.
7. Possibly reduces the incidence of adjacent motion degeneration as frequently happens in rigid fusion.
8. Reoperation rates are comparable with rigid fusion[10]
9. Produces durable pain relief with stability in motion.

Disadvantages

Very few. It cannot be used in high grade degenerative spondylolisthesis. Similarly it will not function properly

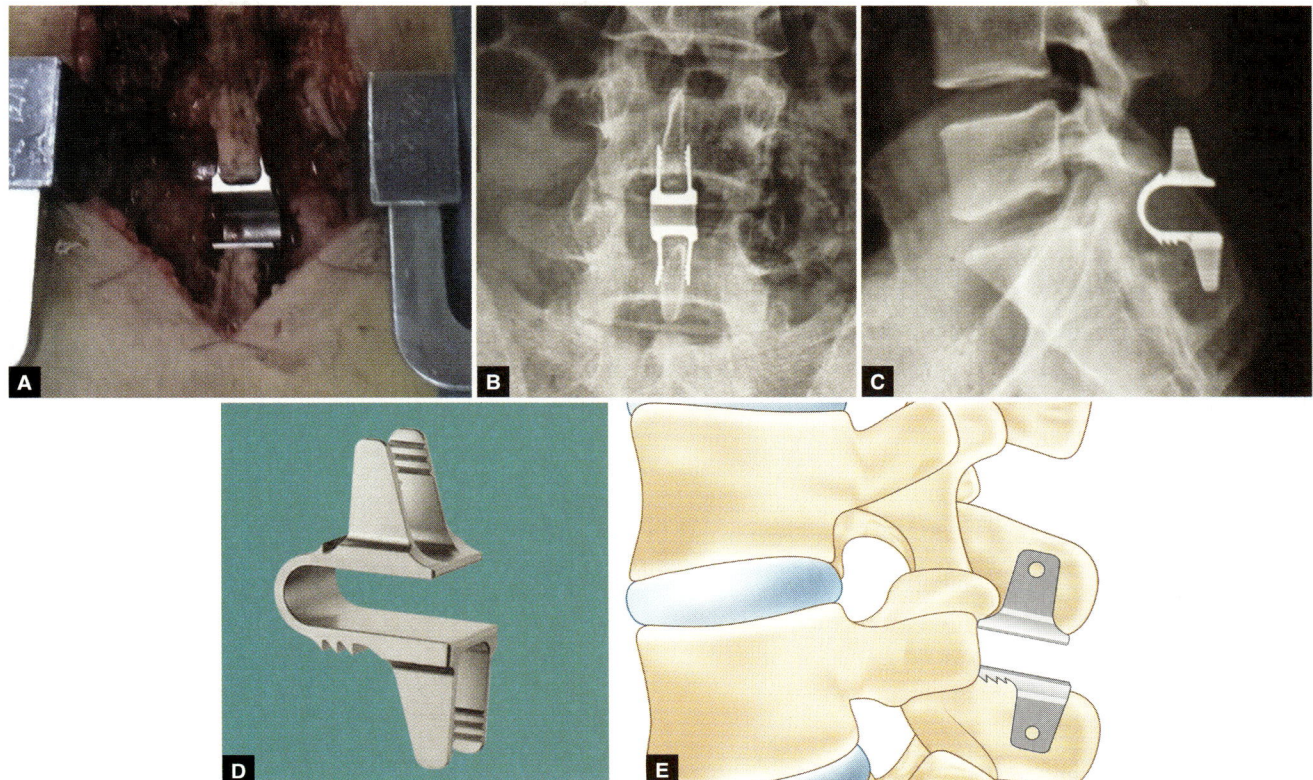

Fig. 18.4A to E: PDS Coflex interlaminar device

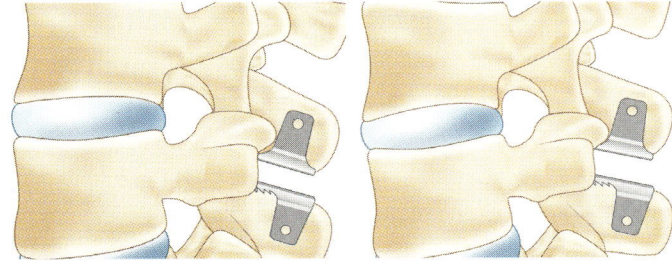

Fig. 18.5: Dynamic X-rays in flexion and extension

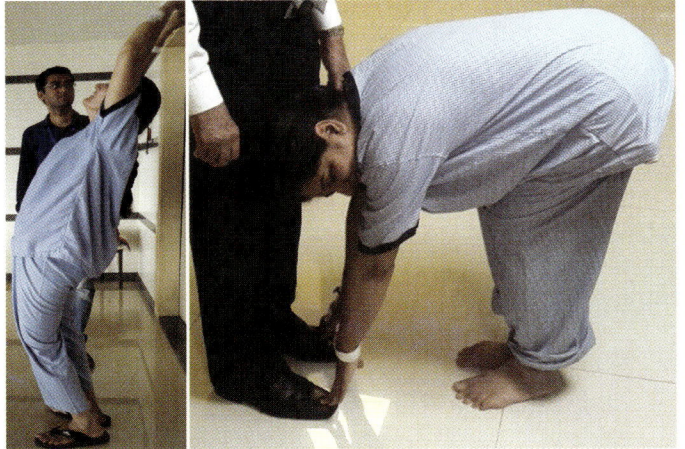

Fig. 18.6: Dynamic position of patient in flexion and extension less than 24 hours after surgery

with gross degenerative changes in the lumbar spine. It works well in one or two segments stabilization although the author has used the device to stabilize up to four levels. Originally, the company did not advocate its use at L5/S1 level. However, the author with direct discourse with the company has used it at that level. The assembly is light and may not work well on obese patient and patients with flabby muscles.

Complications

Over a two year follow up the complications in the author's series were few. This statement has been confirmed by other authors.

At times when patient falls accidently and injures back the spinous process can break and the device can be dislodged. But it is not a cause for concern. One can leave it in that position. Removal is easy and does not alter the outcome.

One patient complained of low back pain and pain in the buttocks six months after surgery. On further questioning, it was realized that he was in the habit of sitting on the floor every day for three hours to perform pooja. He was asked to change his style of performing the pooja. No medicines wee advised. It is necessary that the patient does exercises regularly to tone the back muscles and improve mobility. Dural violation is rare but has been reported by Schmidt et al.[11]

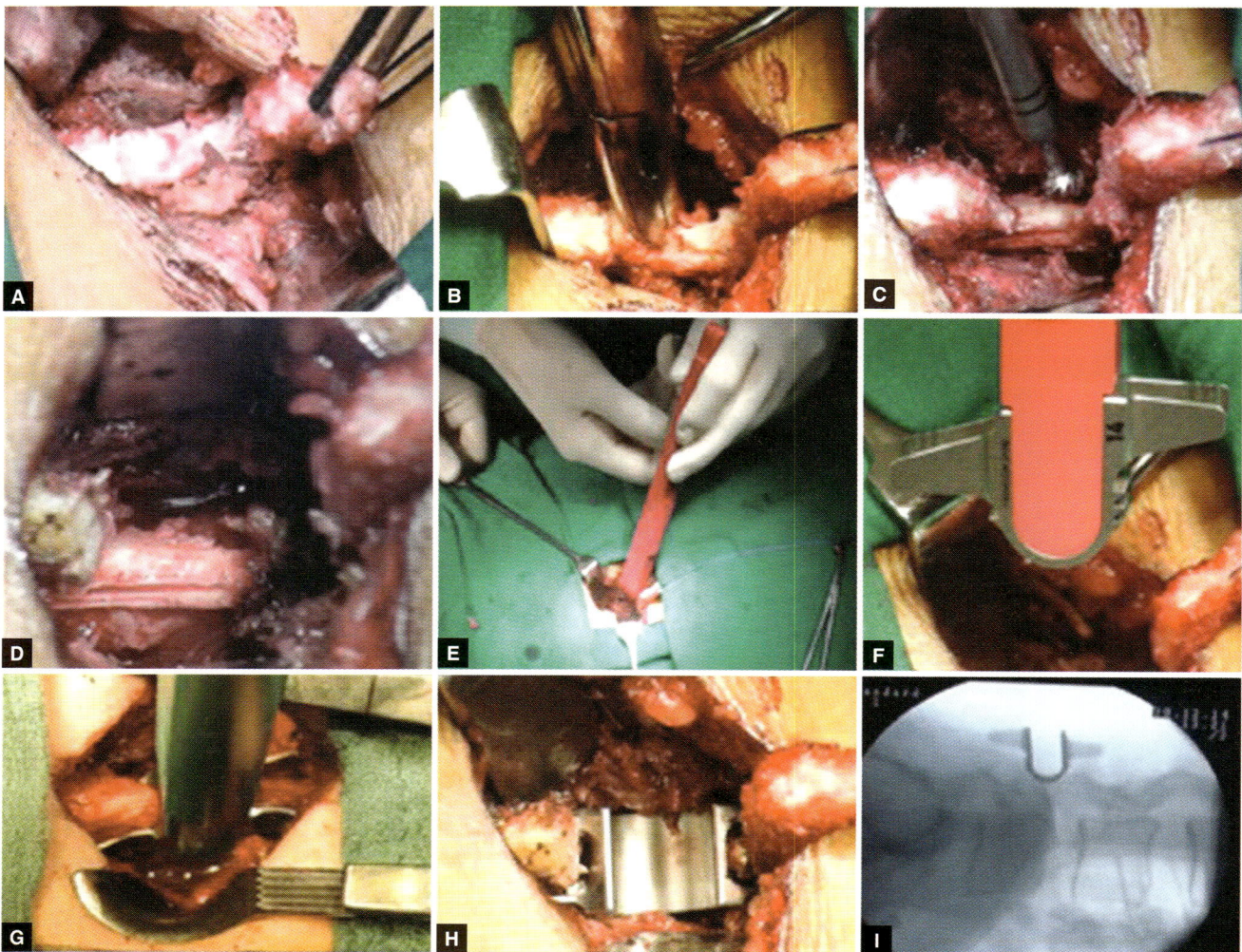

Fig. 18.7: Series of intraoperative photographs describing the steps of implant insertion as given in text

Outcome

In our department, the outcome is assessed by using VAS score, mean ODI and the overall patient satisfaction. In no other technique, the outcome is seen to be more satisfactory than in PDS technique. Other investigators also have confirmed the findings.[1,2,5,11]

The question that arises as to the present procedure is good, better or comparable to rigid fusion with pedicle screws. Studies have shown that the outcome of PDS with IDSS is comparable to rigid fusion and that ASD cannot be guaranteed to have lesser incidence with PDS with IDSS.[2,6]

Discussion

Decompression of neural tissue by using minimally invasive technique of IDSS as described and advocated by the author definitely helps to widen the lateral recesses[9] and thus helps to improve back pain and sciatica in short and midterm outcome reported earlier.[7]

Posterior dynamic stabilization using devices such as coflex aims to maintain foraminal height, limit abnormal extension, reduces the incidence of degenerative spondylolisthesis, unload facet joints, increases the disc height and provides dynamic stability in patients with degenerative spondylotic changes. Its utility is more felt in elderly patients due to its minimally invasive nature and ease of application.[9]

Conclusions

Coflex device is easy to apply, less invasive, prevents adjacent segment degeneration and shows clinical efficiency on midterm follow-up in indicated cases of lumbar canal stenosis.

REFERENCES

1. Bae HW, Lauryssen C, Maislin G, et al. Therapeutic sustainability and durability of coflex interlaminar stabilization after decompression for lumbar spinal stenosis: a four year assessment. Int J Spine Surg 2015;9:15.

2. Davis RJ, Errico TJ, Bae H, et al. Decompression and Coflex interlaminar stabilization compared with decompression and instrumented spinal fusion for spinal stenosis and low-grade degenerative spondylolisthesis: two-year results from the prospective, randomized, multicentre, Food and Drug Administration Investigational Device Exemption Trial. Spine 2013;38:1529–1539.

3. Hobart J, Gilkes C, Adams W, Germon T. Interspinous spacers for lumbar foraminal stenosis: formal trials are justified. Eur Spine J. 22 Suppl 2013;1:S47–53.

4. Kim HJ, Jeong JH, Cho HG, et al. Comparative observational study of surgical outocome of LCS using microsurgical extraforaminal decompression versus posterio lumbar interbody fusion. Eur Spine J 2015;24:388–95 .

5. Kumar N, Shah SM, Ng YH, et al. Role of Coflex as an adjunct to decompression for symptomatic lumbar spinal stenosis. Asian Spine J 2014;8:161–69.

6. Musacchio MJ, Lauryssen C, Davis RJ, et al. Evaluation of decompression and interlaminar stabilization compared with decompression and fusion for the treatment of lumbar spinal stenosis: 5 year follow-up of a prospective, randomized, controlled trial. Int J Spine Surg 2016;10:6.

7. Ramani PS, Maheshwari S. Surgical technique of internal decopression for spinal stenosis (IDSS). J Spinal Surg 2011;2:566–69.

8. Ramani PS, Pawar S, Dhar A, et al. IDSS and PDS (Coflex) for stabilization in the management of LCS. Neurological research 2017;10;1–6.

9. Ramani PS, Singh A, Cahyadi A, et al. Use of technological adavance in surgical management of interanal decompression for spinal stenosis (IDSS) in lumbar canal stenosis. J Spinal Surg 2012;4:992–5.

10. Resnik DK, Choudhri TF, Dailey AT, et al. Guidelines for the performance of fusion procedures for degenerative disease of lumbar spine. Part 9: fusion in patients with stenosis and spndylolisthesis. J. N eurosurg Spine 2005;2;679–85.

11. Schmidt S, Franke J, Rauschmann M, et al. Prospective, randomized, multicenter study with 2-year follow-up to compare the performance of decompression with and without interlaminar stabilization. JNS Spine 2018;28; 406–15.

Role of Virtual Navigation in the Surgery of Lumbar Canal Stenosis

Siddhartha Ghosh, Nidhikumar Patel, Anil Pande

INTRODUCTION

Fusion Surgery for Lumbar Canal Stenosis

Lumbar canal stenosis is a very common condition in elderly and in most patients decompression surgery becomes mandatory. Between 2002 and 2007, the use of surgical decompression alone to treat lumbar spinal stenosis declined slightly but the use of decompression with fusion increased by a factor of 15.[15] It has been reported that the rate of decompression surgery is being superseded by decompression plus fusion.[21,24] Wu, et al based on their analysis of studies advocating fusion for lumbar canal stenosis, concluded that the indications of fusion should be restricted to the lumbar stenosis patients accompanied with spinal instability or deformity.[24] Tye, et al also pointed out that unless indicated to treat instability or deformity, instrumented fusion should not be considered in surgery for lumbar canal stenosis.[21] In such patients presenting with deformity and instability, use of navigation as a device to correctly localize the screw position is a definite advantage and is likely to become the best practice. Ghogawala et al in a randomized controlled trial concluded that in patients with lumbar canal stenosis with or without degenerative spondylolisthesis, decompression surgery plus fusion surgery did not result in better clinical outcomes at 2 years and 5 years than did the decompression surgery alone.[5]

Pedicle screws insertion is a very important technique to stabilize all the 3 columns of the vertebral column. They have replaced most of the other methods of instrumentation utilizing hooks, sublaminar wires, rods and rectangles. Biomechanics of the normal spine are complex, multifactorial and varies with respect to each level.[14] The normal biomechanics and stability can be disrupted or compromised by a wide spectrum of pathologies and this entails that all neurosurgeons are competent and have this important skill in their armamentarium. Free hand technique uses anatomical landmarks and surgeon's anatomical knowledge and experience to place the screws. But the rates of malposition of the pedicle screws in best of experienced surgical hands ranges from 5 to 41% in the lumbar spine and 3–55% in the dorsal spine.[3] 7% of these misplaced screws cause a neurological injury.[3] To reduce this significant rate of incorrect pedicle screw accuracy and ease of placement can be improved with navigation which was introduced in 1995.[1,10] Shin et al in a meta-analysis found that there is a significant decrease in screw misplacement in navigated instrumentation in all levels and with no significant increase in theater time or blood loss.[19] The computer-based navigation and fluoroscopy-based navigation are commonly used. The fluoroscopy-based system may be a 2D or a 3 D version. This becomes even more useful especially when the anatomy is complex, e.g. CV Junction,[8,23] Cervical[23] and thoracic pedicles,[2,17] and in pathological obscured, altered anatomy.[11] Screws that perforate the pedicle cortex may increase the risk of nerve root injury (mild to severe) and dural tear. Less commonly vascular and visceral complications can occur. Malposition of pedicle screws may result in the loss of fixation, especially, if it occurs at the lower end of a construct thus accurate proper pedicle screws placement is important not only for the prevention of neurological injury, but also for the maintenance of the long-term spinal stability. Fluoroscopic virtual navigation is an important advance in spine surgery that allows surgeons to track their instruments and placement of hardware such as pedicle screws, interbody cages, and when manipulating rods for percutaneous pedicle screws in real time relative to multiplanar fluoroscopic images. In comparison to traditional fluoroscopy, the virtual fluoroscopic navigation results in reduction in anatomic shift error, automatic registration, reduced patient radiation exposure, improved ergonomics in comparison to conventional C-arm fluoroscopy.

Factors Contributing to Errors in Pedicle Screw Placement

The placement of the pedicular screw has a steep learning curve and this skill is compounded by varying anatomy and width of cervical, dorsal and lumbar pedicles and also associated complicating deformity and instability. There are special concerns in the CV junction, cervical and dorsal spine where the pedicle morphology and vascular and visceral factors compound the problem.

Rationale for use of Technology

Why do we need navigation?

It is a delicate operation because of great variability in the width, height and spatial orientation of the spinal pedicles and associated complex neurovascular structures. A slight error in direction may result in a significant error in the position of the tip of the screw leading to a breach in the walls which may cause neural, vascular or visceral injury beside leading to implant failure and instability. The earlier misgivings that it does not significantly reduce incidence of misplaced screws, takes much longer, increases theater time and blood loss are now confirmed to be false.[19] It reduces operating time and reduces the learning curve for junior neurosurgeons aiding them without risking patient outcomes.[17,18] Routine use of navigation and electrophysiology allows the theater staff to pick up the nuances thereby establishing protocols and eventually have efficient checklist to prevent lapses. Many recent meta-analyses have supported the usability, applications and advantages of these emerging technology.[9,20,22,25] The era of minimally invasive spine neurosurgery is already here[12] and neuronavigation is probably the most important adjunct that would allow its spectrum to widen.

Equipment and Software

Standard neurosurgical theater set up, navigation system (Fig. 19.1) with spine software and instrumentation (Fig. 19.2). Brain lab, Medtronic and Stryker are the popular systems. The fluoroscopy can be 2D or 3D, e.g. Zheim or an O arm. Certain systems come with compatible instrumentations like navigable screws and screw drivers. Advantages of compatible screws versus non-compatible titanium screws are that screws can be navigable by every thread (Figs 19.3 and 19.4). Non-compatible screws can be made partially compatible by using the navigable screw driver.

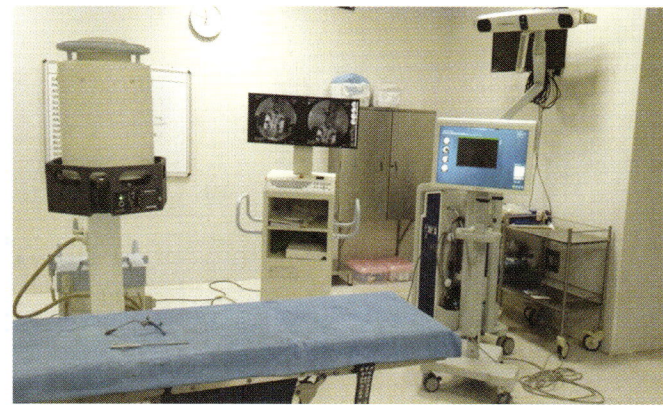

Fig. 19.1: Navigation system

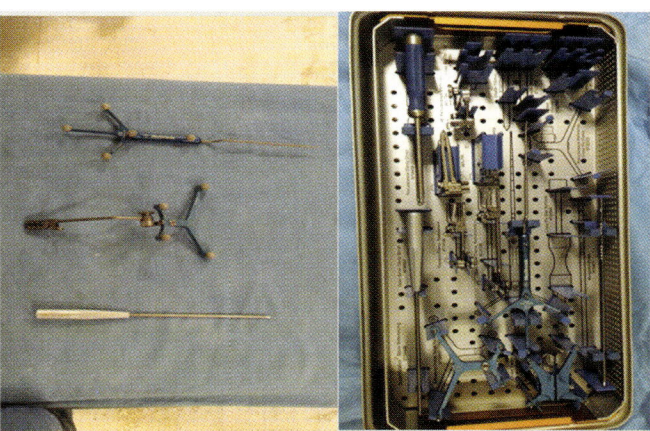

Fig. 19.2: Instruments used

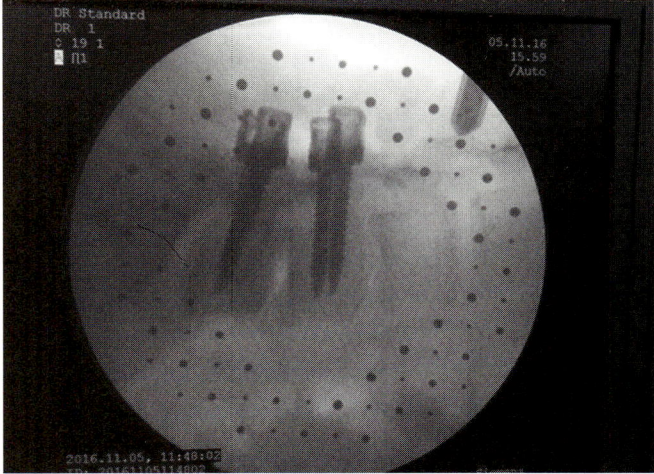

Fig. 19.3: Noncompatible titanium screws at L4 and L5 levels

Through mathematical calculation of geometric projection and back projection, the navigation system can afterwards visualize tracked surgical instruments, which are also equipped with reference bases, in respect to the fluoroscopic image. The camera system integrates the isolated image into the spatial correlation between the patient's pedicular anatomy and image intensifier, and tracks the position of the patients anatomy by

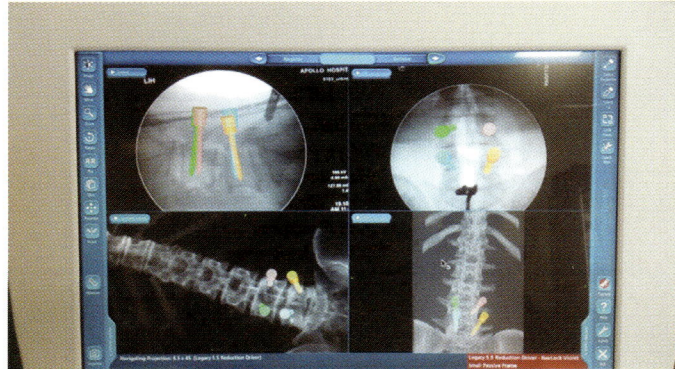

Fig. 19.4: Compatible titanium screws

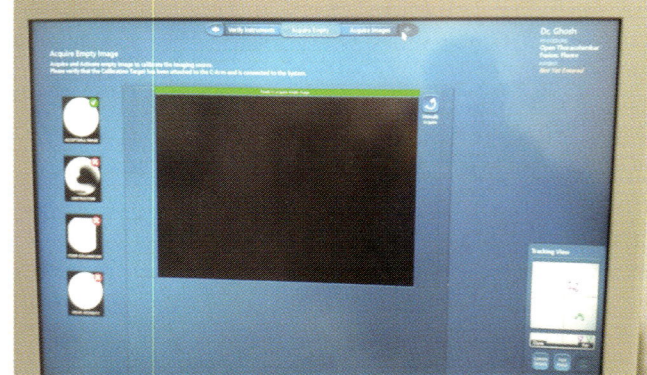

Fig. 19.5: Empty shot

means of a reference base attached to the spinous process as well as the position of the image intensifier by means of another attached reference base. Our 2D Fluoroscopy model did not have inbuilt compatibility with our navigation system. So, we used a calibration grid (tracker) which can be attached to the non-compatible C-arm and make it compatible for navigation system. Compatible C-arms can reduce the set-up time by automatic archiving than manual archiving.

Presurgical Planning

Patients present with intractable pain, neurological symptoms and signs, or both. A detailed neurological examination and radiological evaluation with X-rays static and dynamic, MRI imaging and CT scans in selected cases. Neuronavigation, e.g. medtronic system and C-arm is required. MEP and SSEP must be done for all the patients by the same experienced neurophysiologist.

Surgical Technique

The procedures is done through a standard posterior approach. Spinous processes and laminae of degenerated vertebra are exposed. Additional exposure of spine one level below or above to fix the patient's reference frame is necessary. After connecting the calibration grid to the C-arm three X-rays—(1) empty shot (Fig. 19.5), (2) AP, (3) lateral view are taken and manually archived to the navigation system. All retractors are then removed and the wound cavity is filled with saline. During X-ray shots the anesthetist should be requested to keep the patient in apnea to prevent movement artifacts. In order to avoid multiple shots, an experienced technician is absolutely necessary. The image acquisition and registration process occur simultaneously. Sources of error can occur during image acquisition (poor quality, e.g. in obese patients, inadequate adjustment of the C-arm in regard to the true AP/Lat. plane), image calibration, and finally also

computation of the calibrated images. The navigation probe is verified and accuracy is rechecked. In order to minimize accuracy during the entire procedure steps were taken to prevent the inadvertent movement of the frame (directly or indirectly). Intraoperative imaging is no alternative to sound anatomical knowledge and orientation and is supplemented by haptic, i.e. direct visual and tactile feel.

Neurophysiological monitoring—MEP and SSEP are essential and they complement the visuospatial feedback with real time neural anatomical and functional continuity. A 15% decrease in amplitude may be significant and a 30% decrease points towards a high probability of getting neural deficits. Decrease in amplitude suggests pedicle breach. But it can be within the safe zone medially. On correction the amplitude instantly comes back to normal levels. In all cases X-rays/CT scans should be done postoperatively (Figs 19.6 and 19.7).

Results

We evaluated the feasibility and accuracy of pedicle screw insertion assisted by a realtime, C-arm 2-dimensional (2D) image-guided navigation system in 30 patients who underwent thoracolumbar and/or lumbar stabilization for a period of one year (August 2015–December 2016). The accuracy of pedicle screw placement was assessed by postoperative imaging

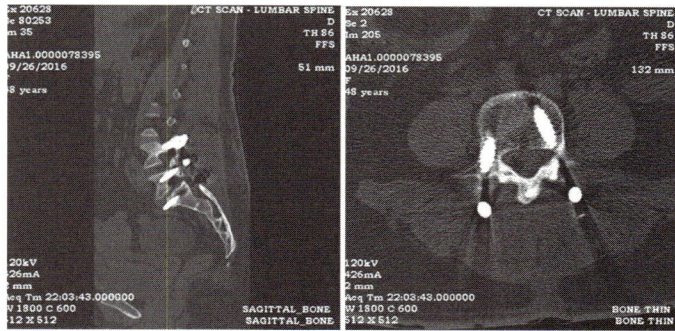

Fig. 19.6: Postoperative CT LS spine

(Figs 19.8 and 19.9). There were minor breaches in pedicle in three screws (4%) (without any injury to

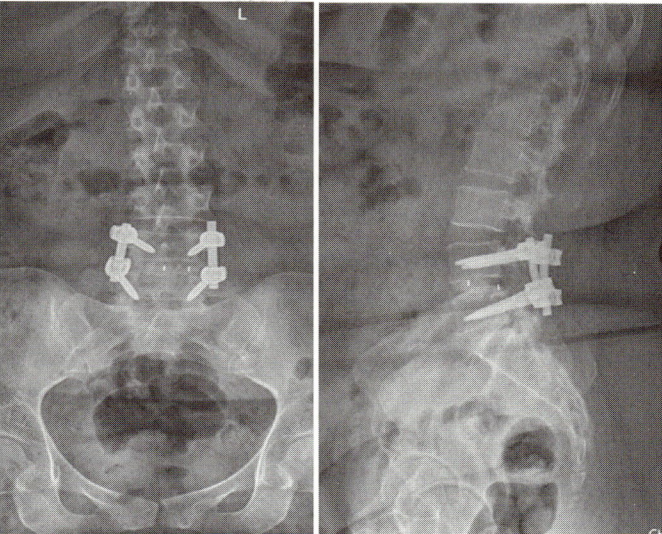

Fig. 19.7: Postoperative X-rays

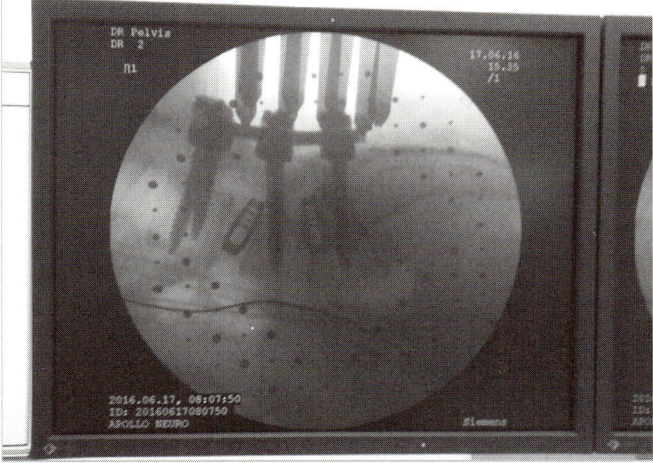

Fig. 19.8: L4, L5, S1 levels

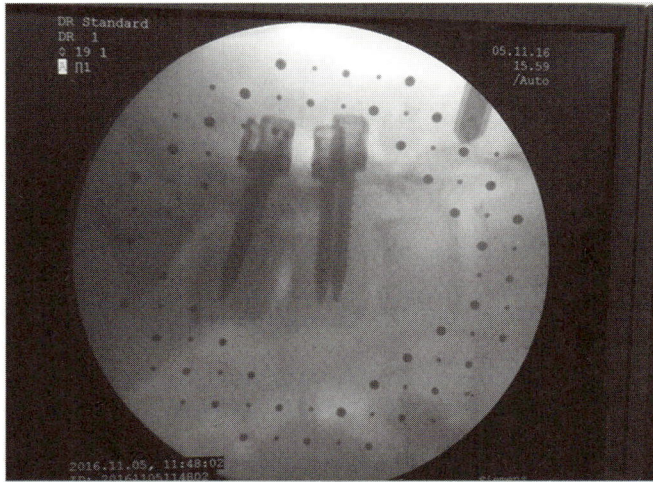

Fig. 19.9: L4, L5, LIF

nerve roots pedicle that is insignificant). There were no lumbar spine anterolateral cortical perforations occurred. There was no structural violation of screw or nerve injury/pain reported. A total of 164 screws were inserted. Two patients had worsening of neurological deficits but later it improved during the follow up. There were minor breaches in pedicle in three screws (without any injury to nerve roots pedicle that is insignificant). Two screws had medial breaches of 5 mm but patient did not have any neurological symptoms or signs.[1] Screws had a lateral breach of 4 mm without any sequale. There were no lumbar spine anterior cortical perforations occurred.

Tricks of the Trade

Rahamathulla et al emphasize that we must not ignore the important point that the images on the screen are not shown in realtime.[16] They further point that polyaxial screwdrivers will have some inherent movement at the instrument tip, and thinner-diameter taps may have some flexibility and caution that care must be taken to insert these instruments as straight as possible to avoid errors in trajectory. Concept of safe zone-has been based on previous assertions by Gertzbein, et al. that there is a total of 4 mm of allowable medial pedicle screw encroachment within the lower thoracic spine and lumbar spine consisting of 2 mm of epidural space and 2 mm of subarachnoid space (Tables 19.1 and 19.2).[4]

Complications and Cost

Lengthy learning curve to use the navigation and its application to spine, in fact is cumbersome and many

Table 19.1: Gertzbein classification	
Grade	Breach distance
0	0 mm (no breach)
1	Less than 2 mm
2	2–4 mm
3	More than 4 mm

Gertzbein and Robbins that cortical breaches of greater than 4 mm were associated with neurological deficits, leading them to conclude that this 4 mm range may constitute a "saft zone" for screws placed from 10 to 14.

Table 19.2: Heary classification	
Grade	Breach
1	None
2	Lateral but screw tip is within VB
3	Anterior or lateral breach of screw tip
4	Medical or inferior breach
5	Breach that immediate revision (due toproximity to sensitive structures)

centers ignore the use of their Brain lab, Medtronic or Stryker spinal navigation capacity.[6] The calibration errors should be addressed as that can lead to misplaced confidence and increased liability to erroneous pedicle screw trajectories defeating the very objective of this expensive technology. Occasional blocking of the surgical field and camera can lead to tracking failure. Inadvertently touching or hitting reference frame by suction tubes instrument or the surgeon displacing it can jeopardize the operation precision. On-rigid connection between reference base and actual surgical site rests the precision. The other minor hitches can be due to inexperienced radiographers taking unnecessary multiple shots during set-up time thereby increasing radiation exposure and operation time. Disturbance of work flow leads to increased time in setting up and thereby operating time but this rapidly reduces as we gain experience and confidence. There is an increased risk of radiation exposure to patients and OT personnel (surgeons, OT nurses, technicians) but less when compared to conventional surgeries but this should be addressed by taking all precautions and avoiding unnecessary shots. Assessment of accuracy of pedicle screw by postoperative X-ray has a lower accuracy compared to CT which is the gold standard now, a few and not all of our patients were assessed by CT. Longer follow-up is required for long-term stability and actual patient reported outcomes. A more realistic measure would be revision rates or patient morbidity which are direct clinical entities that are not reflected in reported accuracy rates.

Conclusions

The era of image guided neurosurgery is already here and as always neurosurgery has lead from the front.[1,7,11,13] Frame based and frameless navigation has become routine and its extension from cranial to spinal and peripheral nerve surgery is just a matter of time. The capability of these technologies to give you precise wanted detail and anatomy is remarkable.[13] The fusion of CT MRI and other modalities to a 3D fused image showing neural, vascular visceral relationship to instrumentation and pedicle screw is no longer imaginative. The use of navigation to guide pedicle screw placement is allowing the higher accuracy and familiarity with use and this rapidly evolving technology will make it indispensable to any neurosurgery procedure and will have tremendous impact in surgical and patient reported outcomes. This is likely to become an indispensable tool and when coupled with routine electrophysiological monitoring during surgery will increase safety and acceptance of spinal surgery. With 2D fluoroscopic image navigation, it is possible to achieve reliable and accurate pedicle

screw insertion during low thoracic and lumbar spinal surgery. In addition, it offers advantages such as minimising radiation exposure in comparison to using traditional fluoroscopy that is reported to be almost 10 times higher. The confidence of surgeon is increased attributed to the immediate feedback on the trajectory of the screw that remains within the confines of the pedicle. With the given feasibility, accuracy, less operating time and safety the C-arm neuronavigation imaging ensures accurate placement of screws as compared to traditional 2D fluoroscopy.

Acknowledgement

Ms Sapline Prabha, prepared the manuscript.

REFERENCES

1. Brodwater BK, Roberts DW, Nakajima T, Friets EM, Strohbehn JW. Extracranial application of the frameless stereotactic operating microscope: experience with lumbar spine. Neurosurgery. 1993;32(2):209–13.
2. Fisher CG, Sahajpal V, Keynan O, Boyd M, Graeb D, Bailey C, et al. Accuracy and safety of pedicle screw fixation in thoracic spine trauma. J Neurosurg Spine. Dec 2006 ;5(6):520–6.
3. Gelalis ID, Paschos NK, Pakos EE, Politis AN, Arnaoutoglou CM, Karageorgos AC, et al. Accuracy of pedicle screw placement: a systematic review of prospective in vivo studies comparing free hand, fluoroscopy guidance and navigation techniques. Eur Spine J: 2012 ;21(2):247–55.
4. Gertzbein SD, Robbins SE. Accuracy of pedicular screw placement in vivo. Spine. 1990;15(1):11–4.
5. Ghogawala Z, Dziura J, Butler WE, Dai F, Terrin N, Magge SN, et al. Laminectomy plus Fusion versus Laminectomy Alone for Lumbar Spondylolisthesis. N Engl J Med. Apr 2016;14;374(15):1424–34.
6. Härtl R, Lam KS, Wang J, Korge A, Kandziora F, Audigé L. Worldwide survey on the use of navigation in spine surgery. World Neurosurg. Jan; 2013;79(1):162–72.
7. Hott JS, Deshmukh VR, Klopfenstein JD, Sonntag VKH, Dickman CA, Spetzler RF, et al. Intraoperative Iso-C C-arm navigation in craniospinal surgery: the first 60 cases. Neurosurgery. May;54(5):1131-6; discussion 2004;1136–37.
8. Hurlbert RJ. Frameless stereotactic guidance for surgery of the upper cervical spine. Neurosurgery. 1997;41(6):1448–49.
9. Kosmopoulos V, Schizas C. Pedicle screw placement accuracy: a meta-analysis. Spine. 2007;32(3):E111-E120 .
10. Nolte L, Zamorano L, Arm E, Visarius H, Jiang Z, Berlerman U, et al. Image-guided computer-assisted spine surgery: a pilot study on pedicle screw fixation. Stereotact Funct Neurosurg. 1996;66(1-3):108-17.
11. Nottmeier EW. A review of image-guided spinal surgery. J Neurosurg Sci. 2012;56(1):35–47.
12. O'Toole JE. The Future of Minimally Invasive Spine Surgery. Neurosurgery 2013;Aug 1;60(CN_suppl_1):13–9.
13. Overley SC, Cho SK, Mehta AI, Arnold PM. Navigation and Robotics in Spinal Surgery: Where Are We Now? Neurosurgery. 2017 Mar 2017;1;80(3S):S86–99.
14. Pande A, Cugati G. Biomechanics of the spine. In: Tandon P, Ramamurthi R, editors., Textbook of Neurosurgery. 3 edition. New Delhi: Jaypee Brothers Medical Pub; cited 2018;550–1.
15. Peul WC, Moojen WA. Fusion for Lumbar Spinal Stenosis—Safeguard or Superfluous Surgical Implant? https://doi.org/101056/NEJMe1600955 [Internet]. 2016 Apr

16. Rahmathulla G, Nottmeier EW, Pirris SM, Deen HG, Pichelmann MA. Intraoperative image-guided spinal navigation: technical pitfalls and their avoidance. Neurosurg Focus. Mar 2014;1;36(3):E3.

17. Rajasekaran S, Vidyadhara S, Ramesh P, Shetty AP. Randomized clinical study to compare the accuracy of navigated and non-navigated thoracic pedicle screws in deformity correction surgeries. Spine. Jan 2007;15;32(2):E56-64.

18. Rampersaud YR. Editorial: Computed tomography and pedicle screws. J Neurosurg Spine. 2014;Jun 13;21(3):317–9.

19. Shin BJ, James AR, Njoku IU, Härtl R. Pedicle screw navigation: a systematic review and meta-analysis of perforation risk for computer-navigated versus freehand insertion. J Neurosurg Spine 2012 Aug;17(2):113–22.

20. Tian N-F, Huang Q-S, Zhou P, Zhou Y, Wu R-K, Lou Y, et al. Pedicle screw insertion accuracy with different assisted methods: a systematic review and meta-analysis of comparative studies. Eur Spine J Off Publ Eur Spine Soc Eur Spinal Deform Soc Eur Sect Cerv Spine Res Soc. 2011;Jun;20(6):846–59.

21. Tye EY, Anderson JT, Haas AR, Percy R, Woods ST, Ahn UM, et al. Decompression versus Decompression and Fusion for Degenerative Lumbar Stenosis in a Workers' Compensation Setting. Spine 2017; 01;42(13):1017–23.

22. Verma R, Krishan S, Haendlmayer K, Mohsen A. Functional outcome of computer-assisted spinal pedicle screw placement: a systematic review and meta-analysis of 23 studies including 5,992 pedicle screws. Eur Spine J Off Publ Eur Spine Soc Eur Spinal Deform Soc Eur Sect Cerv Spine Res Soc 2010;19(3):370–5.

23. Welch WC, Subach BR, Pollack IF, Jacobs GB. Frameless stereotactic guidance for surgery of the upper cervical spine. Neurosurgery 1997;40(5):958–63.

24. Wu A-M Tong T-J, Wang X-Y. A rethink of fusion surgery for lumbar spinal stenosis. J Evid-Based Med 2016;9(4):166–9.

25. Youkilis AS, Quint DJ, McGillicuddy JE, Papadopoulos SM. Stereotactic navigation for placement of pedicle screws in the thoracic spine. Neurosurgery. 2001;48(4):771–8; discussion 778–79.

Minimally Invasive Tubular Decompression Technique in Lumbar Spinal

Kulkarni AG, Patel A, Ruparel S, Mewara N

INTRODUCTION

Lumbar canal stenosis, which is defined as narrowing of spinal canal, is the most common cause for spinal surgery in elderly patients.[1–3] Failure of conservative treatment is one of the main indications for operative intervention in this condition.

Unless associated with instability, these patients were treated with lumbar decompression surgery alone. However, several new and minimally invasive techniques of treating this condition have evolved over the past few decades. Laminectomy is an excellent procedure and has historically been the gold standard. The procedure involves extensive resection of posterior spinal elements, possibly leading to postoperative iatrogenic pain and sowing the seeds of progressive segmental instability. With an aim to preserve as much bony and soft tissue integrity as possible and to prevent iatrogenic instability, the science of MISS (minimally invasive spinal surgery) such as laminotomy, lamino-foraminotomy and bilateral microlumbar decompression technique came into vogue. The advent of tubular retractors was a revolution when it was introduced in the surgical arena for management of lumbar canal stenosis. The ability to perform a thorough ipsilateral/contralateral decompression through a small unilateral portal with preservation of the paraspinal muscles and the stabilizing structures make MISS a unique technique compared to other procedures.

Tubular decompression surgical procedures involve smaller incisions, lesser blood loss, better visualization of pathological site and faster rehabilitation without compromising the surgical outcome. The following chapter discusses the technique of tubular decompression in detail and highlights several points, which are necessary to be considered before clinical application of this procedure in day-to-day practice.

Indications and Contraindications

Indications for doing tubular decompression are not quite different from any other technique used for lumbar spinal stenosis. Central and lateral recess stenosis can be decompressed using this technique with minimal bone removal, thus maintaining stability of the motion segment.[4–9] The technique can be used to decompress multi-level lumbar canal stenosis using the same portal or multiple portals depending upon the anatomy. The indication for spinal canal decompression using microendoscopic technique can be extended for decompression of synovial cysts[10–12] and selected cases of stenosis associated with degenerative spondylolisthesis.[13]

For this technique to be successful, the surgeon must have an access to the facilities like surgical microscope, C/O-arm, high speed drill, etc. The technique is not very useful for mobile degenerative spondylolisthetic stenosis, narrow bony canal with small facets in the sagittal plane.

Advantages

The advantages of MED (microendoscopic decompression) fall into two categories—biomechanical and clinical. MED serves to keep the biomechanics and stability of spinal motion segment intact. The amount of soft tissue trauma as compared to conventional decompression is quite less. Decompression of the central canal, bilateral lateral recesses and foramina can be achieved through one keyhole preserving the contralateral anatomy. The side of port of entry is chosen based on patient symptoms, facet inclination on the axial MRI and spinal alignment.

Minimal morbidity and pain are hallmarks of this procedure. There is minimal blood loss, almost zero infection rate[14] and reduced hospital stay as compared to open laminectomy procedures. Patients can be mobilized in a few hours following the surgery. It is cosmetically more appealing whilst accomplishing the same goal. The greatest advantage of this procedure is for patients with high BMI, who would otherwise need long incisions even for a single level surgery. It also avoids a wrong level surgery as the entry of the tubular retractor is done under image-intensifier guidance[15] (Fig. 20.1).

Disadvantages

There is a steep learning curve to this procedure. Initially, the surgical time and complications may be higher. However, with experience decompression can be safely and quickly performed. Technical challenges include working through a tube wherein there is small operative corridor and focused vision. This would make it difficult to identify proper anatomical landmarks. Working with tube would not allow much of instrument angulation during decompression and one will have to train him to work with use of parallel instruments and if angulation is required the whole tube needs to be angulated.

Surgical Technique

Instruments for tubular decompression:
1. Tubular dilators and retractors (Fig. 20.2)
2. Operating table that can tilt in all directions.
3. Specialized long bayonet instruments for use in MIS
4. Curved Kerrison ronguer
5. Long cautery tip
6. High speed cutting burr
7. Nerve root retractor and nerve hooks and probe
8. Gel foam, bone wax, neurosurgical patties
9. Fibrin glue (TISSEL®)

Preoperative Work-up

The surgeon should be precise about the location of the pathology as the exposure is limited. MR films should be examined to locate the level, site and side/s of pathology, the orientations of the facet joints and subtle signs of instability like the vacuum sign, facet fullness and presence of spondylolisthesis at the

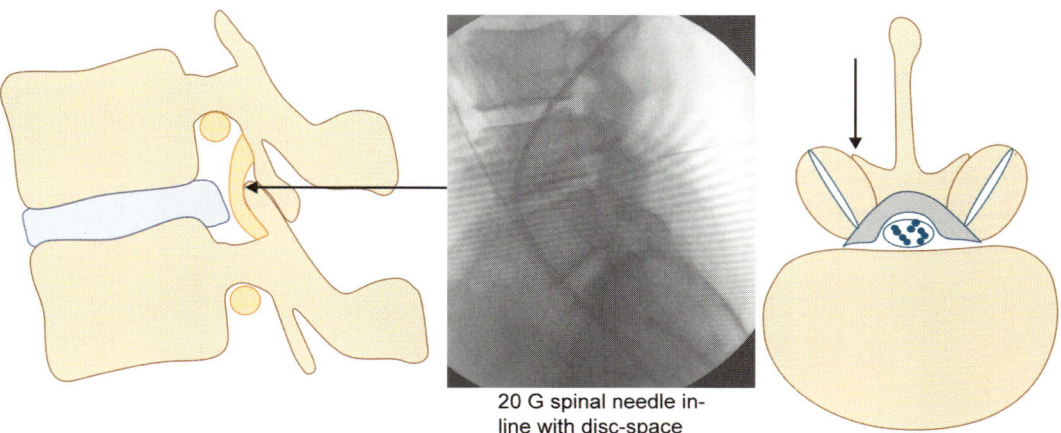

20 G spinal needle in-line with disc-space

Fig. 20.1: Level marking with 20 G spinal needle and IITV guidance. The needle is placed in-line with the disc-space of interest

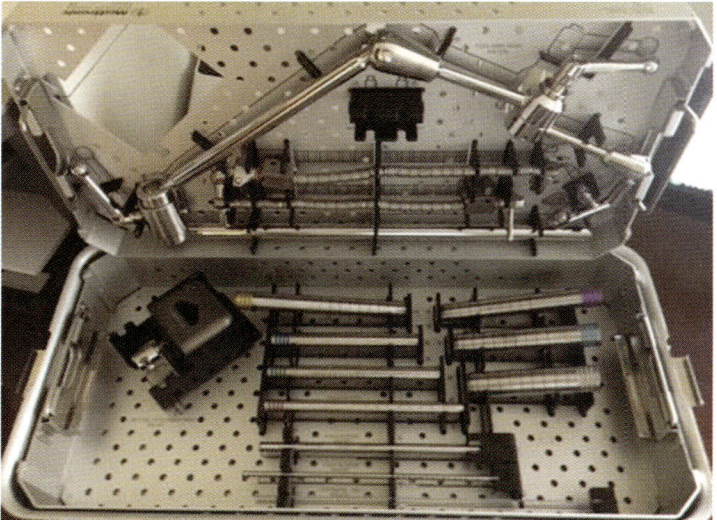

Fig. 20.2: Tubular dilators and retractors in METRx™ system (Medtronic Sofamor Danek)

affected segments. Dynamic radiographs confirm any dynamic instability. Patient with good clinico-radiological correlation and without dynamic instability is a good candidate for MED.

All symptomatic levels need to be decompressed. When operating more than one level the author prefers a single incision at the lower lumbar levels, taking advantage of the natural lordosis at this level that make wandering from one level to the other quiet smooth. At higher levels incisions can be taken on contralateral sides or the same incision can be extended by another centimeter to achieve decompression at both levels.

In the presence of sagittal facet orientation, it is important to remember to dock the tube in less of inclination to avoid inadvertent damage to the ipsilateral facet joint.

In case of unilateral symptoms and no stenosis on the other side author prefers to enter from the contralateral side and hence avoid encroaching into the facet joints of both sides. In patients with bilateral symptomatic stenosis and symptoms, a bilateral decompression is possible from any of the sides. In general, right-sided approach is more comfortable for a right-handed surgeon. Decompression of the lateral recess and foramina is quite easy from the contralateral side as the inclination of the tube allows direct visualization of the opposite side, thus the tube can be docked contralateral to the more stenotic side. The side from which facets can be spared should be chosen.

Anesthesia

The procedure is always performed under general anesthesia.

Positioning

Patient is positioned on a radiolucent table in prone position with bolsters below the chest and iliac crest, keeping the abdomen free to reduce intravenous pressure in the epidural plexus. This position helps to put the patient in natural lordosis, thus facilitating decompression of the canal in its narrowest dimension. The head-side of the table is raised by 10–15° to avoid venous engorgement in the eyes. The foot end of the table should be flexed as the patient may slip-off as the head end of the table is raised. Pressure points should be well padded. Patient should be firmly strapped to the table to avoid slipping while turning the table. The surgeon should stand on the side that he chooses to decompress depending on the MRI findings and the leg symptoms. The table mount and flexible arm of the tubular system should be tightly secured before the incision.

Site Identification

Using lateral fluoroscopy imaging a 20 G spinal needle is inserted at the level of the involved disc space and parallel to both the end plates. The needle is inserted about 1 cm lateral to the midline and position confirmed with a lateral image in the image intensifier (Fig. 20.2)

Sequential dilator insertion and tube docking (Figs 20.3 and 20.4).

About 5 cc of 0.5% bupivacaine diluted in 15 cc of saline is infiltrated for pre-emptive analgesia. A 2 cm incision is then centered over the needle and deepened till the fascia. Although the diameter of the tube (working portal) is 18 mm, it is better to take a slightly longer (2 cm) incision to allow for wandering of the

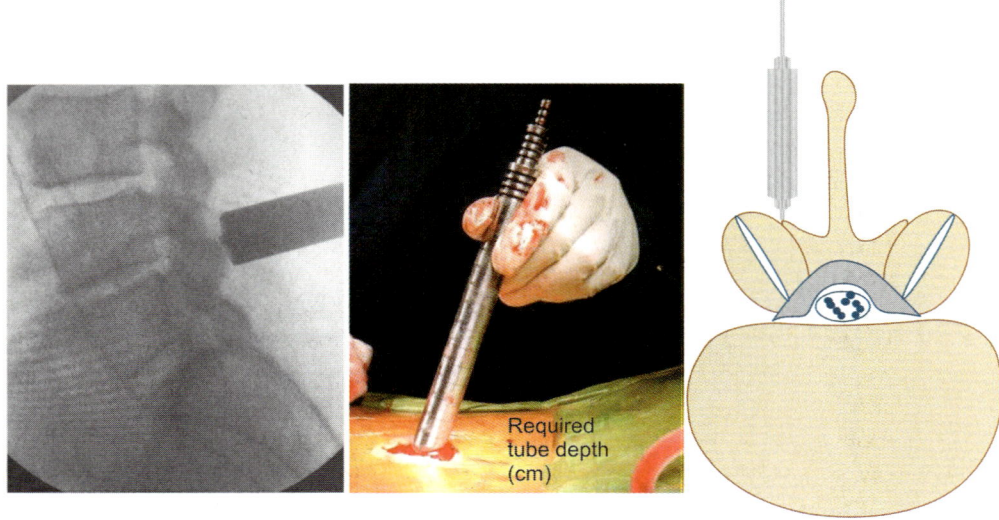

Fig. 20.3: Serial dilatation of muscles with sequential dilators. Each successive dilator has to be rotated and kept firmly over bone to achieve adequate muscle separation

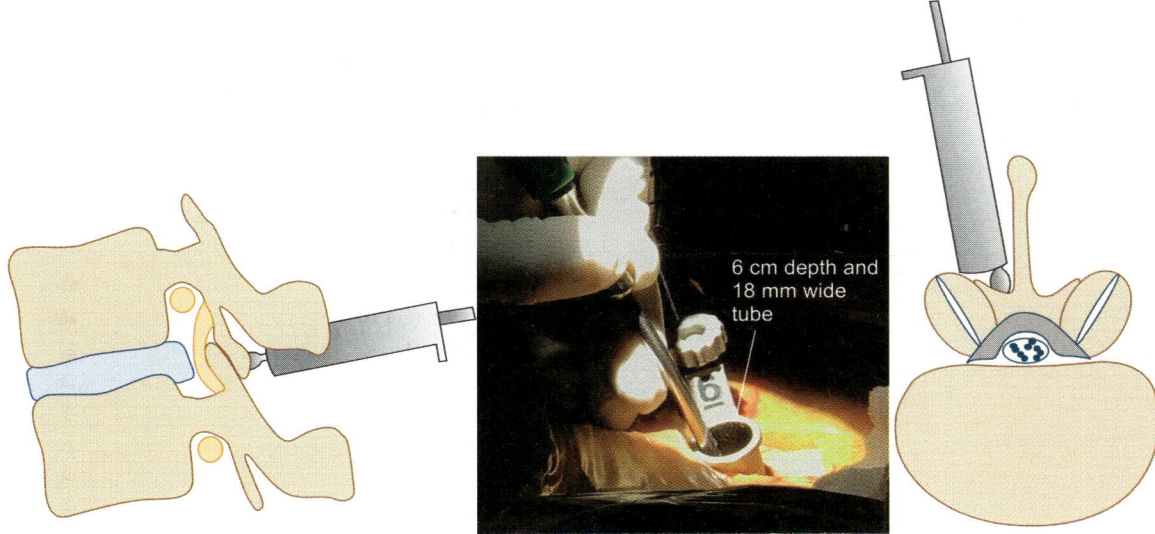

6 cm depth and
18 mm wide
tube

Fig. 20.4: Appropriate length (3–9 cm) and wide (18 mm) tube docking. The reading is taken off the last dilator and tube matching the diameter of last dilator is passed over them and affixed to the flexible arm

tube and prevent maceration of the skin. To avoid injury related to guide wire the author has stopped using the same, and uses the initial dilator to locate the inferior lamina of the superior vertebra. The initial dilator is then used to sweep off the paraspinal muscle mass and palpate the bony landmarks. The spinous process medially and the facet joint complex laterally are felt as two mountains with the lamina as the valley in-between. Sequential dilators are then inserted while confirming the target site under fluoroscopy. The dilators have graduations marked on them to determine the depth of the tube. The marking on the final dilator at the level of skin provides the length of the tubular retractor. If the marking is between 4 and 5 then a number 5 tubular retractor should be used. 18 mm diameter tubular retractor is then docked with the flexible arm as the final working channel. The dilators should be deeply seated on the lamina to avoid "muscle creeping" into the working field. The working channel should be kept as perpendicular to the floor to maintain an easy working position for the surgeon. This can be achieved by raising the head end of the table. This is essential for decompressing the L4–5 and L5–S1 levels owing to the lumbar lordosis. Microscope is then brought into the field. As an alternative, an endoscopic camera can also be attached to the tubular retractor.

Visualization of the Anatomical Landmarks

Soft tissue is separated using a long cautery tip till the lamina can be visualized. An excellent exposure is one, wherein the inferior part of superior lamina and flavum are visualized.

Ipsilateral Laminotomy (Fig. 20.5)

Lamina is then burred using a 4 mm cutting burr, till the junction of the inner cortex and ligamentum flavum is encountered. Ligamentum flavum is separated from the lamina by using a bayonet-handle angled curette. Ipsilateral laminotomy is completed using a no 2 Kerrison ronguer, leaving the flavum intact. Intact flavum protects the dural sac from injury whilst drilling the opposite side.

Going Over the Top (Fig. 20.6)

In order to decompress the opposite side, the line of vision must extend underneath the spinous process and interspinous ligament across the midline. This is achieved by, aiming the tubular retractor medially and tilting the table away from the operating surgeon towards the opposite side. This helps in providing a better visualization of the lateral recess of the contra-lateral side. The inner cortex of the contralateral lamina till the hypertrophied medial margins of the opposite facet joint is drilled with a high-speed burr, beginning at the base of the spinous process and proceeding laterally within the canal. This de-roofs the canal and exposes the flavum entirely.

Contralateral Decompression (Fig. 20.7)

The insertion of the flavum is then detached using a no 4 Penfield. The intervening ligamentum flavum is then removed piece-meal thus decompressing the dural sac and the opposite side nerve root. This successive resection is carried until the contralateral caudal pedicle is visualized. Using a curved Kerrison, the lateral recess and foramen are decompressed effectively.

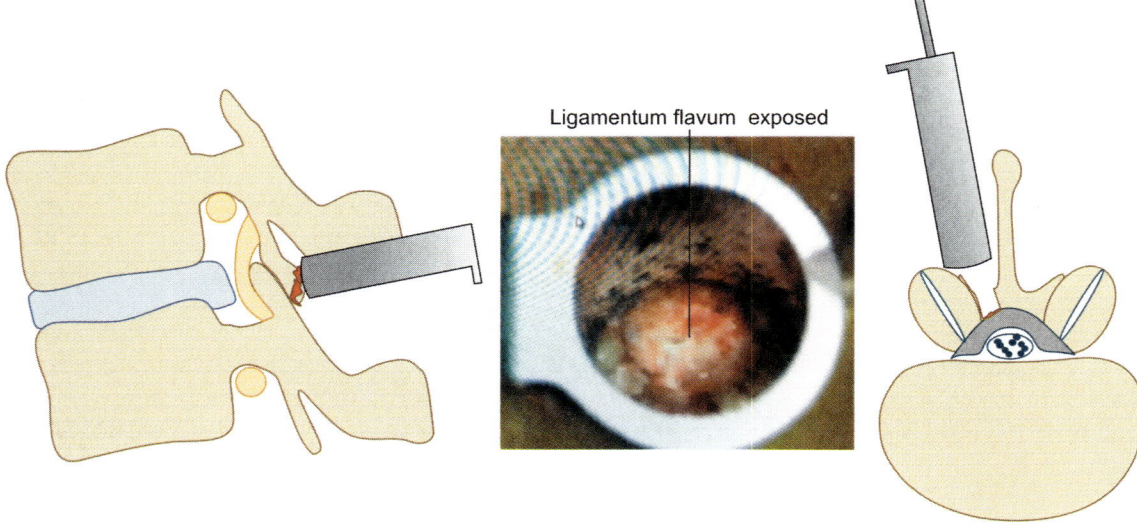

Fig. 20.5: Ipsilateral laminotomy

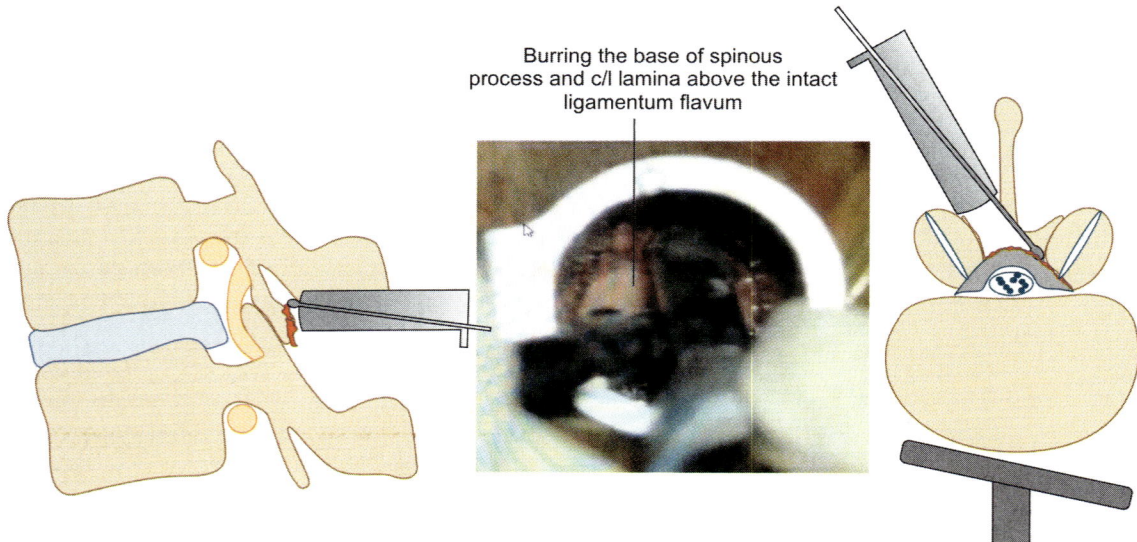

Fig. 20.6: Over the top decompression

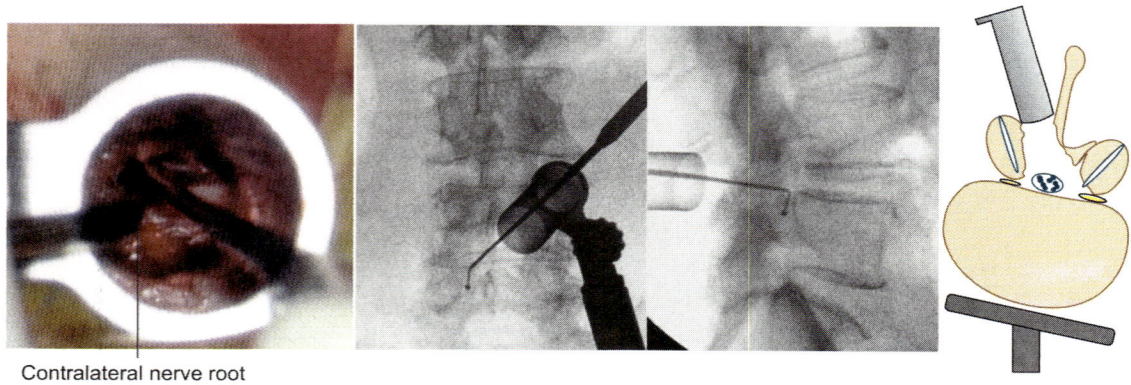

Fig. 20.7: Contralateral nerve root decompression

A dural retractor or a nerve hook is used to confirm if adequate decompression has been achieved. The nerve root is traced from its exit from the dura till it exits out of the foramen. Changing the direction of the tube superiorly and inferiorly and tilting the operating table aids in achieving this.

Ipsilateral Decompression (Fig. 20.8)

The tube is then turned back laterally and table turned towards the surgeon and the ipsilateral side is decompressed similarly. The nerve root on this side is similarly traced.

Hemostasis and Closure

Bleeding is controlled using a combination of bipolar cautery, bone wax and gel-foam. Fascia and subcutaneous tissue are closed using 2-0 Vicryl. Skin is closed using 3-0 Monocryl. Steri-strips are applied to hold the skin edges together. Waterproof dressing is applied. If another level is to be decompressed the same

	Pearls	Pitfalls
Table 20.1: Tubular decompression—pearls and pitfalls		
Preoperative evaluation	1. Proper clinicoradiological co-relation 2. Get instability X-rays 3. Evaluate for facetal orientations 4. Decide the side of approach	1. Chances of incomplete decompression or violation of the stable facet (especially ipsilateral): If proper note of anatomy not taken preoperatively
Surgical Tube docking	1. Get perfect lateral image 2. Start with spinal needle 1 cm away from midline parallel to the disc 3. Avoid use of sharp instruments 4. Use the first dilator to precisely feel the anatomical landmarks 5. Proper docking: Inferior part of superior lamina superiorly, interlaminar space inferiorly, spinous process medially and facet joint laterally and the tube should be precisely in line with the surgical corridor	1. Sharp guide wire may penetrate and cause dural injury 2. Lateral docking may cause injury to pars or facetal violation 3. Radiation hazard—use all possible protection gears like the lead apron and thyroid shield
Working through tube	1. Bony work first, keeping flavum intact to act as a shield 2. Tilting the table and angulations of tube for contralatral decompression: Adequately strap the patient 3. Use curved kerrison for decompression of difficult sites like the foramina 4. Bilateral pedicle to pedicle decompression 5. Avoid going too lateral 6. Use long and bayoneted instruments, specifically designed for MIS 7. Learn the art of proper use of burr	1. Learning curve—need training 2. Orientation of anatomy through the tube 3. In difficult situations like revision decompression/ severe stenosis/facetal cyst, the risk of inadvertent durotomy is high: Precisely and patiently separate the tissues adherent to the dura 4. Dural punctures—difficult to suture 5. Ipsilateral foraminotomy: Difficult to achieve

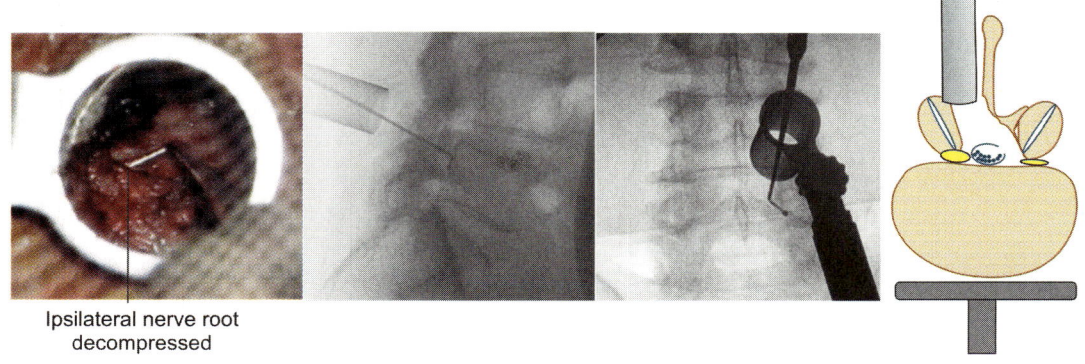

Ipsilateral nerve root decompressed

Fig. 20.8: Ipsilateral nerve root decompression, confirmation on C-arm and diagramatic representation

procedure is repeated with a separate incision on the contralateral side or it is sometimes possible to decompress L4–5 and L5–S1 levels through the same incision owing to the lordosis.

Technical Tips for Contralateral Decompression

1. Adequate contralateral decompression can be achieved through the same incision
2. L4–5 and L5–S1 levels may be approached through a single skin incision.
3. Patient should be tightly secured to the table to safely tilt the table on to the sides
4. Avoid using guide wires.
5. Select appropriate size of the tube so that it sits on the lamina properly to avoid muscle creep and can be freely angulated in all directions.
6. Long-bayonet instruments are required for an unobtructive visual field through the microscope.
7. Use of burr is mandatory to drill the base of the spinous process to approach contralateral side
8. Curved Kerrison ronguers aids in opposite lateral recess decompression.

Postoperative Management

Patient is mobilized the same evening and is discharged the next day. Only one dose of intravenous antibiotic is given the same night. Injectable analgesics are given on the day of surgery and oral analgesics the next day onwards. Patient is weaned off oral analgesics by the 5th day postoperatively. Bathing is allowed immediately. Patient can go back to light-duty work after 10 days and is not allowed to lift heavy weights. A gradual back strengthening program is started after 6 weeks. The scar usually shrinks to a size of 1.0 to 1.5 cm after healing (about 3 months).

Case example: A 62-year-old lady had bilateral lower limb radiating pain for 6 months. Claudication distance was less than 500 meters with paresthesia's both lower limbs. Patient did not get adequate relief with conservative treatment. Preoperative images (Fig. 20.9) revealed L5–S1 lumbar canal stenosis without instability. Patient was operated with microendoscopic decompression (MED). Intraoperative images show docking of tubular retractor for decompression of ipsilateral and contralateral nerve roots (over the top decompression) (Fig. 20.10). Note the relative position of the retractor and patient with C-arm images. Adequate decompression of nerve roots on the contralateral (Fig. 20.11) and ipsilateral side (Fig. 20.12) can be seen. The procedure was done through a very small incision (Fig. 20.13). Patient was adequately relived of her symptoms at follow up with MRI images showing adequacy of decompression (Fig. 20.14).

Complications

The most commonly reported complication is durotomy. Other complications include neurological injuries, inadvertent facet violation, postoperative hematoma and wrong level surgeries.[16–18] Small dural tears can be managed with masterly inactivity[19] but large tears may need the usage of fibrin glue to seal the tear. Use of sharp (Trocar tip) guide wires can lead to neurological injuries and dural tears and should be avoided. A laterally placed portal can lead to violation of the medial facet while executing ipsilateral decompression, requiring fusion. Spinous process fracture may occur while drilling the base. Inadequate decompression leading to an unfavorable outcome is a disappointing complication. One of the ways of avoiding this is to learn the technique from a master, by assisting a few simple and difficult cases. A good way of learning from mistakes is to perform a post-operative MRI and to keep a check on the locations of stenosis that one tends to miss and concentrate on them the next time.

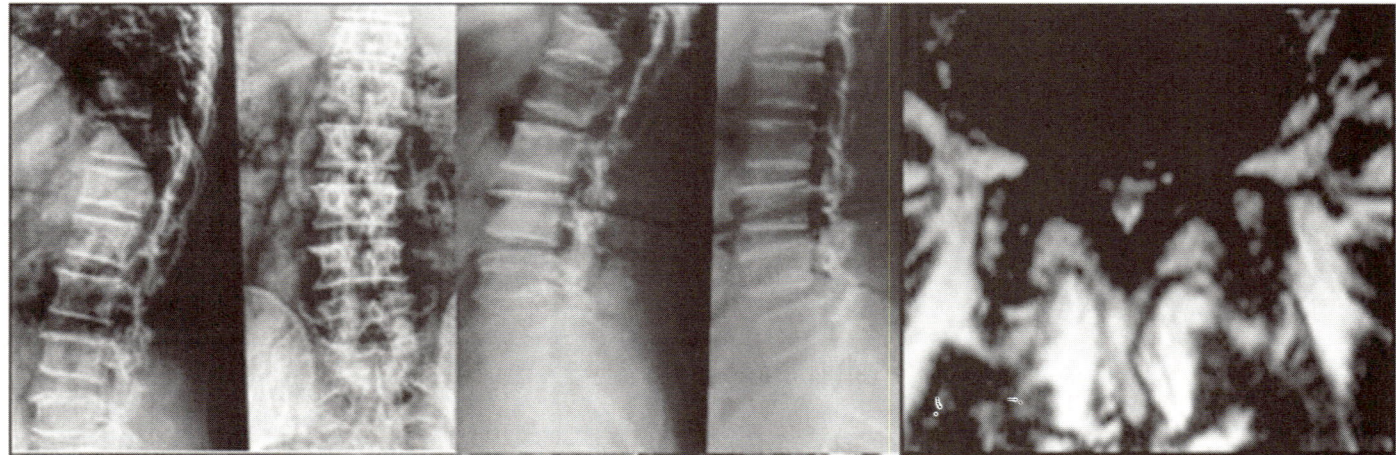

Fig. 20.9: Preoperative radiological images

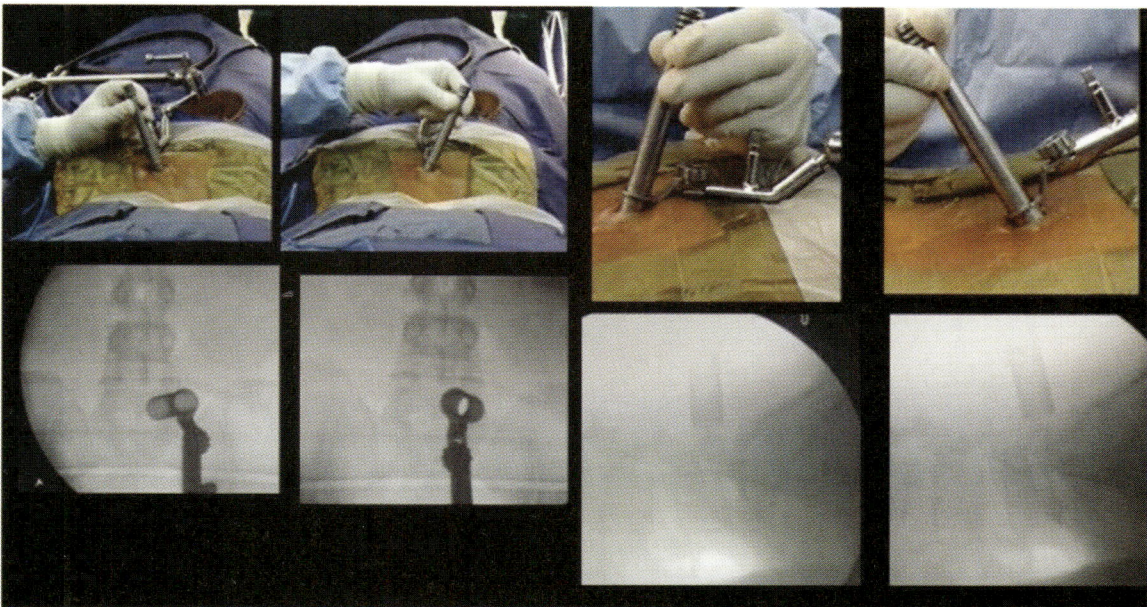

Fig. 20.10: Docking of tubular retractor for ipsilateral and over the top decompression

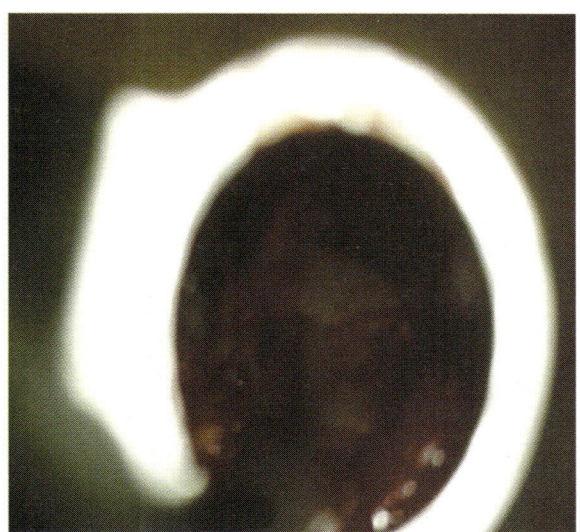

Fig. 20.11: Contralateral nerve root decompression

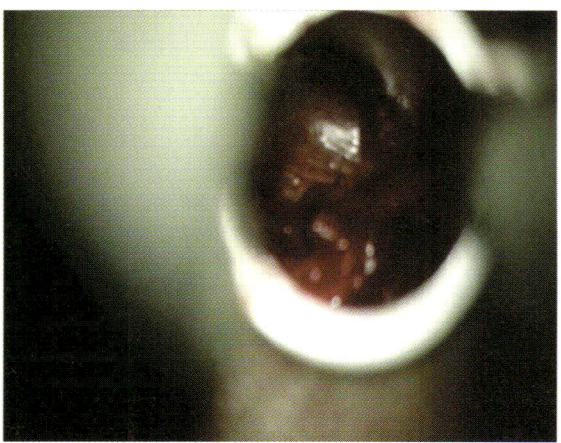

Fig. 20.12: Ipsilateral nerve root decompression

Surgeon's anatomical knowledge and painstaking attention to details helps in reducing the complication rates. The author prefers to complete the bony decompression first, with the intact ligamentum serving as a shield reducing the risk of durotomy as well as neurological injury. The sharp ends of the instruments should be directed away from dura and suction tip can be used as effective protection for the neural structures. The spinous process and the inferior edge of the lamina can be used as anatomical landmarks to prevent injury to critical supporting structures, such as the facets. Meticulous hemostasis should be used to prevent postoperative hematoma. Intraoperative fluoroscopy and proper assessment of the preoperative films (especially in the presence of transitional vertebrae) can prevent surgeries at wrong levels.

Author's Experience

At author's institution, almost all cases of single, two levels and occasionally 3-level lumbar canal stenosis without instability are operated with microendoscopic lumbar decompressive (MELD) technique. With vast experience in minimally invasive techniques, we found that MISS is associated with less postoperative infection rates[2] as compared to open techniques. In author's study of 1043 patients treated with MISS techniques, 763 underwent non-instrumented surgeries and 280 underwent instrumentation over a period of 8 years. The overall infection rate after MISS was 0.29% with surgical site infections (SSI) of 0% in non-instrumented cases. Authors concluded that MISS can markedly reduce the SSI rate and can be an effective tool to minimize hospital costs.[14]

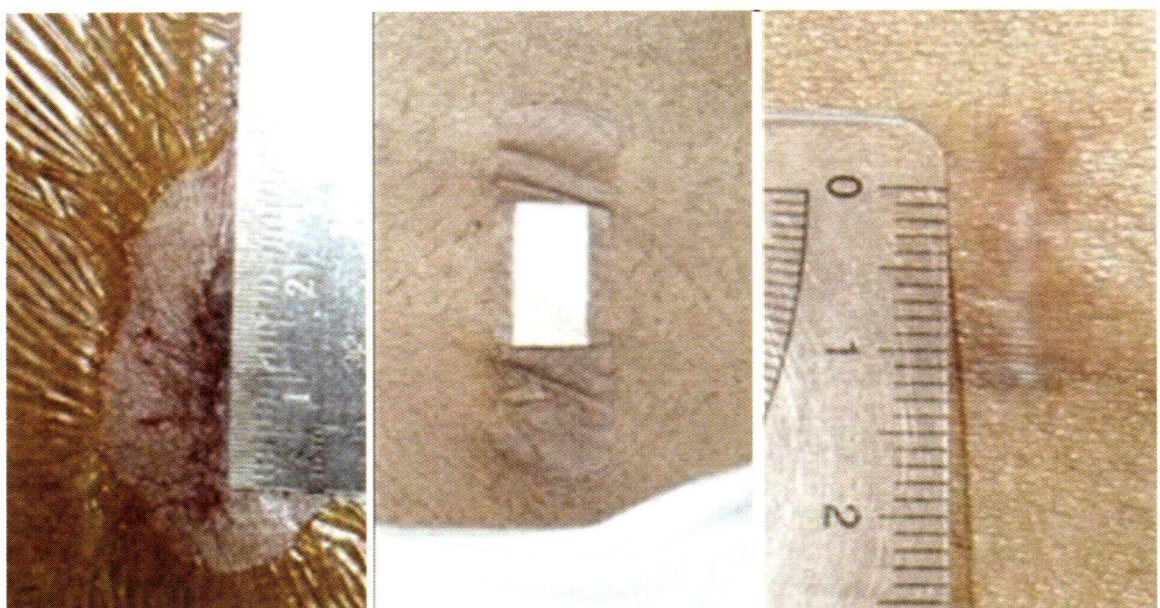

Fig. 20.13: Skin incision

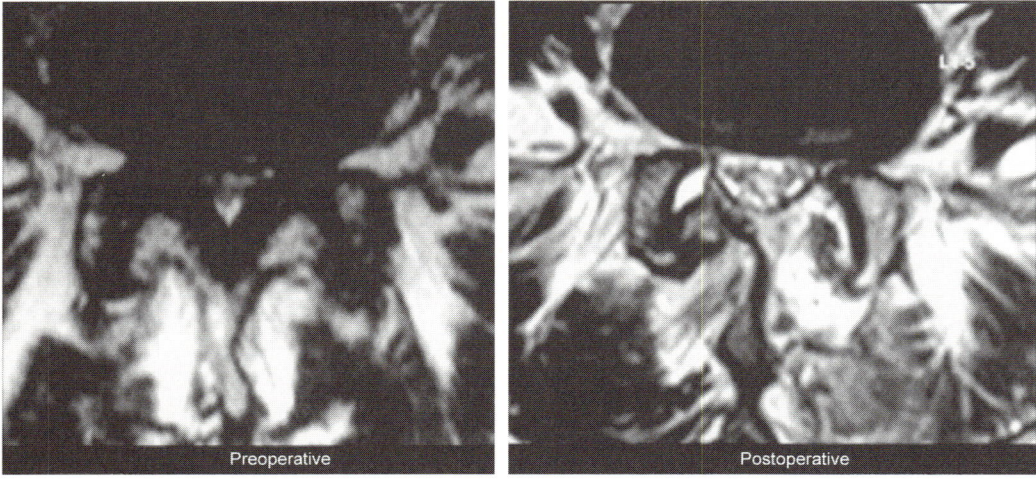

Fig. 20.14: Comparison of pre- and postoperative MRI images

The use of tubular retractor system for decompression can be extended to numerous pathological conditions. The traditional approach for treatment of lumbar intraspinal synovial cysts (LISC) is with decompression with or without fusion.[30,31] The authors believe that stand-alone decompression is sufficient in selected patients unless associated with gross instability. In a total of 30 patients with LISCs treated with isolated microdecompression technique at author's institution over a period of 6 years and a minimum follow up of 3 years, all patients reported good to excellent results with no cases of recurrence or reoperation.[28]

Similarly, in patients with stable degenerative spondylolisthesis (DS), MELD has little influence on the natural history of DS and can be done as stand-alone procedure without adding fusion. Authors conducted a study[13] wherein patients with DS were divided into 2 groups (stable DS and unstable DS) based on multiple clinical, morphological factors and functional expectations. Out of 329 patients, 41 patients were classified as having stable DS and underwent stand-alone decompression. At a minimum follow up of 3 years, 39 patients reported significant improvement in their symptoms. The author believes that this would have significant economic implications.

Conclusions

Tubular decompression technique for lumbar canal stenosis has significant advantage of decreasing the collateral tissue damage reflecting clinically as decreased postoperative pain, less bleeding, less infection rate, early rehabilitation and early return to work. There is a learning curve associated with this technique but once the expertise is achieved, the results are better than traditional open decompression technique.

REFERENCES

1. Atlas SJ, Keller RB, Robson D, et al. Surgical and non-surgical management of lumbar spinal stenosis: four year outcomes from Maine Lumbar Spine Study. Spine 2000;25:556–62.

2. Hurri H, Slatis P, Soini K, et al. Lumbar spinal stenosis: Assessment of long-term outcome 12 years after operative and conservative treatment. J Spinal Disord 1998;11:110–5.

3. Katz JN, Stucki G, Lipson SJ, et al. Predictors of surgical outcome in degenerative spinal stenosis. Spine 1999;21:2229–33.

4. Houten JK, Tandon A. Comparison of postoperative values for C-reactive protein in minimally invasive and open lumbar spinal fusion surgery. Surg Neurol Int 2011;2:94.

5. Schick U, et al. Microendoscopic Lumbar Discectomy versus open surgery: an introp EMG study. European Spine J 2002;Vol 11:20–26.

6. Khoo LT, Fessler RG. Microendoscopic decompressive laminotomy for the treatment of lumbar stenosis. Neurosurgery 2002;51:S146–S154.

7. Katayama Y, Matsuyama Y, Yoshihara H, Sakai Y, Nakamura H, Nakashima S, et al. Comparison of surgical outcomes between macro discectomy and micro discectomy for lumbar disc herniation: A prospective randomized study with surgery performed by the same spine surgeon. J Spinal Disord Tech 2006;19:344–7.

8. Larry Khoo, Fessler Richard. Microendoscopic Decompressive Laminotomy for the Treatment of Stenosis. Neurosurgery. Suppl 2002;51:146–54.

9. David Rosen, John O, et al. Minimally invasive Lumbar Spinal Decompression in the Elderly. Outcomes of 50 patients aged 75 years and older. Neurosurgery. Suppl 2007;60:503–10.

10. Sandhu FA1, Santiago P, Fessler RG, Palmer S Minimally invasive surgical treatment of lumbar synovial cysts. Neurosurgery. Jan 2004;54(1):107–11; discussion 111–2 .

11. Sehati N, Khoo LT, Holly LT. Treatment of lumbar synovial cysts using minimally invasive surgical techniques. Neurosurg Focus. 2006;Mar 15;20(3): E2.

12. Lumbar juxtafacet cyst resection: the facet sparing contralateral minimally invasive surgical approach. James A, Laufer I, Parikh K, Nagineni VV, Saleh TO, Härtl R. J Spinal Disord Tech. 2012;25:0–17.

13. Kulkarni AG, et al. Degenerative spondylolisthesis. Is it always unstable? A new scoring system to aid decision making and apply value based spine care. Podium presentation at VTI gold medal session at Association of Spine Surgeons of India [ASSICON] Conference, 2017.

14. Kulkarni AG, et al. Does Minimally Invasive Spine Surgery Minimize Surgical Site Infections?Asian Spine J. Dec 2016;10(6):1000–1006.

15. Kulkarni AG. The 'Nightmare' Of Wrong Level In Spine Surgery: Is Minimally Invasive Spine Technique More Forgiving? (Accepted for publication by JMISST, Korea)

16. Ikuta K, Tono O, Tanaka T, et al. Surgical complications of microendoscopic procedures for lumbar spinal stenosis. Minim Invasive Neurosurgery 2007;50(3):145–9.

17. Jhala A, Mistry M. Endoscopic Lumbar discectomy: experience of first 100 cases. Indian J Orthop 2010;44(2):184–90.

18. Podichetty VK, Spears J, Isaacs RE, et al. Complications assosiated with minimally invasive decompression fpr lumbar spinal stenosis. J Spinal Disord Tech 2006;19(3):161–6.

19. Kulkarni AG. Are Dural Tears in Minimal Invasive Spine Surgery of the Lumbar Spine More Forgiving than in Open Spine Surgery? Proceedings of the NASS 29th annual meeting/ The Spine Journal 2014;14;IS 183s.

20. Foley KT, Smith MM. Micro-endoscopic discectomy. Techniques in Neurosurgery 1997;3:301–7.

21. Outpatient spine surgery. In: Perez-Cruet MJ, Fessler RG, editors 1stediction. St. Louis (MO): Quality Medical Publishing; 2002.

22. Guiot BH, Khoo LT, Fessler RG. A minimally invasive technique for decompression of the lumbar spine. Spine 2002;27:432–8.

23. Stevens KJ, Spenciner DB, Griffiths KL, et al. Comparison of minimally invasive and conventional open posterolateral lumbar fusion using magnetic resonance imaging and retraction pressure studies. J Spinal Disord Tech 2006;19:77–86.

24. Kim KT, Lee SH, Suk KS, Bae SC. The quantitative analysis of tissue injury markers after mini open lumbar fusion. Spine (Phila Pa 1976) 2006;31:712–6 .

25. Asgarzadie F, Khoo LT. Minimally invasive operative management for lumbar spinal stenosis: overview of early and long-term outcomes. OrthopClin North Am 2007;38:387–99.

26. Palmer S, Turner R, Palmer R. Bilateral decompression of lumbar spinal stenosis involving a unilateral approach with microscope and tubular retractor system. J Neurosurg x; 2007;97:213–7.

27. Nowitzke AM. Assessment of the learning curve for lumbar microendosopic discectomy. Neurosurgery 2005;56:755–62.

28. Kulkarni AG, Dutta S, Dhruv A, Bassi A. Should we label all synovial cysts as unstable? Acceptd for publication by Global Spine Journal.

29. Kulkarni AG, Patel R, Dutta S, Patil V. Stand-alone Lateral Recess Decompression without Discectomy in Patients Presenting with Claudicant Radicular Pain and MRI Evidence of Lumbar Disc Herniation: A Prospective Study. Accepted for publication by Spine (Phila Pa 1976).

30. Nancy E. Epstein, MD. Lumbar Laminectomy for the Resection of Synovial Cysts and Coexisting Lumbar Spinal Stenosis or Degenerative Spondylolisthesis. SPINE 2004;29:1049–56.

31. Amir M. Khan, Federico Girardi. Spinal lumbar synovial cysts. Diagnosis and management challenge. Eur Spine J 2006;15:1176–82.

Microendoscopic MISS Surgery for Surgical Management of Lumbar Canal Stenosis

YR Yadav, Shailendra Ratre, Vijay Parihar, Amitesh Dubey

INTRODUCTION

Endoscopic surgery in routinely used in several cranial conditions and spine conditions.[7,14,18,38,53-64,66,68,73,75-80,82-84,86,88] The technique is also used in spinal conditions like cervical spine[36,69,70,81] lumbar disc disease,[8,65,72] spinal tumours,[34] and Arnold-Chiari malformations.[39]

Endoscopic surgery is being effectively utilized in the surgical management of lumbar canal stenosis with good results.[85,87] Results of bilateral decompression through unilateral approach have been found to be effective and safe.[5,49] Good dural decompression up to 408.0% (range: 211–774%) could be achieved by a unilateral approach.[46] Better visualization, short hospital stays, reduced morbidity, and lower cost are some of the advantages of endoscopic technique over the conventional open technique. Main advantage of endoscopic procedure is better visualization of contralateral compression on neural tissue with less tissue dissection. Another advantage of the procedure is that assistants and observers along with other operating staff can involve themselves in the procedure. It is good for teaching. This endoscopic spine technique is associated with steep learning curve, and the surgeon must be prepared to convert to an open procedure if needed.

This chapter is based on personal experience of 289 endoscopic surgeries performed for lumbar canal stenosis by the senior author and review of articles published in PubMed and Google in last 20 years.

Indications and Contraindications

The natural history of LCS is highly unpredictive as the symptoms do not necessarily worsen with progressive degeneration. The surgery thus should not be undertaken merely on radiological observations. Careful evaluation of symptoms and neurological signs is necessary before advising surgery. Surgery is indicated for those who do not improve with conservative management including medications like non-steroidal or steroidal anti-inflammatory drugs and or epidural injections. Surgery is indicated in the presence of neurological deficit and or loss of bladder or bowel function. Endoscopic technique can be used to effectively decompress lateral recess along the entire length of the nerve root from the spinal canal to the extra-foraminal space.[16,41,46,93,94] Usually unstable spine, prior lumbar surgery infection and trauma patients are not considered for endoscopic procedure.

Work-up for Surgery

Meticulous history and physical examination should be done to detect correct level of lesion responsible for symptoms. It is possible that the degeneration may appear widespread on radiological investigations. Patient's symptoms must correspond with radiological findings. Various parameters, such as anteroposterior diameter, cross-sectional area of the spinal dura are used for objective diagnosis of stenosis. For lateral stenosis, height and depth of the lateral recess must be measured and for foraminal stenosis the foraminal diameter should be measured.

X-rays in flexion and extension are performed to find out any instability. Upright radiographs usually demonstrate anterolisthesis better as compared with supine magnetic resonance imaging (MRI). The anterolisthesis of 5 mm or more is usually indicative of instability and further work-up should be done with the help of MRI[10] which is considered as the "gold standard" in the evaluation of lumbar canal stenosis (Fig. 21.1). It permits the assessment of the intervertebral disc, neural elements, ligaments and the thecal sac in a non-invasive manner.[50]

Up right MRI, it is useful in patients having neural compression not visualized on conventional MRI but

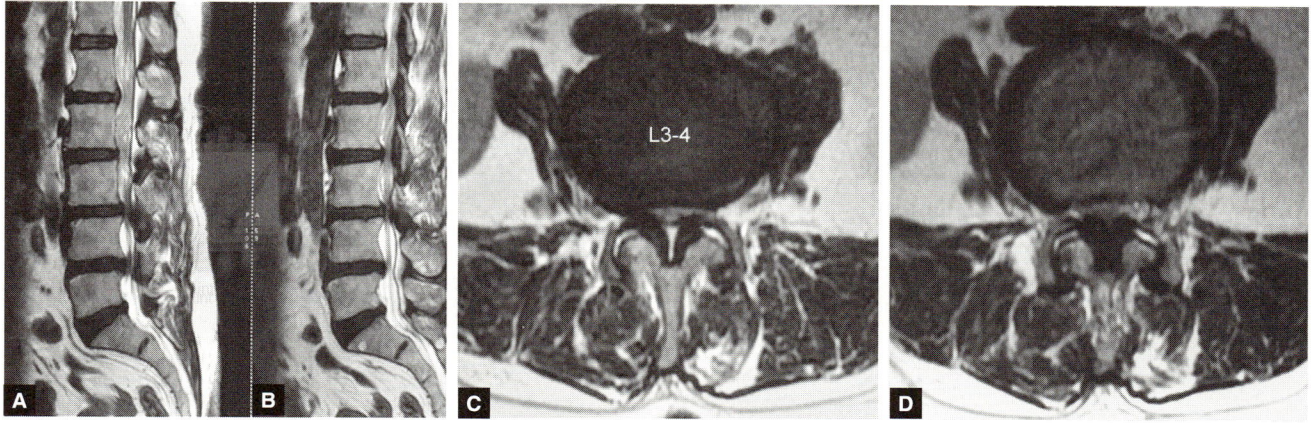

Fig. 21.1: Preoperative MRI showing two-level compression (L3–L4 and L4–L5) in sagittal (A and B) and axial cuts (C and D)

neural compression is suspected. The foraminal dimensions could be overestimated by conventional supine MRI.[23] Up right MRI may increase the diagnostic value in patients with obesity when spinal canal stenosis is suspected.[28] Dural sac cross-sectional area and sagittal AP diameter on standing MRI correlate significantly better than in supine MRI. Standing MRI also demonstrates dynamic changes of dural sac and provides an additional value to supine MRI in correlating clinical symptoms of lumbar spinal stenosis.[24] Although MRI is the standard imaging tool for diagnosis of lumbar spinal stenosis, there is a weak correlation between extent of stenosis and clinical findings.[43] Both ligamentum flavum thickness and the area of dural sac can be measured on MRI.[19]

Computed tomography (CT) scanning provides a more accurate account of the bony anatomy, but is less sensitive in estimating the soft-tissue components and is not usually sufficient as a stand-alone imaging modality. Computerized tomographic myelography and computerized tomographic discography can help in assessment of the prolapsed disc and nerve root. It can help in preventing nerve damage in selected patients. Myelography with water soluble contrast medium is not routinely used. Electrophysiological testing is rarely contributory, unless a diagnosis of peripheral neuropathy is being suspected.

Surgical Technique

Surgery is carried out in the prone position on a radiolucent operating table under general anesthesia. A small skin incision is taken after verifying the correct level under image guidance. Surgeon stands on the more symptomatic side or a right handed surgeon stands on the left side if the compression is similar on both sides. Which side to approach also depends on the position and angulation of spinous process. Approach should be from contralateral side to deviated

spinous process for easy positioning of endoscope.[37] Incision is made about 1–2 cm away from midline. Usually, one incision is adequate to decompress two adjacent levels.

Dilatation technique is used to gain access through subcutaneous fat, fascia and muscles rather than cutting the tissues to reduce surgical trauma. The operative sheath is placed at the desired level over ligamentum flavum and upper lamina. Soft-tissue on the lamina, facet joint and ligamentum flavum is excised. High-speed drill or kerrison punch are used to excise bone. An ultrasonic bone curette can be used for bone resection. Part of superior and inferior lamina along with the medial facet is excised. Removal of base of the spinous process, osteophytes of the opposite facet and under cutting of the opposite side lamina can be achieved by inclining the endoscope (Fig. 21.2). If the stenosis is gross then there is a chance of dural tear. To avoid it the ligamentum flavum is not removed until the bony resection is completed. En bloc flavectomy can then be performed with preservation of facet joints. Piece meal resection should be avoided as the small piece of ligamentum flavum retracts behind superior articular process making its removal difficult with chance of injury to facet joint.[13] Damage to facet joint can be prevented by removing the curled up ligamentum flavum with 45° forward angled curette. The offending disc when present is excised.

Proper hemostasis should be achieved before closure. Although hematomas over the dura can resolve spontaneously, it can result in poor expansion of the sac. It can delay patient recovery and lead to a poorer clinical improvement. The prevention of postoperative hematoma formation can avoid neurological deterioration.[49] Various systems, such as EasyGO (Karl Storz GmbH and Co KG Tuttlingen Germany), Destandau (Karl Storz GmbH and Co KG Tuttlingen Germany), SMART (Karl Storz GmbH and Co KG

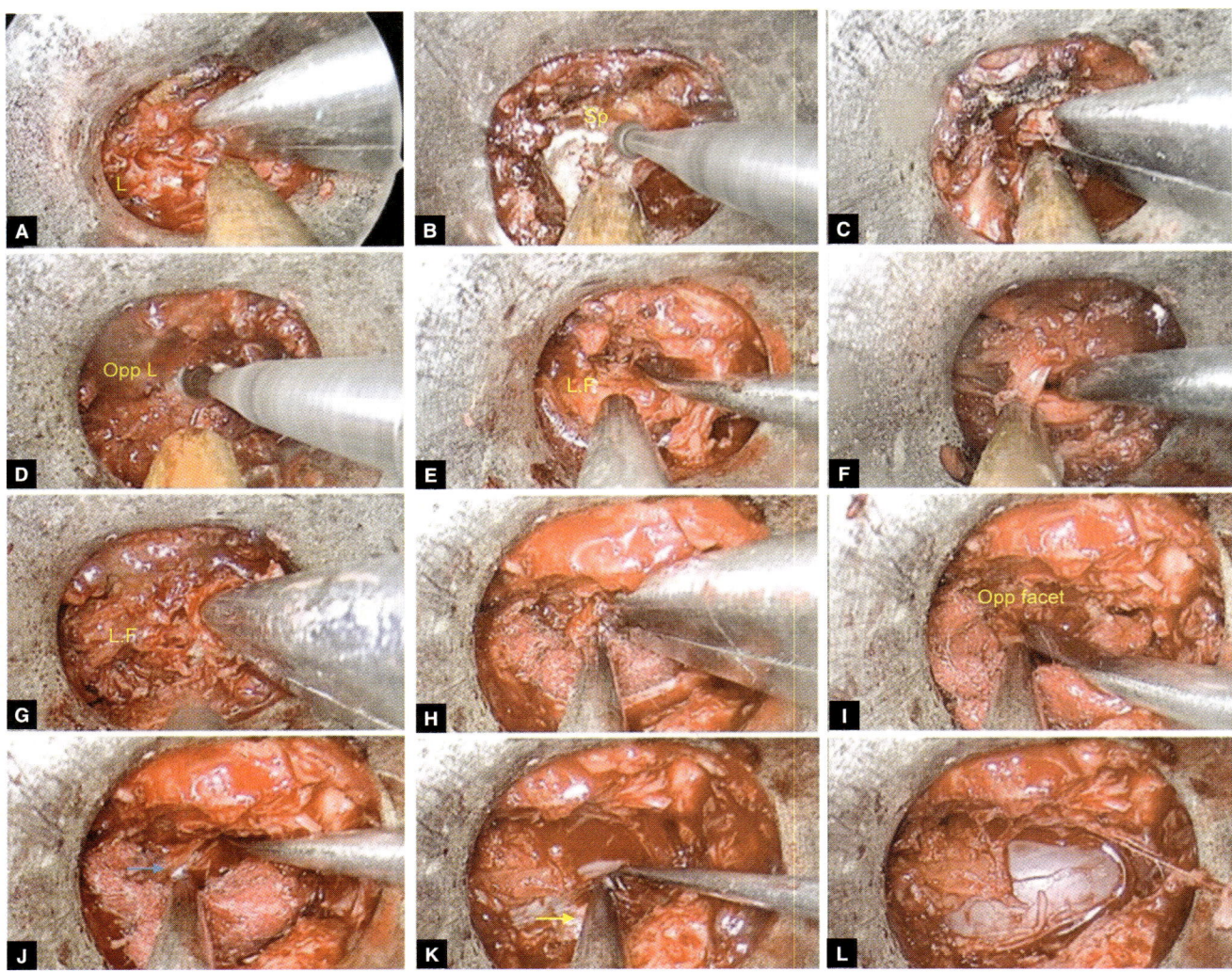

Fig. 21.2: (A) Removal of left hemi lamina, (B) drilling of under surface of spinous process, (C) removal of drilled paper-thin bone. (D) Drilling of under surface of opposite lamina, (E) detachment of ligamentum flavum from opposite facet and lamina and (F, G and H) removal of ligamentum flavum. (I) Visualised medial surface of opposite facet, (J) decompressed opposite root (Blue arrow), (K) decompressed ipsilateral nerve root (Yellow arrow) and (L) well-decompressed thecal sac. (L = Lamina; Sp = Spinous process; L.F = Ligamentum flavum)

Tuttlingen Germany) system, etc. are available commercially. All these systems are effective and safe. The technique can be combined with transforaminal approach for lumbar interbody fusion in selected patients with instability of less than grade 2 listhesis.[95] The combination of inter-spinous process implant fusion and endoscopic decompression can be used for decompression and stabilization of the spine.[27] Endoscopic LCS surgery should be performed after achieving good experience to prevent complications.[8,16,46,65]

Results of Surgery

In our department endoscopic surgery as performed on 289 stenotic levels in 240 patients. There was preponderance of males with 186 patients as against 56 female patients age ranged from 36 to 69 years with

an average of 57 years. In 191 patient the stenosis was at one level and in 49 patients the stenosis was at two levels out of 289 stenotic levels, compression was seen at L4–L5, L5–S1, L3–4, L2–L3 and L1–2 levels in 132, 114, 35, 6 and 2 patients, respectively. Most of our patients (n = 216, 90%) showed good clinical improvement after endoscopic decompression. One hundred eighty (75%) patients did not complain of any pain after surgery and did not require any analgesics. Thirty-six patients (15%) continued to have intermittent pain requiring occasional pain medication. Twenty-four patients (10%) required continuous pain medication for pain relief after decompression. Similar results were observed in other reported series.[4,21,40,96] The clinical results were excellent in Xu et al series with 65.6% and 34.4% patients had excellent and good pain relief respectively according to the Macnab scale.[49] Wada et al also reported improvement in the mean Japanese Orthopaedic Association (JOA) score from 17.0 to 23.3 after surgery.[46]

In our and other series the endoscopic surgical decompression in lumbar canal stenosis has given good results and can be used as a valid alternative to open technique for one and two level stenosis.[44] The procedure is less invasive and more safer than the microscopic procedure.[12,22]

The operative time was 72 minutes for single level and the average blood loss was 30 ml. Similar observations of less operative time (mean 70 min, range, 50–100 min for single level) and the blood loss (mean 150 ml, range, 50–350 ml) was observed in other endoscopic series.[49]

Nerve root canal decompression by microendoscopic disectomy for the treatment of lumbar canal stenosis is an effective procedure.[91] We used uniportal and unilateral approach for bilateral decompression (Figs 21.3 and 21.4).[25] Biportal technique has also been described:[9] We were able to decompress spinal dura satisfactorily.[5] There was significant improvement in AP diameter (4.75–1.75 mm to 10.33–2.11 mm), interfacet distance (12.70–4.86 mm to 18.92–3.53 mm), and dural surface area (76.45–25.36 mm^2 to 187.13–41.04 mm^2) after decompression. Significant improvement was noted in mean height and angle of lateral recess after surgery of both sides suggesting that effective decompression of the canal bilaterally was possible using a unilateral approach.[5] The mean vertebral canal area and sagittal diameter of the lateral recess were significantly larger at 6 months and 2 years follow-up compared with measurements taken before surgery.[96] Bilateral decompression with a unilateral approach can increase the area of the dural tube up to 408.0% (range: 211–774%).[46]

We were satisfies with satisfactory bilateral decompression by unilateral approach.[21] Guiot et al used one of the four procedures (unilateral microendoscopic laminotomy, bilateral microendoscopic laminotomy, unilateral open laminotomy and bilateral open laminotomy) in cadavers. Satisfactory improvement in the spinal canal midsagittal, interpedicular dimensions was achieved in all the four procedures. The exiting nerve roots were well-visualized using any one of these techniques. Complications, including dural tears and facet complex instability, is a possibility.[15]

Endoscopic decompression alone without fusion was associated with good outcome, at 3 years follow up, even in patients with lumbar degenerative spondylolisthesis.[45]

Although we did not do fusion with the help of endoscope, bilateral decompression and fusion could be achieved with good results using unilateral approach when needed.[51]

Complications

Complications like dural tear, hematoma formation, facet joint injury and neural injury are possible but the complication rate was low in the endoscopic group.[15,21] Clinical results in severe bilateral osseous stenosis may not be good using this technique.[41] The result of endoscopic decompression is usually poor if back pain

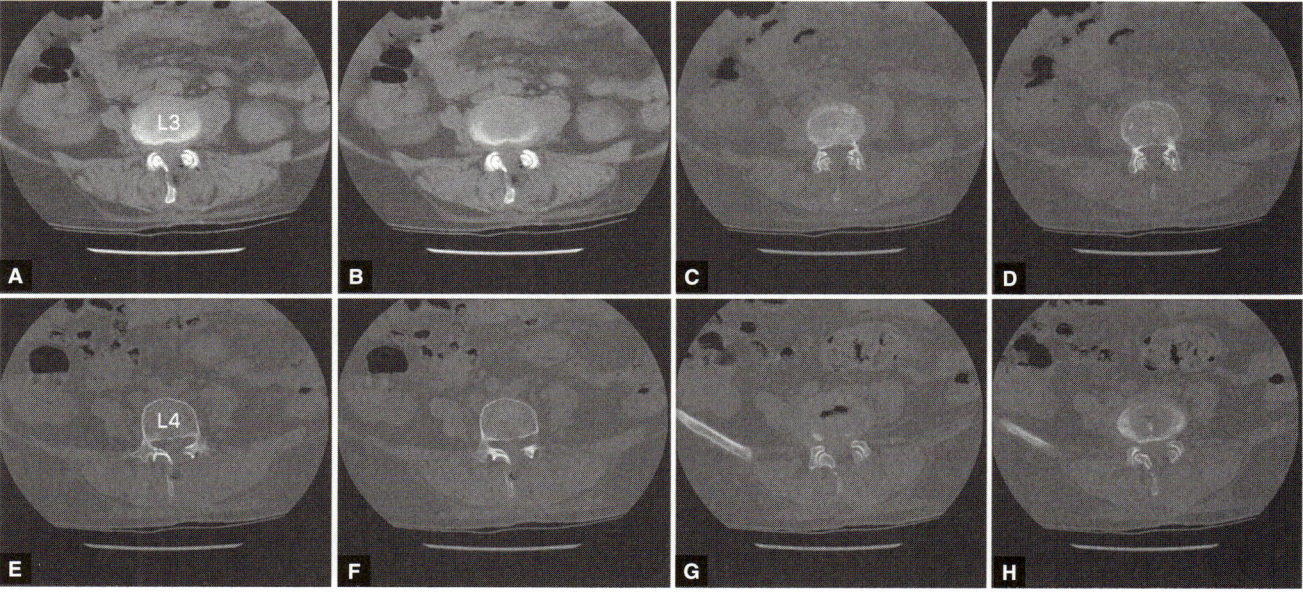

Fig. 21.3: Postoperative CT scan showing drilling of base of spinous process (A, B) with undercutting of opposite side lamina and decompressed canal, (C and D) at L3-4 level. Similarly, base of spinous process, (E and F) and canal, (G and H) at L4-5 level is well decompressed

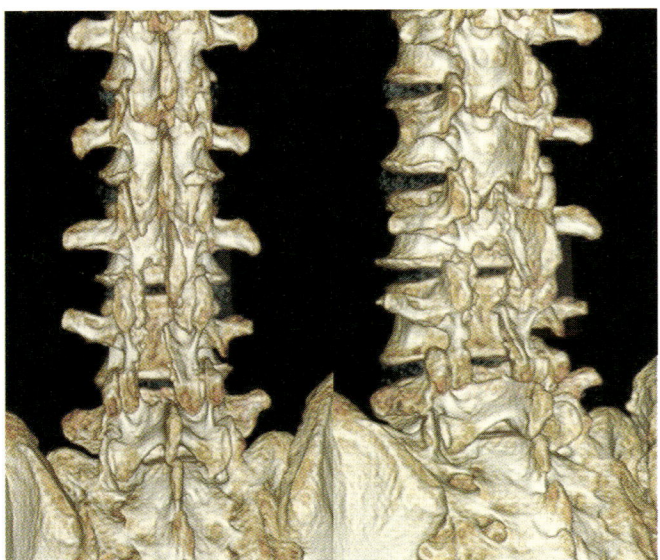

Fig. 21.4: Reconstructed image showing removal of left lower L3, and L4 lamina with sparing of spine and opposite lamina

is out of proportion to the leg symptoms and such patients should be investigated for instability. Preoperative lumbar lordosis is associated with good outcome after decompression.[2] Correction of sagittal balance significantly affected the outcome of patients.[3] Greater multifidus muscle fatty infiltration and decreased cross-sectional area of psoas muscles were associated with poor outcome.[11] Similarly, the prognosis in patients suffering from cervical spondylosis in tandem were not encouraging.[89]

Advantages

Endoscopic techniques can achieve adequate decompression with reduced morbidity to the patient. It is less invasive with less chances of facet joint injury. Less facet injury could be the reason why endoscopic decompression alone without fusion was associated with good outcome, at 3 years follow-up in patients with lumbar degenerative spondylolisthesis.[45] Although the size of skin incision can be comparable in the endoscopic technique and microscopic approach, main advantage of endoscopic procedure is better visualization and excision of contralateral compressive pathology.[15]

Limitations

The limitations of this procedure are more operating time for multiple level compressions and steep learning curve. Complication rate could be more in the initial learning curve.[41,65] The learning curve for this surgery could be 30 cases. The learning curve of microendoscopic decompression surgery for LCS was defined by a single surgeon in an institution as follows: The operating time seems to decrease along a natural logarithmic function. The intraoperative blood loss gets lesser after the first 30 cases.[31] All the same perioperative complications can occur at any time even after mastering the technique.[31]

Avoiding Complication

Bleeding improper positioning of the patient and increase in the resistance during ventilation can cause excessive bleeding. Gentle pressure by surgical patties and warm saline irrigation helps in stopping such bleeding. Sometime there may be the problem during surgery when brisk bleeding causes staining of lens tip. Keeping telescope away from the bleeding site allows proper visualization and control of bleeding. Bimanual technique using bipolar electrocautery and suction can be used to control bleeding. Normally compression by the sheath of the endoscope on the surrounding tissues helps in preventing small oozing. Minor ooze may occur from adjoining operative site when more than one incision is used for multi level compression. Gentle gauze packing of the other operative site can prevent such bleeding. Cranial and caudal gauze packing can also prevent bleeding.

Tissue coming inside the tube: Excessive cranial or caudal angulations of the operative sheath can allow unwanted tissues (muscle, fat or ligament, etc.) to come inside the tube, which may obscure visualization and proper execution of the surgery. Some angulations (up to 20–30°) may be allowed. Keeping sheath as vertical as possible prevents entry of such tissues. If the tube needs to be moved cranially or caudally it has to be pushed cranially or caudally respectively keeping it as vertical as possible.

Dural tear: Dural tear may occur in any lumbar surgery. Incidence is high in the beginning of the learning curve. Severe canal stenosis and in multiple level compressions the dura can get injured. This can be prevented by keeping ligamentum flavum intact until all the bony decompression is over. This can also be prevented by keeping surgical patties between the dura mater and ligamentum flavum or the bone. It can also be prevented by partially retracting the Kerrison punch after nibbling of the bone or excision of ligamentum flavum. Holding the proximal part of the tissue before it is completely detached and removed can prevent dural injury. Cerebrospinal fluid leak due to the dural tears can be stopped by sealing the rent with a fascia patch and tissue glue or by using dura synthetic patch and tissue glue.

Visual obscuration: There are several causes of poor vision during surgery, such as incorrect system assembly, damaged lenses, fogging of lenses and scope out of focus. Fogging of the lens and visual obscuration may occur due to excessive moisture in the media, staining of lens by blood, bone dust or any tissue, etc. The lens fogging usually occurs when there is an imbalance between the temperature of the lens, temperature of the airway cavity and humidity of the environment. Telescope can be removed and cleaned. Warm saline irrigation can also be used to clean lens tip. Suction of air containing excessive moisture from the operative area can improve vision. Anti-fogging agents, such as baby shampoo, savlon and provodine scrub are very effective agents. Sometime undesired tissue may come in front of the lens and obscure visualization of desired structures. Proper positioning of telescope (slight withdrawal from the obstructing tissue), moving telescope cranial, caudal or to the side, away from the obstructing object, can improve visualization. Obstructing tissue can be removed. Bone drilling in LCS can prolong operative time due to frequently staining of telescope tip by bone dust or saline. This problem can be partly avoided by keeping telescope as far away as possible from the drilling site and by using intermittent irrigation in between the short period of drilling. It is helpful to use lower revolutions per minute to reduce staining during the drilling.

Steep learning curve: This technique is associated with a steep learning curve. This learning curve can be improved by attending live operative workshops, practice on models and hands on cadaveric dissection.[63,65] Training in laboratory can help in learning endoscopic surgery.[52,67,71,74] An exoscope system (video telescopic operating monitor) can be used for learning endoscopy.[35] Training with indigenous Inexpensive models can be used for skill development in neuroendoscopy.[1]

Other minimally invasive technique for LCS: Midline microendoscopic decompression technique was associated with improved outcome in terms of the VAS score from 3 months and JOA scores over 3 years of follow-up. This technique enables preservation of paravertebral muscles and bilateral facet joints.[29] The results of decompression using paramedian approach were comparable to the midline approach in lumbar spinal canal stenosis.[20]

The chimney sublaminar decompression technique for the degenerative LCS can be used, which do not require stripping of the paravertebral muscles. Excellent, good and fair outcomes were achieved in 61%, 28%, and 11% patients, respectively. No patient required any brace and there was no worsening of pre-existing spondylolisthesis. The spinal canal was increased to 2- to 6.8-fold (mean 4.2 fold) of the pre-operative size.[26]

Microscopic bilateral decompression via a unilateral approach was also found to be effective with prevention of postoperative spinal instability due to preservation of the posterior elements including the facet joints.[6] Similarly, microscopic discectomy using tubular retractor have been found to be safe and effective.[33]

Two 0.5 cm port technique with one for the endoscope and the other for instruments can be used. This technique with irrigation allows the surgeon to safely perform effective central and foraminal decompression in LCS. Substituting long surgical incisions with 0.5 cm stabs and direct placement of instruments without dissection or dilatation could result in an improved postoperative course, shortened time for hospitalization, and reduced infection rate. However, still multicenter studies and randomized trials are needed before making final conclusions about this technique.[42]

Conclusions

The percutaneous endoscopic transforaminal lumbar spinal canal decompression was found to be simple, safe, and effective minimally invasive surgery for patients with lumbar spinal stenosis.[32,47,92] It was also used in foraminal stenosis.[90] On the other hand Xiong et al found that although transforaminal technique has been reported to be safe and minimally-invasive to treat lumbar spinal stenosis associated with disk herniation, potential complications still should be given a careful consideration.[48] Nellensteijn et al observed that there was no valid evidence from randomized controlled trials on the effectiveness of transforaminal endoscopic surgery for lumbar stenosis.[30] Two approaches of transforaminal decompression and oblique lateral lumbar interbody fusion can be combined.[17]

REFERENCES

1. Bajaj J, Yadav YR, Pateriya A, Parihar V, Ratre S, Dubey A. Indigenous Inexpensive practice models for skill development in Neuroendoscopy. J Neurosci Rural Pract 2017;8(2):170–3.
2. Chang HS. Influence of Lumbar Lordosis on the Outcome of Decompression Surgery for Lumbar Canal Stenosis. World Neurosurg 2018;109:e684–90.
3. Chang HS. Effect of Sagittal Spinal Balance on the Outcome of Decompression Surgery for Lumbar Canal Stenosis. World Neurosurg. pii: 2018 Jul 20;S1878–8750(18)31582–1.
4. Choi G, Pophale CS, Patel B, Uniyal P. Endoscopic Spine Surgery. J Korean Neurosurg Soc 2017;60(5):485–97.
5. Dewangan NK, Yadav YR, Parihar V, Ratre S, Kher Y, Bhatele PR. Extent of decompression of lumbar spinal canal after endoscopic surgery. J Neurol Surg A Cent Eur Neurosurg 2017;78(6):541–7.
6. Dohzono S, Matsumura A, Terai H, Toyoda H, Suzuki A, Nakamura H. Radiographic evaluation of postoperative bone re-

growth after microscopic bilateral decompression via a unilateral approach for degenerative lumbar spondylolisthesis. J Neurosurg Spine 2013;18(5):472–8.

7. Dubey A, Yadav N, Ratre S, Parihar VS, Yadav YR. Full endoscopic vascular decompression in trigeminal neuralgia: Experience of 230 Patients. World Neurosurg. pii: 2018 Feb 24;S1878-8750(18)30381–4.

8. Dubey A, Yadav N, Ratre S, Parihar VS, Yadav YR. Lumbar Microendoscopic Discectomy: Clinical Results of 920 Patients? The Journal of Spinal Surgery 2018;5(1):1–6.

9. Eun SS, Eum JH, Lee SH, Sabal LA. Biportal Endoscopic Lumbar Decompression for Lumbar Disk Herniation and Spinal Canal Stenosis: A Technical Note. J Neurol Surg A Cent Eur Neurosurg. 2017;78(4):390–6.

10. Finkenstaedt T, Del Grande F, Bolog N, Ulrich NH, Tok S, Burgstaller JM, Steurer J, Chung CB, Andreisek G, Winklhofer S; LSOS working group. Correlation of listhesis on upright radiographs and central lumbar spinal canal stenosis on supine MRI: is it possible to predict lumbar spinal canal stenosis? Skeletal Radiol. 2018;47(9):1269–75.

11. Fortin M, Lazáry À, Varga PP, Battié MC. Association between paraspinal muscle morphology, clinical symptoms and functional status in patients with lumbar spinal stenosis. Eur Spine J. 2017;26(10):2543–51.

12. Fujimoto T, Taniwaki T, Tahata S, Nakamura T, Mizuta H. Patient outcomes for a minimally invasive approach to treat lumbar spinal canal stenosis: is microendoscopic or microscopic decompressive laminotomy the less invasive surgery? Clin Neurol Neurosurg. 2015;131:21–5.

13. Fujiwara Y, Manabe H, Sumida T, Izumi B, Nakanishi K, Tanaka N, Adachi N. Facet Preserving Technique by En Bloc Flavectomy in Microscopic Posterior Decompression Surgery for Lumbar Spinal Stenosis: Semicircumferential Decompression (SCD). Clin Spine Surg 2017;30(5):197–203.

14. Gajdhar M, Yadav YR. A case of thalamic abscess treated by endoscopic surgery. Neurology India 2005;53:345–6.

15. Guiot BH, Khoo LT, Fessler RG. A minimally invasive technique for decompression of the lumbar spine. Spine (Phila Pa 1976) 2002; 27:432–8.

16. Ikuta K, Tono O, Tanaka T, Arima J, Nakano S, Sasaki K, Oga M. Surgical complications of microendoscopic procedures for lumbar spinal stenosis. Minim Invasive Neurosurg 2007;50:145–9.

17. Katzell J. Endoscopic foraminal decompression preceding oblique lateral lumbar interbody fusion to decrease the incidence of post operative dysaesthesia. Int J Spine Surg. 8, 2014 Dec 1; doi: 10.14444/1019. eCollection 2014.

18. Kher Y, Yadav N, Yadav YR, Parihar V, Ratre S, Bajaj J. Endoscopic Vascular Decompression in trigeminal Neuralgia. Turk Neurosurg. 2016 May 25. doi: 10.5137/1019-5149.JTN.17046–16.1. [Epub ahead of print]

19. Kim YU, Park JY, Kim DH, Karm MH, Lee JY, Yoo JI, Chon SW, Suh JH. The Role of the Ligamentum Flavum Area as a Morphological Parameter of Lumbar Central Spinal Stenosis. Pain Physician 2017;20(3):E419–4.

20. Komatsu J, Muta T, Nagura N, Iwabuchi M, Fukuda H, Kaneko K, Shirado O. Tubular surgery with the assistance of endoscopic surgery via a paramedian or midline approach for lumbar spinal canal stenosis at the L4/5 level. J Orthop Surg (Hong Kong). 26(2):2309499018782546, 2018. doi: 10.1177/2309499018782546.

21. Komp M, Hahn P, Merk H, Godolias G, Ruetten S. Bilateral operation of lumbar degenerative central spinal stenosis in full-endoscopic interlaminar technique with unilateral approach: Prospective 2-year results of 74 patients. J Spinal Disord Tech 2011;24:281–7.

22. Komp M, Hahn P, Oezdemir S, Giannakopoulos A, Heikenfeld R, Kasch R, Merk H, Godolias G, Ruetten S. Bilateral spinal decompression of lumbar central stenosis with the full-endoscopic interlaminar versus microsurgical laminotomy technique: a pro-

spective, randomized, controlled study. Pain Physician 2015; 18(1):61–70.

23. Lang G, Vicari M, Siller A, Kubosch EJ, Hennig J, Südkamp NP, Izadpanah K, Kubosch D. Preoperative Assessment of Neural Elements in Lumbar Spinal Stenosis by Upright Magnetic Resonance Imaging: An Implication for Routine Practice? Cureus. 10(4):e2440, 2018 Apr 6. doi: 10.7759/cureus.2440.

24. Lau YYO, Lee RKL, Griffith JF, Chan CLY, Law SW, Kwok KO. Changes in dural sac caliber with standing MRI improve correlation with symptoms of lumbar spinal stenosis. Eur Spine J 2017; 26(10):2666–75.

25. Lee CW, Yoon KJ, Jun JH. Percutaneous Endoscopic Laminotomy with Flavectomy by Uniportal, Unilateral Approach for the Lumbar Canal or Lateral Recess Stenosis. World Neurosurg 2018; 113:e129-37.

26. Lin SM, Tseng SH, Yang JC, Tu CC. Chimney sublaminar decompression for degenerative lumbar spinal stenosis. J Neurosurg Spine 2006;4:359–64.

27. Liu G, Zhao JN, Dezawa A. Endoscopic decompression combined with interspinous process implant fusion for lumbar spinal stenosis. Chin J Traumatol 2008;11:364–7.

28. Lorenc T, Palczewski P, Wójcik D, Glinkowski W, Go?e?biowski M. Diagnostic Benefits of Axial-Loaded MRI Over Recumbent MRI in Obese LBP Patients. Spine (Phila Pa 1976). 2017 Dec 26. doi: 10.1097/BRS.02532. [Epub ahead of print]

29. Mikami Y, Nagae M, Ikeda T, Tonomura H, Fujiwara H, Kubo T. Tubular surgery with the assistance of endoscopic surgery via midline approach for lumbar spinal canal stenosis: a technical note. Eur Spine J 2013;22(9):2105–12.

30. Nellensteijn J, Ostelo R, Bartels R, Peul W, van Royen B, van Tulder M. Transforaminal endoscopic surgery for lumbar stenosis: A systematic review. Eur Spine J 2010;19:879–86.

31. Nomura K, Yoshida M. Assessment of the Learning Curve for Microendoscopic Decompression Surgery for Lumbar Spinal Canal Stenosis through an Analysis of 480 Cases Involving a Single Surgeon. Global Spine J 2017;7(1):54–8.

32. Oyelese AA, Fridley J, Choi DB, Telfeian A, Gokaslan ZL. Minimally invasive direct lateral, retroperitoneal transforaminal approach for large L1-2 disc herniations with intraoperative CT navigational assistance: technical note and report of 3 cases. J Neurosurg Spine 2018;29(1):46–53.

33. Palmer S. Use of a tubular retractor system in microscopic lumbar discectomy: 1 year prospective results in 135 patients. Neurosurg Focus 2002;13:e5.

34. Parihar VS, Yadav N, Yadav YR, Ratre S, Bajaj J, Kher Y. Endoscopic management of spinal intradural extra-medullary tumors. J Neurol Surg A Cent Eur Neurosurg 2017;78(3):219–26.

35. Parihar V, Yadav YR, Kher Y, Ratre S, Sethi A, Sharma D. Learning neuroendoscopy with an exoscope system (video telescopic operating monitor): Early clinical results. Asian J Neurosurg 2016;11:421–6.

36. Parihar VS, Yadav N, Ratre S, Amitesh Dubey M, Yadav YR. Endoscopic anterior approach for cervical disc disease (disc preserving surgery). World Neurosurg. 2018 Apr 24. pii: S1878-8750(18)30827-1. doi: 10.1016/j.wneu.2018.04.107. [Epub ahead of print]

37. Phan K, Teng I, Schultz K, Mobbs RJ. Treatment of Lumbar Spinal Stenosis by Microscopic Unilateral Laminectomy for Bilateral Decompression: A Technical Note. Orthop Surg 2017;9(2):241–6.

38. Ratre S, Yadav YR, Parihar VS, Kher Y. Micro-endoscopic removal of deep-seated brain tumors using tubular retraction system. J Neurol Surg A Cent Eur Neurosurg 2016;77(4):312–20.

39. Ratre S, Yadav N, Yadav YR, Parihar V, Bajaj J, Kher Y. Endoscopic management of Arnold Chiari Malformation type 1 with or without syringomyelia. J Neurol Surg A Cent Eur Neurosurg 2018; 79(1):45–51.

40. Ruetten S. Full-endoscopic Operations of the Spine in Disk Herniations and Spinal Stenosis. Surg Technol Int. 2011;21:284–98.

41. Sairyo K, Sakai T, Higashino K, Inoue M, Yasui N, Dezawa A. Complications of endoscopic lumbar decompression surgery. Minim Invasive Neurosurg 2010;53:175–8.

42. Soliman HM. Irrigation endoscopic decompressive laminotomy. A new endoscopic approach for spinal stenosis decompression. Spine J. 2015;15(10):2282–9.

43. Splettstößer A, Khan MF, Zimmermann B, Vogl TJ, Ackermann H, Middendorp M, Maataoui A. Correlation of lumbar lateral recess stenosis in magnetic resonance imaging and clinical symptoms. World J Radiol 2017;9(5):223–9.

44. Tacconi L, Spinelli R. Lumbar canal stenosis: can we treat it endoscopically? Our experience. J Neurosurg Sci. 2018 May 28. doi: 10.23736/S0390-5616.18.04416-8. [Epub ahead of print]?

45. Ulrich NH, Gravestock I, Held U, Schawkat K, Pichierri G, Wertli MM, Winklhofer S, Farshad M, Porchet F, Steurer J, Burgstaller JM. Does Preoperative Degenerative Spondylolisthesis Influence Outcome in Degenerative Lumbar Spinal Stenosis? Three-Year Results of a Swiss Prospective Multicenter Cohort Study. World Neurosurg. 114:e1275–83, 2018 Jun.

46. Wada K, Sairyo K, Sakai T, Yasui N. Minimally invasive endoscopic bilateral decompression with a unilateral approach (endo-BiDUA) for elderly patients with lumbar spinal canal stenosis. Minim Invasive Neurosurg 2010;53:65–8.

47. Wen B, Zhang X, Zhang L, Huang P, Zheng G. Percutaneous endoscopic transforaminal lumbar spinal canal decompression for lumbar spinal stenosis. Medicine (Baltimore). 2016;95(50): e5186.

48. Xiong C, Li T, Kang H, Hu H, Han J, Xu F. Early outcomes of 270-degree spinal canal decompression by using TESSYS-ISEE technique in patients with lumbar spinal stenosis combined with disk herniation. Eur Spine J. 2018 Jun 16. doi: 10.1007/s00586-018-5655-4. [Epub ahead of print]

49. Xu BS, Tan QS, Xia Q, Ji N, Hu YC. Bilateral decompression via unilateral fenestration using mobile microendoscopic discectomy technique for lumbar spinal stenosis. Orthop Surg 2010;2:106–10.

50. Xu BS, Xia Q, Ma XL, Yang Q, Ji N, Shah S, He J, Liu Y. The usefulness of magnetic resonance imaging for sequestered lumbar disc herniation treated with endoscopic surgery. J Xray Sci Technol 2012;20:373–81.

51. Xu B, Xu H, Ma X, Liu Y, Yang Q, Jiang H, Li N, Ji N. Bilateral decompression and intervertebral fusion via unilateral fenestration for complex lumbar spinal stenosis with a mobile microendoscopic technique. Medicine (Baltimore). 97(4):e9715, 2018. doi: 10.1097/MD.0000000000009715.

52. Yadav YR, Bajaj J, Parihar VS, Ratre S, Pateriya A. Practical aspects in neuroendoscopic techniques and complication avoidance: A systematic review. Turk Neurosurg. 2018;28(3):329–40.

53. Yadav YR, Basoor A, Todorov M, Parihar V. Endoscopic management of large multicompartmental intraventricular arachnoid cyst extending from foramen magnum to foramen of Monro. Neurol India 2010;58:481–84.

54. Yadav YR, Jaiswal S, Adam N, Basoor A, Jain G. Endoscopic third ventriculostomy in infants. Neurol India. 2006;54(2):161–3.

55. Yadav YR, Madhariya SN, Parihar VS, Namdev H, Bhatele PR. Endoscopic Transoral Excision of Odontoid Process in Irreducible Atlantoaxial Dislocation: Our Experience of 34 Patients. J Neurol Surg A Cent Eur Neurosurg. 2013;74(3):162–7.

56. Yadav YR, Mukerji G, Parihar V, Sinha M, Pandey S. Complex hydrocephalus (combination of communicating and obstructive type): an important cause of failed endoscopic third ventriculostomy. BMC Res Notes 2009 Jul 16;2:137.

57. Yadav YR, Mukerji G, Shenoy R, Basoor A, Jain G, Nelson A Endoscopic management of hypertensive intraventricular haemorrhage with obstructive hydrocephalus. BMC Neurol 2007 Jan 47:1.

58. Yadav YR, Nishtha Y, Vijay P, Shailendra R, Yatin K. Endoscopic endonasal trans-sphenoid management of craniopharyngiomas. Asian J Neurosurg 2015;10:106.

59. Yadav YR, Parihar V, Sinha M, Jain N. Endoscopic treatment of the suprasellar arachnoid cyst. Neurol India 2010;58(2):280–3.

60. Yadav YR, Parihar V, Agrawal M, Bhatele PR. Endoscopic third ventriculostomy in tubercular meningitis with hydrocephalus. Neurol India 2011;59:855–60.

61. Yadav YR, Parihar V, Agarwal M, Sherekar S, Bhatele PR. Endoscopic vascular decompression of the trigeminal nerve. Minim Invasive Neurosurg 2011;54(3):110–4.

62. Yadav YR, Parihar V, Pande S, Namdev H, Agarwal M. Endoscopic third ventriculostomy. J Neurosci Rural Pract. 2012;3(2);163–73.

63. Yadav Y, Sachdev S, Parihar V, Namdev H, Bhatele PR. Endoscopic endonasal trans-sphenoid surgery of pituitary adenoma. J Neurosci Rural Pract 2012;3:328–37.

64. Yadav YR, Parihar V. The endoscopic trans-fourth ventricle aqueductoplasty and stent placement for the treatment of trapped fourth ventricle; stent blockage complications under estimated? Neurol India 2012;60:455.

65. Yadav YR, Parihar V, Namdev H, Agarwal M, Bhatele PR. Endoscopic inter laminar management of lumbar disc disease. J Neurol Surg A Cent Eur Neurosurg 2013;74(2):77–81.

66. Yadav YR, Parihar V, Bhatele P. Endoscopic Treatment of Arachnoid Cyst. Proceedings of All India Seminar on Biomedical Engineering 2012 (AISOBE 2012) Lecture Notes in Bioengineering 2013, pp 29–35. Publisher Springer India Editors Veerendra Kumar, Mukta Bhatele. DOI 10.1007/978-81-322-0970-6_4 Print ISBN 978-81-322-0969-0 Online ISBN 978-81-322-0970-6.

67. Yadav YR, Parihar V, Kher Y. Complication avoidance and its management in endoscopic neurosurgery. Neurol India 2013;61:217–25.

68. Yadav YR, Parihar V, Pande S, Namdev H. Endoscopic management of colloid cysts. J Neurol Surg A 2014;75:376–80.

69. Yadav YR, Parihar V, Ratre S, Kher Y. Endoscopic anterior decompression in cervical disc disease. Neurol India 2014;62:417–22.

70. Yadav YR, Parihar V, Ratre S, Kher Y, Bhatele P. Endoscopic decompression of cervical spondylotic myelopathy using posterior approach. Neurol India. 2014;62:640–5.

71. Yadav YR, Parihar VS, Ratre S, Kher Y. Avoiding Complications in Endoscopic Third Ventriculostomy. J Neurol Surg A Cent Eur Neurosurg 2015;76(6):483–494.

72. Yadav YR, Parihar V, Kher Y, Bhatele PR. Endoscopic inter laminar management of lumbar disease. Asian J Neurosurg 2016;11:1–7.

73. Yadav YR, Parihar VS, Todorov M, Kher Y, Chaurasia ID, Pande S, Namdev H. Role of endoscopic third ventriculostomy in tuberculous meningitis with hydrocephalus. Asian J Neurosurg 2016;11:325–9.

74. Yadav YR, Parihar V, Ratre S, Iqbal M. Microneurosurgical skills training. J Neurol Surg A Cent Eur Neurosurg 2016;77(02):146–54.

75. Yadav YR, Parihar V, Janakiram N, Pande S, Bajaj J, Namdev H. Endoscopic management of cerebrospinal fluid rhinorrhea. Asian J Neurosurg 2016;11:183–93.

76. Yadav YR, Parihar VS, Ratre S. Letter to the Editor Regarding "Endoscopic Submandibular Retropharyngeal Approach to the Craniocervical Junction and Clivus: An Anatomic Study". World Neurosurg. 111:420, 2018. doi: 10.1016/j.wneu.2017.10.084.

77. Yadav YR, Parihar V, Ratre S. Endoscopic microvascular decompression for trigeminal neuralgia: Is it what we should aim for? World Neurosurg 114:436-437, 2018. DOI: https://doi.org/10.1016/j.wneu.2018.03.154.

78. Yadav YR, Parihar V and Ratre S Endoscopic Transoral Odontoidectomy. Pp. 25-32 (8) In Frontiers in Neurosurgery, Volume 2--[Video Atlas of Spine Surgical Techniques]" Editor(s):

Federico A. Landriel and Eduardo Vecchi. Bentham science Publishers. DOI: 10.2174/9781681081229116020008, eISBN:978-1-68108-122-9, 2016, eISSN:2405-741X, ISBN:978-1-68108-123-6, ISSN:2405-7401.

79. Yadav YR, Parihar V, Ratre S and Dubey A. Endoscopic anterior approaches to the craniovertebral junction. Pages 103–16 in Progress in clinical neurosciences. Editors: N Muthukumar, Vinay Goyal. Thieme publishers Delhi ISBN: 978-93-86293-37-4, 2017.

80. Yadav YR, Ratre S, Parhihar V, Dubey A, Dubey NM. Endoscopic technique for single-stage anterior decompression and anterior fusion by transcervical approach in atlantoaxial dislocation. Neurol India 2017;65:341–7.

81. Yadav YR, Ratre S, Parihar V, Dubey A, Dubey MN. Endoscopic partial corpectomy using anterior decompression for cervical myelopathy. Neurol India. 2018;66(2):444–51.

82. Yadav YR, Shenoy R, Mukerji G, Sherekar S, Parihar V. Endoscopic transoral excision of odontoid process in irreducible atlanto-axial dislocation. In Progress in Clinical Neurosciences. Volume 24. Deepu Banerji, Apoorva Pauranik (ed). New Delhi, Byword Books Private Limited and Neurological society of India. pages 159–169. 2010. ISBN 818193055X, ISBN13: 978-81-81930-552 pages 159–69.

83. Yadav YR, Shenoy R, Mukerji G, Parihar V. Water jet dissection technique for endoscopic third ventriculostomy minimises the risk of bleeding and neurological complications in obstructive hydrocephalus with a thick and opaque third ventricle floor. Minim Invasive Neurosurg. 2010;53(4):155–8. Epub 2010 Dec 3.

84. Yadav YR, Sinha M, Neha, Parihar V. Endoscopic management of brain abscesses. Neurol India. 2008;56(1):13–6.

85. Yadav YR, Yadav N, Parihar V, Kher Y, Ratre S. Endoscopic management of lumbar canal stenosis using posterior approach. In clinical Neuroendoscopy: Current Status by Neuroendoscopy Group of India Editors C Deopujari, Ashish Suri, Venkatraman Publishers Thieme India 2013. ISBN; 978-93-82076-52-0 93-820-76-522.

86. Yadav YR, Yadav N, Parihar V, Ratre S, Bajaj J. Role of endoscopic third ventriculostomy in tuberculous meningitis with hydrocephalus. In tuberculosis of the central nervous system: Pathogenesis, imaging, and Management. editors Mehmet Turgut, Ali Akhaddar, Ahmet T. Turgut, Ravindra K. Garg. Published by Springer International Publishing AG; 1st ed. 2017 edition (26 June 2017) Pages 429–446 ISBN-10: 33-19507-11-7, ISBN-13: 978-33-195-0711-8.

87. Yadav YR, Yadav N, Parihar V, Kher Y,Ratre S. Endoscopic posterior decompression of lumbar canal stenosis. Indian J Neurosurg 2013;2:124–30.

88. Yadav YR, Yadav S, Sherekar S, Parihar V. A new minimally invasive tubular brain retractor system for surgery of deep intracerebral hematoma. Neurol India 2011;59(1):74–77.

89. Yamada T, Yoshii T, Yamamoto N, Hirai T, Inose H, Kato T, Kawabata S, Okawa A. Clinical Outcomes of Cervical Spinal Surgery for Cervical Myelopathic Patients With Coexisting Lumbar Spinal Canal Stenosis (Tandem Spinal Stenosis): A Retrospective Analysis of 297 Cases. Spine (Phila Pa 1976). 43(4):E234-E241, 2018 Feb 15;

90. Yamashita K, Higashino K, Sakai T, Takata Y, Hayashi F, Tezuka F, Morimoto M, Chikawa T, Nagamachi A, Sairyo K. Percutaneous full endoscopic lumbar foraminoplasty for adjacent level foraminal stenosis following vertebral intersegmental fusion in an awake and aware patient under local anesthesia: A case report. J Med Invest. 2017;64(3.4):291–295.

91. Ye CP, Zhu JJ. [Treatment of senile lumbar nerve root canal stenosis with ?micro-endoscope discectomy]. Zhongguo Gu Shang. 2013 Oct;26(10):805–9.

92. Yokosuka J, Oshima Y, Kaneko T, Takano Y, Inanami H, Koga H. Advantages and disadvantages of posterolateral approach for percutaneous endoscopic lumbar discectomy. J Spine Surg. 2016; 2(3):158–166.

93. Yoshimoto M, Takebayashi T, Kawaguchi S, Tsuda H, Ida K, Wada T, Suzuki D, Yamashita T.Minimally invasive technique for decompression of lumbar foraminal stenosis using a spinal microendoscope: Technical note. Minim Invasive Neurosurg 2011;54:142–6.

94. Zhai XJ, Bi DW, Fu H, Zu G. Treatment of lumbar disc herniation with lateral recess stenosis by microendoscopic discectomy. Zhongguo Gu Shang 2008;21:120–1.

95. Zhou W, Li LJ, Tan J. Treatment of degenerative lumbar spondylolisthesis by transforaminal lumbar interbody fusion with microendoscopic surgery. Zhongguo Gu Shang 2010;23:251–3.

96. Zhou X, Zhang L, Zhang HL, He SS, Gu X, Gu GF, Fu QS. Clinical Outcome and Postoperative CT Measurements of Microendoscopic Decompression for Lumbar Spinal Stenosis. Clin Spine Surg. 2017; 30(6):243–250.

Percutaneous Stabilisation of the Lumbar Spine in LCS

PD Kulkarni, Irfan Malik, Gordan Grahovac

INTRODUCTION

Pedicle screws and rods for spinal stabilisation is a widely used procedure but usual open technique involves extensive muscle dissection. A similar construct can be achieved by minimally invasive percutaneous technique. It is commonly used in thoracic, thoracolumbar and lumbosacral vertebrae. The length of the construct depends on the spinal anatomy, pathology, type of operation and the experience of the operating surgeon.

When lumbar fusion is indicated in lumbar canal stenosis, percutaneous pedicle screws (PPS) can be used as they are minimally invasive. PPS can be used in MIS TLIF, MIS PLIF, XLIF and ALIF operations. The percutaneous pedicle screws can be put using navigational system or standard C-arm. The method of putting PPS in MIS TLIF is described here.

Clinical symptoms and evaluation, neuroradiology and other aspects of management (conservative and surgical) are discussed in other parts of this manual. Therefore, I have focussed on the topic of percutaneous pedicle screws in the management of LCS (lumbar canal stenosis).

Management of LCS could be conservative or surgical. Surgical treatment includes minimal decompression surgery, e.g. foraminotomy, unilateral foraminotomy with bilateral decompression crossing over the dura, hemilaminectomy, laminectomy with or without discectomy (Flowchart 22.1).

When there is increased back pain or instability lumbar fusion operation is considered. Instability could be due to facet joint degeneration or spondylolisthesis. This instability could be at one or two levels. Some patients who had previous lumbar spinal fusion develop stenosis above or below the level of fusion called adjacent segment disease (ASD). Lumbar fusion

Flowchart 22.1: TLIF with PPS

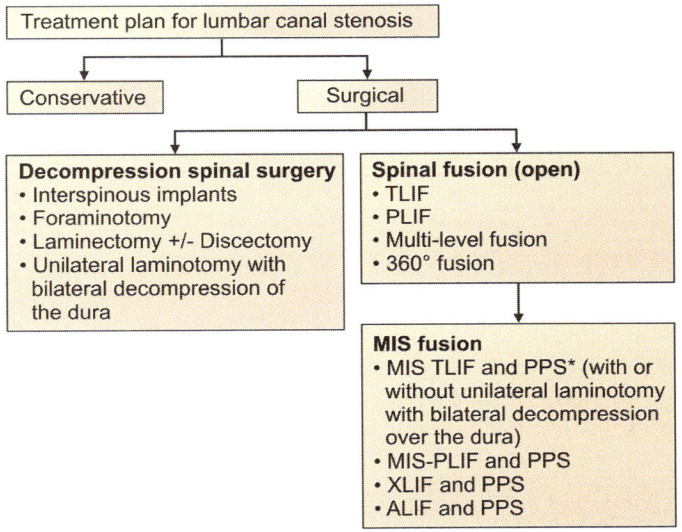

*PPS — Percutaneous pedicle screws

can be done using open technique in various ways, e.g. PLIF, TLIF, XLIF or ALIF.[2]

MIS TLIF: This operation is becoming more popular where percutaneous pedicle screws are put in and TLIF cage is put in the disc space after facetectomy on one side.

MIS PLIF: In this procedure a cage is put in on either side after facetectomy, in addition to the percutaneous pedicle screws. So, there will be 2 cages in MIS PLIF.

Surgery is indicated when conservative treatment fails, or symptoms become more severe. This conservative period could be between 3 months and 1 year period. The aim of the surgery is to give pain relief, stop further neurological deterioration and give chance for neurological improvement.

While considering surgery consideration should be given to age, severity of symptoms, number of previous surgeries, adjacent segment disease (ASD) and comorbidities.

Spondylolisthesis: Degenerative, isthmic type of spondylolisthesis are considered here. Spondylolisthesis also could be due to previous lumbar decompression surgery. Though lumbar instability due to lumbar laminectomy is rare (1% of all laminectomies for stenosis will develop progressive subluxation), fusion is rarely required to prevent progression of subluxation with degenerative stenosis. Stability without fusion is thought to be maintained, if >50–66% of the facets are preserved during surgery and disc space is not violated. These are responsible for maintaining integrity of the anterior and middle column. Active and younger patients are at higher risk of subluxation.

Flexion extension X-rays of the lumbosacral spine after decompression surgery are useful to diagnose symptomatic slippage (instability). These could be treated by fusion using spinal instrumentation.[4]

Here we are considering only minimally invasive technique for spinal fusion in lumbar canal stenosis using percutaneous pedicle screws (PPS). Usually this operation is MIS PLIF or MIS TLIF. We have used PPS in XLIF and ALIF, which are supposed to increase dimensions of the spinal canal and the neural foramina.

Indications of PPS (in same sitting or separately) with lumbar fusion in LCS in cases of instability associated with back pain and radicular symptoms are:

1. MIS TLIF (Fig. 22.1)
2. MIS PLIF (Fig. 22.2A and B)
3. XLIF (Fig. 22.3)
4. ALIF (Fig. 22.4)

Indications of Lumbar Fusion

- Degenerative or recurrent disc disease, instability
- Persisting back pain and leg pain not relieved by conservative methods

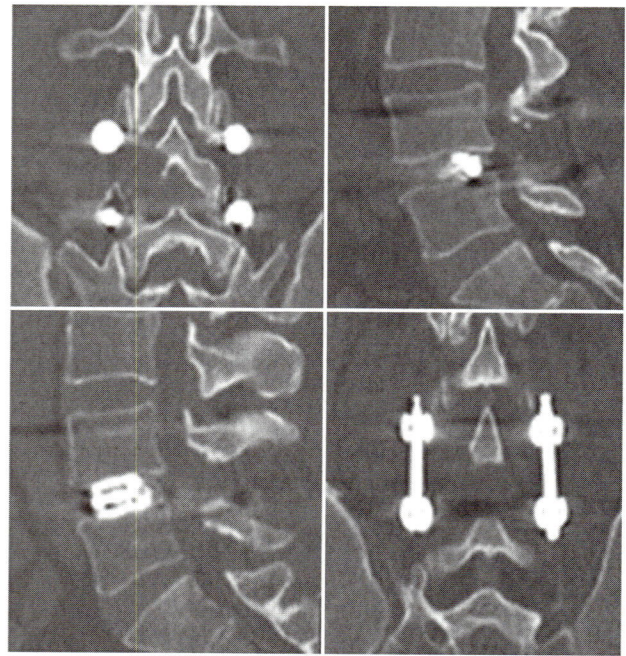

Fig. 22.2A: TLIF with PPS at L4/5. Please note unilateral facetectomy, R L4 unilateral laminotomy and bilateral decompression of the canal over the dura

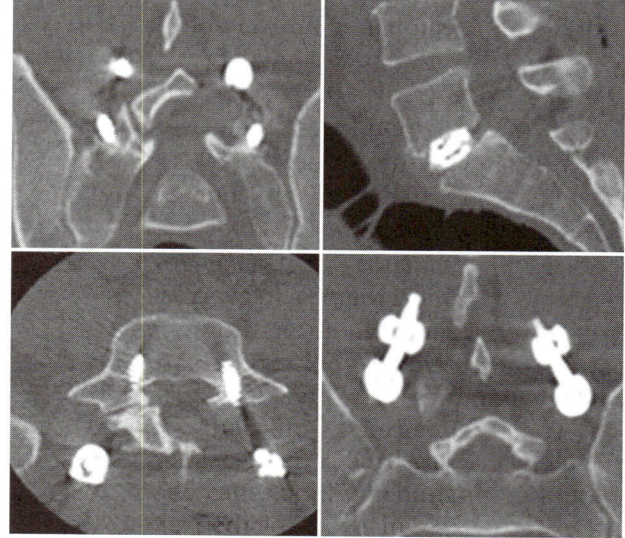

Fig. 22.2B: TLIF with PPS at L5/S1. Please note unilateral facetectomy, R L4 unilateral laminotomy and bilateral decompression of the canal over the dura

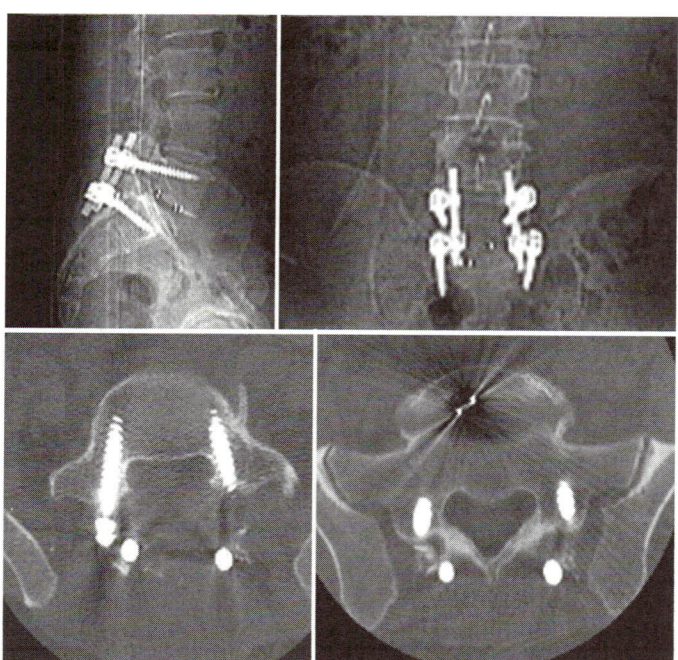

Fig. 22.1: TLIF with PPS

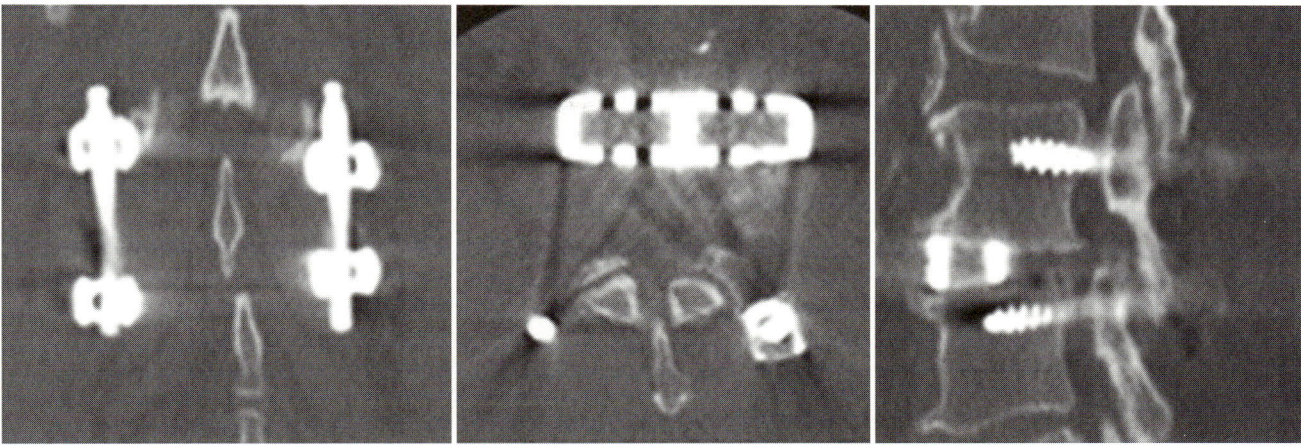

Fig. 22.3: TXLIF with PPS. Please note XLIF cage and PPS at L4/5

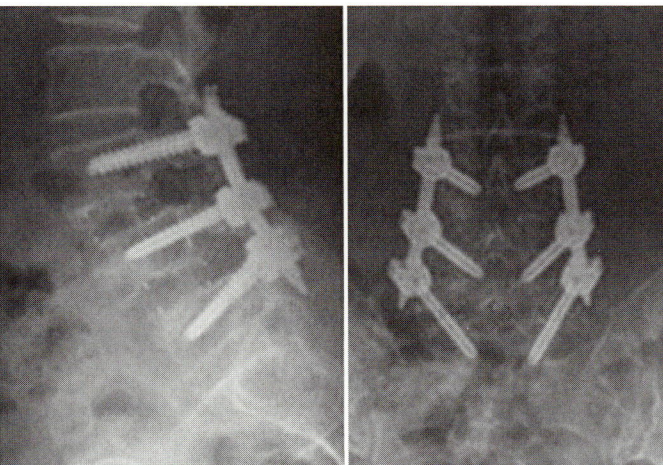

Fig. 22.4: ALIF with PPS

- Affecting job and income
- Cannot continue with analgesics
- Progressive neurological deficit with instability
- Do not forget to consider psychological and social status, e.g. income support

Assessment of the patient before considering fusion operation:

1. Age-fusion operation should be avoided above the age of 75 years.
2. VAS score for back and leg pain, chronicity of pain, e.g. 1 yr, 5 yr, 10 yr as results of operation will vary.
3. Previous conservative treatment with reviews from physiotherapy and pain team.
4. Psychological assessment.
5. Patient with a job or jobless.
6. Failed back (previous multiple lumbar surgeries)
7. Imaging: MRI, CT scan, flexion-extension X-rays, radioisotope scans, discography
8. Kyphoscoliosis, sagittal and coronal balance and its rectification should be considered
9. Comorbidities and preanesthetic check up

Multidisciplinary Team (MDT)

It is also very important to discuss the patient in complex spine MDT or peer-group discussion to get multiple views on management to come to an appropriate operation decision-making process.

Special operation considerations in lumbar canal stenosis:

PPS can be put in the same operation sitting or as separate procedure. Operative procedure of putting PPS is similar in all operation procedures of MIS TLIF, MIS PLIF, XLIF and ALIF. There are various types of cages available for lumbar fusion and we have used PEEK, carbon, titanium and titanium expandable cages.[5]

Usually when there is back pain and unilateral leg pain TLIF operation is considered. When canal is narrow and there are bilateral leg symptoms PLIF is considered.

MIS TLIF is a popular operation. When there is canal stenosis at the level of surgery, then unilateral laminotomy and bilateral internal decompression can be carried out. After ipsilateral laminotomy, base of spinous process is drilled out. One may have to tilt table or angulate the muscle retractor so as to look over the dura to the other side for decompression. Preservation of ligamentum flavum initially helps to protect the dura while drilling the facet on the other side. By this way nerve root on the other side can be decompressed. It is also possible to do discectomy on the other side when required. This technique needs to be understood and popularised. This technique could be used without spinal instrumentation and laminectomy could be avoided in selected cases.[6]

Due to minimal invasive operation technique there is:

- Less tissue dissection
- Less blood loss

- Preservation of normal tissue
- Less pain
- Early recovery and therefore less hospital stay
- More cosmetic and gives more satisfaction to the patient.

Examples of percutaneous pedicle screws (PPS) with lumbar fusion: PPS is common to all operative procedures, e.g. MIS TLIF, MIS PLIF, XLIF and ALIF.

Operative technique of putting percutaneous pedicle screws (Fig. 22.5A to C):

a. Using navigational technique
b. Using C-arm

Neuro-navigational technique using O-arm or Ziehm vision (Stryker) could be used. This avoids more exposure to the radiation but they are more expensive.

Intraoperative neurophysiology monitoring could be used for safety. I have used O-arm before but nowadays we use Ziehm Vision (Stryker) in Kings College Hospital, London regularly (Fig. 22. 6A and B). Patient is positioned prone on the operation table (Alan or Jackson). O-arm or 3D C-arm (Ziehm Vision) goes around the patient's waist. All theatre staff goes out of the operation theater when the patient is scanned to prevent radiation exposure. This helps to create sagittal, coronal and axial images on the monitor. A calibrated tool attached to the spinal instrument, e.g. Jamshidi needle. When it is put on to the entry point of the pedicle, its trajectory will be seen in the sagittal, coronal and axial images on the monitor as shown. With the help of these image Jamshidi needle is passed through the pedicle. Once the needle is accurately placed, guide wire is passed through the Jamshidi needle. Pedicle

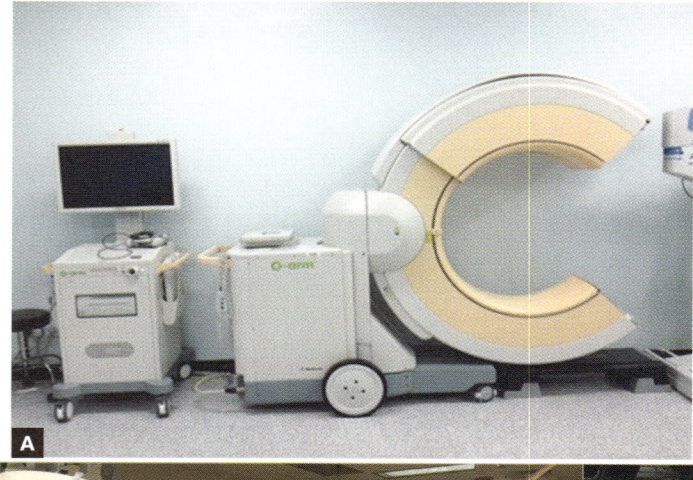

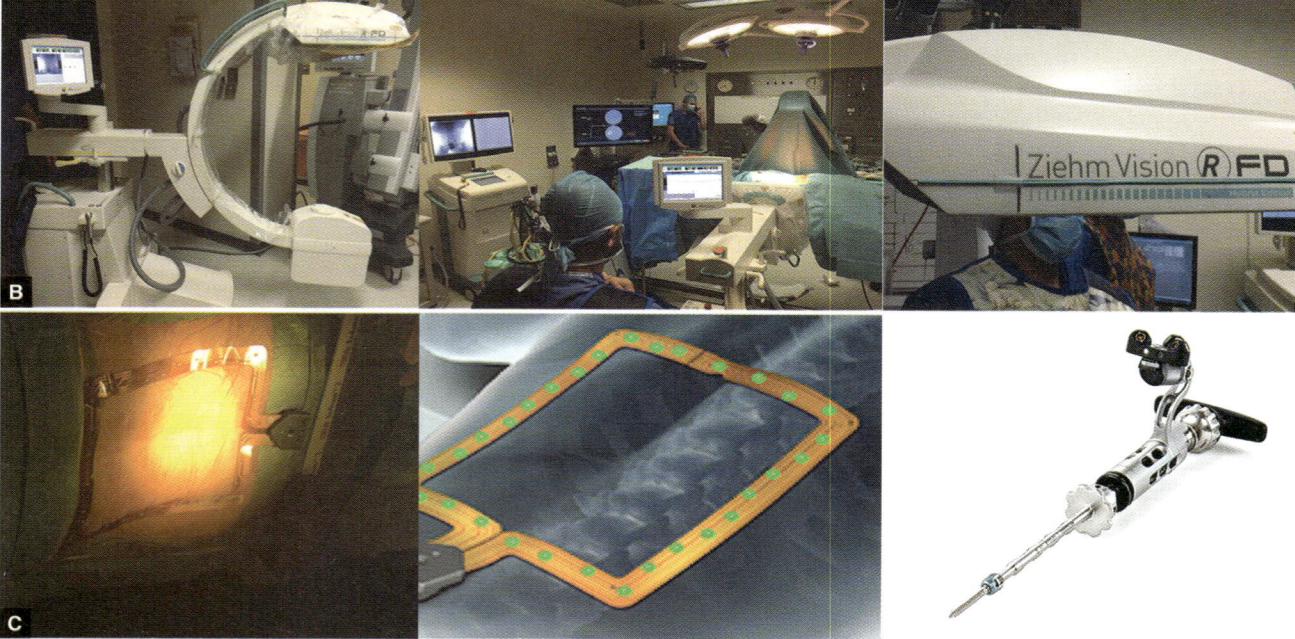

Fig. 22.5A to C: PPS using various navigational technique: (A) O-arm (navigation tool); (B) NAV 3i platform—Stryker; (C) Spine map 3D software, adhesive spine mask tracer

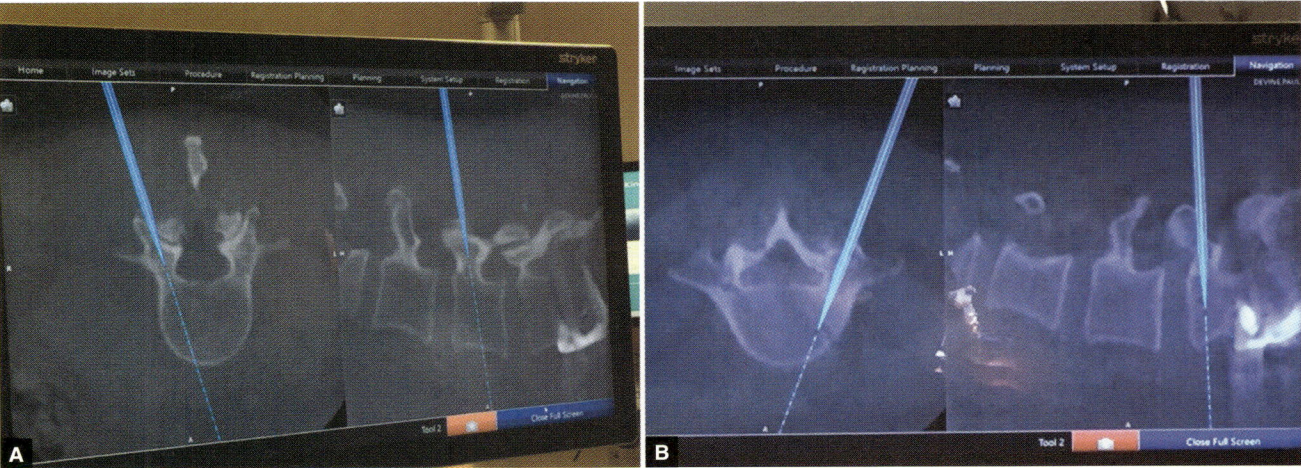

Fig. 22.6A and B: Various navigation techniques: (A) Stryker-navigation tool; (B) Ziehm Vision

screw is then rail rolled on the guidewire into the vertebral body. This process is repeated at all pedicle screw insertion sites. Patient is re-scanned to check the accuracy of the pedicle screws. The technique of putting the rods and tightening them with screws is same as described later using C-arm technique.

PPS using C-arm Technique (Fig. 22.7)

C-arms are available everywhere but there is risk of exposure to more radiation. One needs experienced radiographer for this procedure.

Percutaneous Pedicle Screw Systems

There are approximately 20 different percutaneous pedicle screw systems in the market. We have used Mantis (Stryker) and Viper 2 (DePuy) extensively[3] (Fig. 22.8A and B).

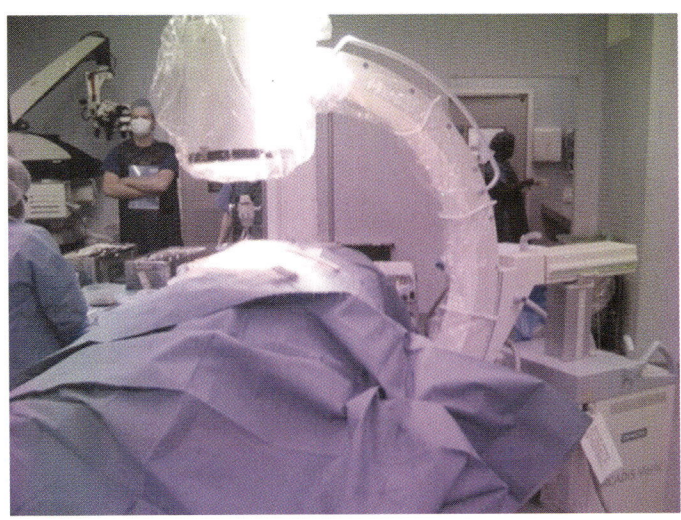

Fig. 22.7: Standard C-arm

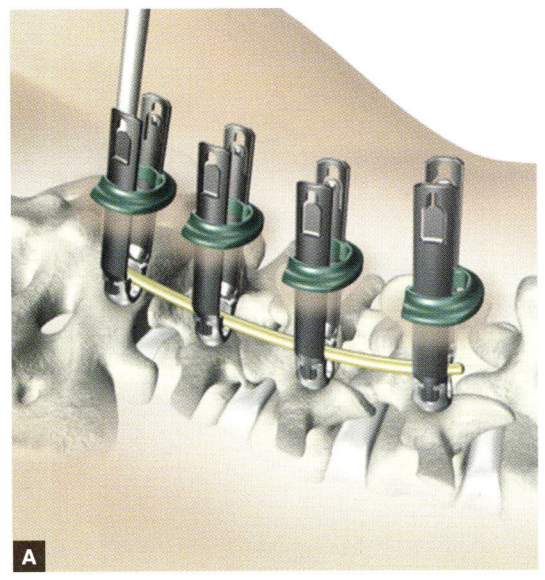

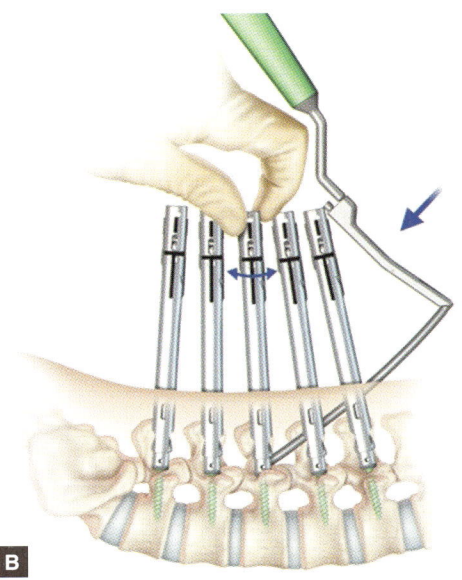

Fig. 22.8A and B: (A) Mantis (Stryker); (B) Viper 2 (DePuy)

Limitations

- Poor anatomy due to deformity, e.g. high-grade spondylolisthesis
- Poor X-ray quality or severe osteoporosis

Advantages

- Smaller incisions and minimal dissection
- Less trauma to tissues and less blood loss
- Less postoperative pain
- Earlier recovery and therefore short hospital stay
- Decreased incidence of infection

Disadvantages

- Long learning curve
- More surgical time during learning curve
- Radiation exposure

Applied Anatomy and Radiology

This is mainly a fluoroscopy (radiology) dependant procedure. Clear visualisation of pedicles in AP and lateral view of the vertebra is extremely vital before putting pedicle screws.

Preoperative Overview

- Pre-anesthetic check-up
- CT scan of spine including 3D view to delineate anatomy of the spine. It helps to measure the pedicle diameter and pedicle angle.

Operative Technique

Steps
1. Patient positioning
2. Pedicle targeting
3. Jamshidi needle and guide wire placement
4. Screw placement
5. Rod insertion, reduction and final tightening

1. *Patient Positioning*

Position—prone, neutral.

Use radiolucent table and mattress (we use Montreal mattress). Alan or Jackson table can be used. Check AP and lateral views of the appropriate vertebrae with C-arm and check that the pedicle anatomy is satisfactory (Fig. 22.9A to E). A radiographer well-trained in this procedure will help to reduce operation time and

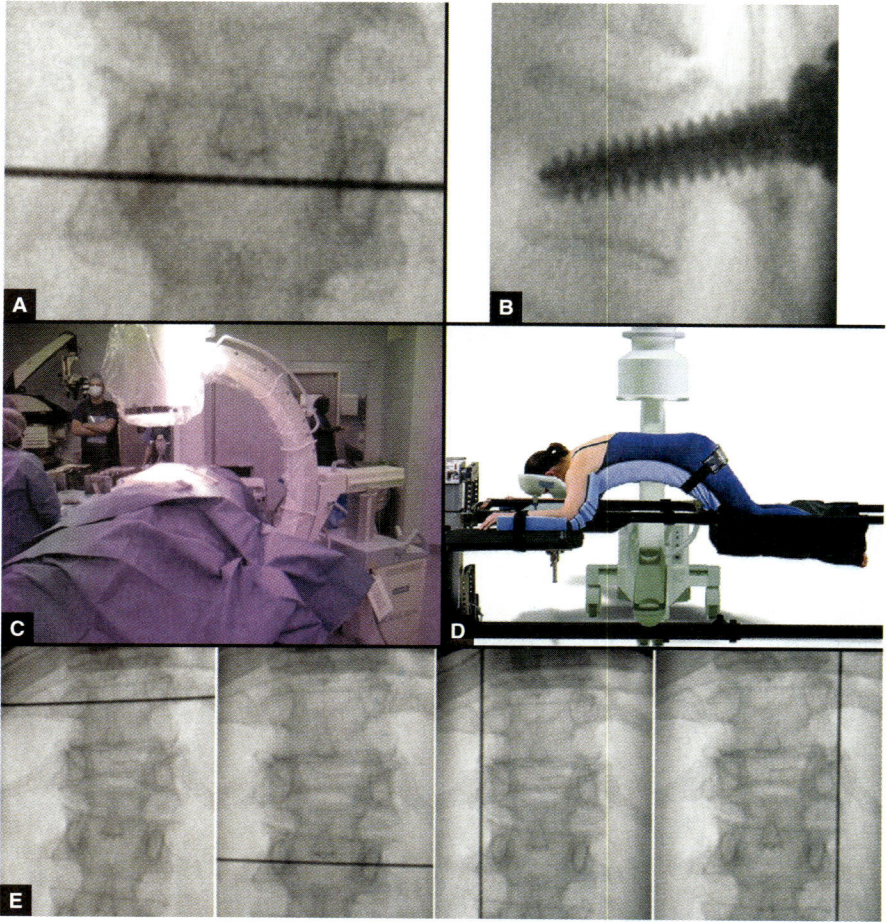

Fig. 22.9A to E: AP and lateral views of the pedicle to mark incision

radiation exposure to the theater staff. Previously we have used two C-arms, but now we use single C-arm.

2. Pedicle Targeting

Use AP view of the desired vertebrae and mark the pedicles across the midline transversely as shown with the help of the guide wire. Then use the guide wire to mark the lateral border of the desired pedicles as shown in Fig. 22.10. These lines are well marked on the patient's skin as shown. The insertion point of the Jamshidi needle lays 1 to 2 cm lateral to the point of intersection depending upon the angulation of the pedicle.

3. Jamshidi Needle and Guide Wire Placement

As shown in the image below, the Jamshidi needle insertion starts at the 3 or 9 o'clock position on the AP view involving the middle and lateral third of the pedicle in the lumbar region. Particularly in the thoracic region, we prefer to use the upper outer quadrant of the pedicle and the needle insertion point at 1 or 11 o'clock. The needle should not cross the medial border of the pedicle.[8]

Always remain inside the pedicle and advance the needle as shown in Fig. 22.11A to D.

The Jamshidi needle should not cross the medial border of the pedicle until it enters the body of the vertebra. This is well confirmed using a lateral view X-ray. The needle is marked approximately 20 mm above the skin before insertion. This is the approximate length of the pedicle. Now remove the trocar of the needle and insert a sharp guide wire through it into the pedicle (Fig. 22. 12A to F).

Throughout the procedure, precaution is taken not to allow the guide wire to come out of the pedicle until the screw is inserted. Also, while tapping the pedicle or inserting the screw, see that the guide wire does not pierce the anterior cortex of the body of the vertebra and injure great vessels in front of the spine.

4. Screw Placement

Approximately 15 mm of the skin needs to be incised to allow a cannula, tap and screw to go easily over the guide wire without causing damage to the surrounding

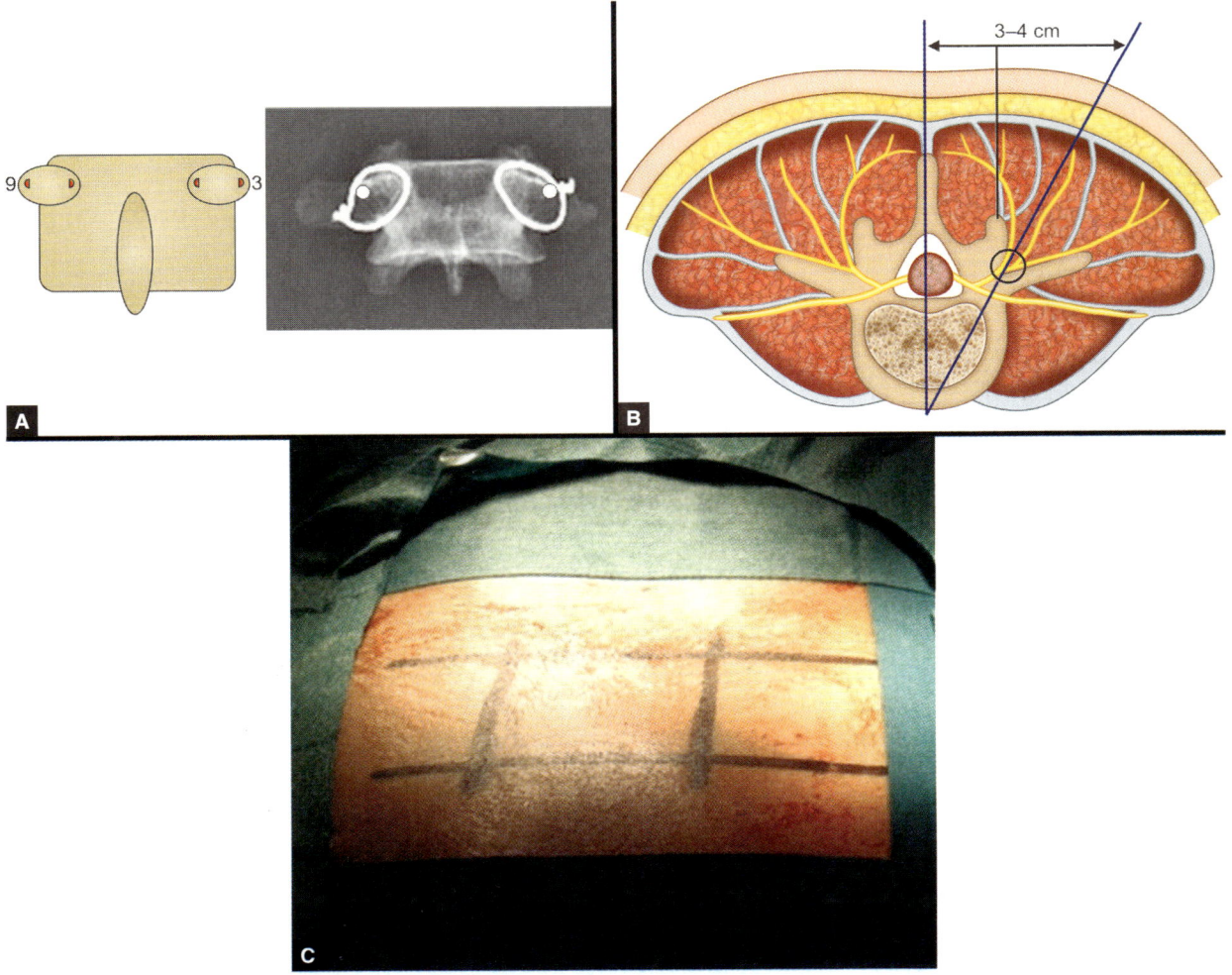

Fig. 22.10A to C: Marking pedicle entry to skin

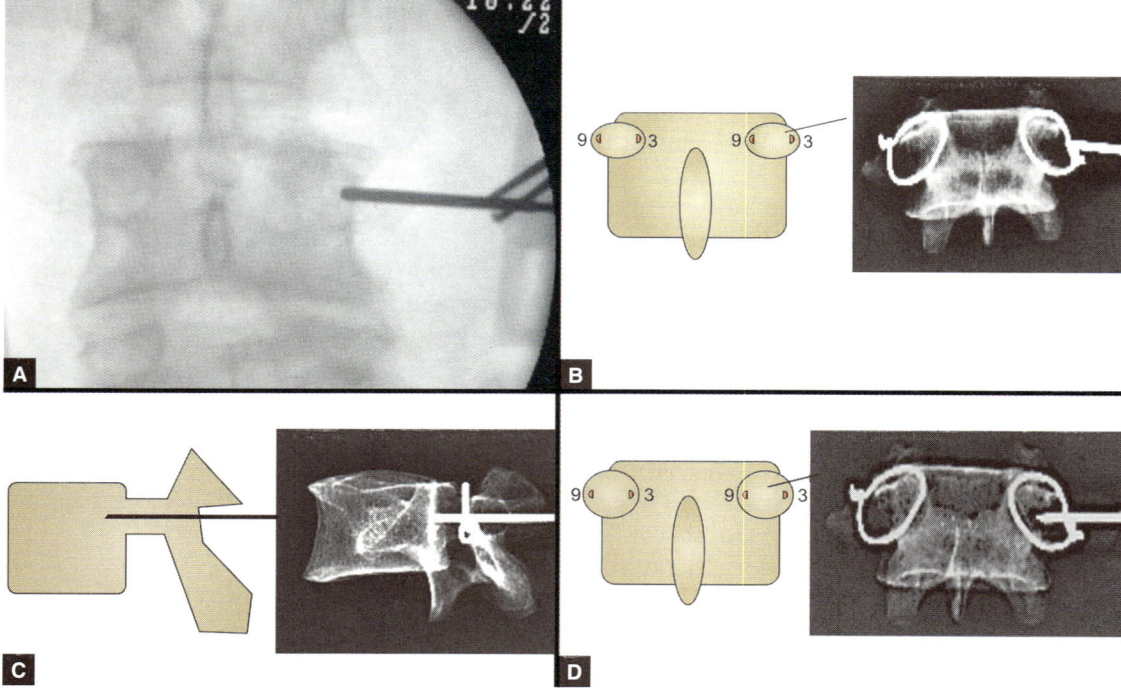

Fig. 22.11A to D: Lateral X-ray confirms the needle tip into the vertebral body

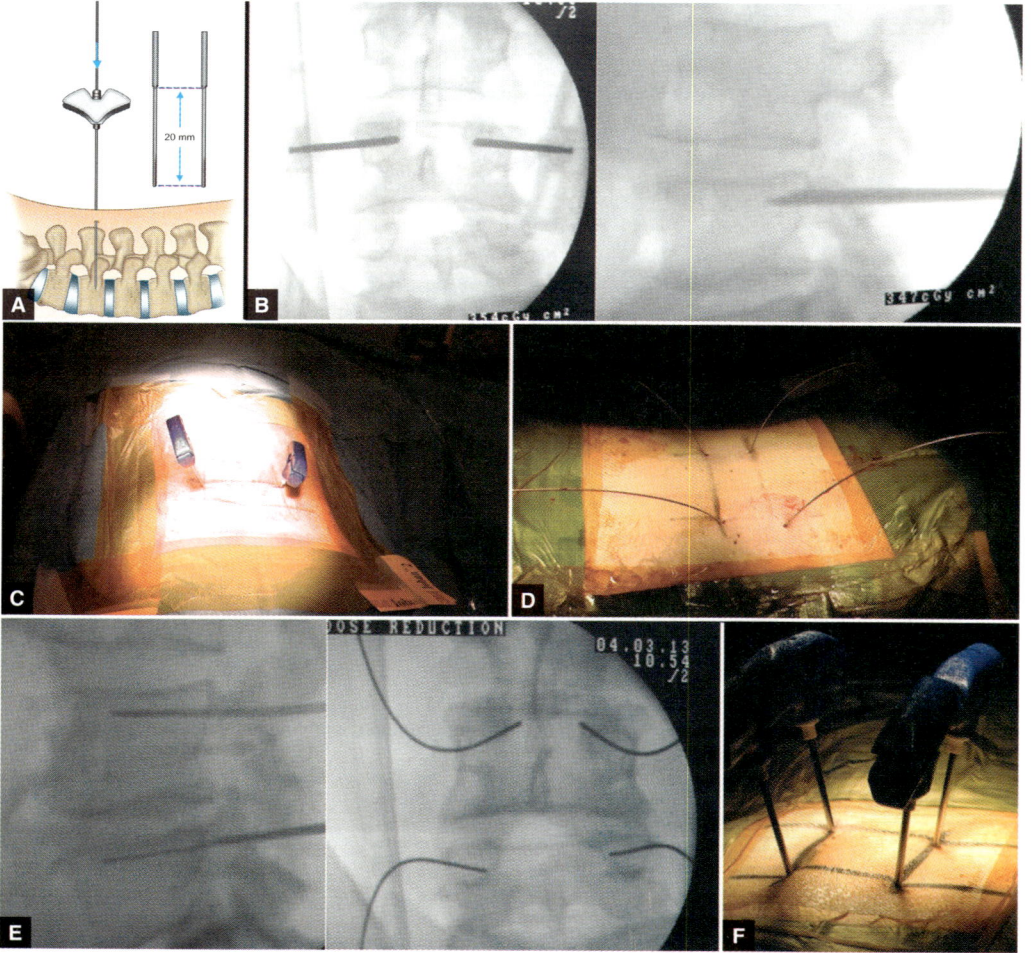

Fig. 22.12A to F: Insertion of Jamshidi needles into the pedicle J

skin. Dilators (blunt and hollow) are then used along the guide wire. A hollow cannula is inserted and the dilator is removed. The hollow cannula prevents injury to surrounding muscles during tapping or inserting screws through the pedicle. A cannulated modular tap is then used to tap the pedicle and body. This is again checked with the fluoroscopy. We have used neurophysiology monitoring to prevent neural damage.

Screw assembly is prepared using the appropriate length of screw. We find that the presence of a company representative is very useful to the surgeon and the theater nurse in getting the appropriate instruments. The screw is guided over the wire to penetrate the pedicle and body. A fluoroscopy is used again to confirm the correct position. After removing the screw driver, a green sliding ring is left around the blades. Other screws are inserted in a similar manner[7] (Fig. 22.13A to G).

At this stage, MIS TLIF or MIS PLIF can be done by extending the incisions over the facet joint. Special MIS TLIF retractors are used as shown. Unilateral drilling of facet joint, discectomy and insertion of titanium

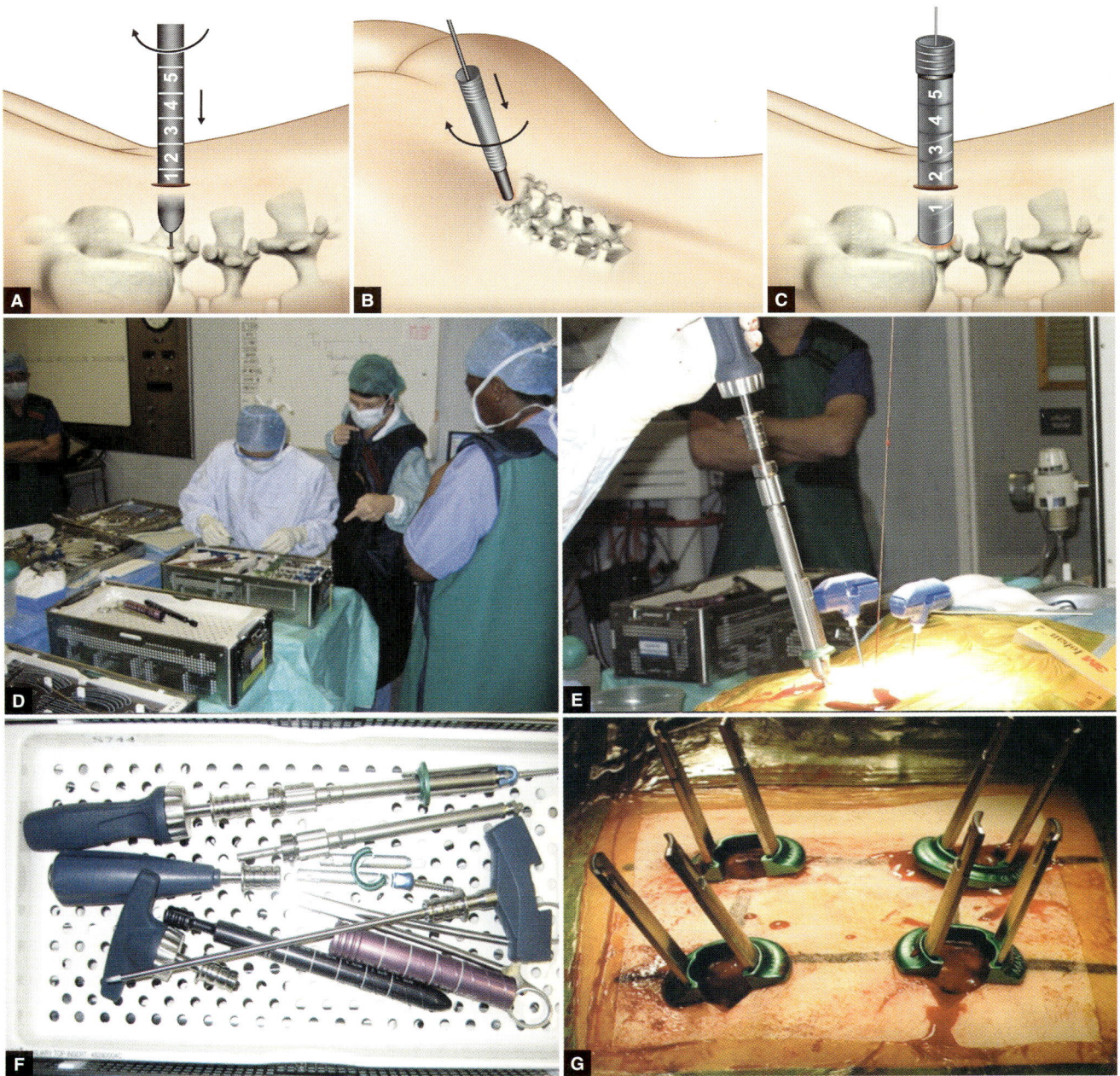

Fig. 22.13A to G: Steps of screws insertion: (A) Blunt dilator; (B) Hollow dilator goes over blunt dilator; (C) Hollow cannula; (D) A company representative directing the nurse; (E) First screw in position; (F) Screw assembly; (G) All screws are inserted and then the screw driver is removed showing blades and green sliding rings

simple or expandable cage is used in MIS TLIF. When similar cage is put on the other side it will be called MIS PLIF (Fig. 22.14A to I).

4. Rod Insertion, Reduction and Final Tightening

Rod contouring shafts and rod contouring linkages are used to measure the length and assess the curvature of the rod. This rod is attached to a rod inserter and passed through the retractor blades from the open side of the sliding ring. The position of the rod is confirmed clinically and with a fluoroscopy. Blockers are used initially to hold the rod on the screw heads. Compression and distraction devices are used when desired, and finally blockers are tightened. Green sliding rings and retractor blades are removed and the wound is closed after good irrigation[1] (Fig. 22.15A to D).

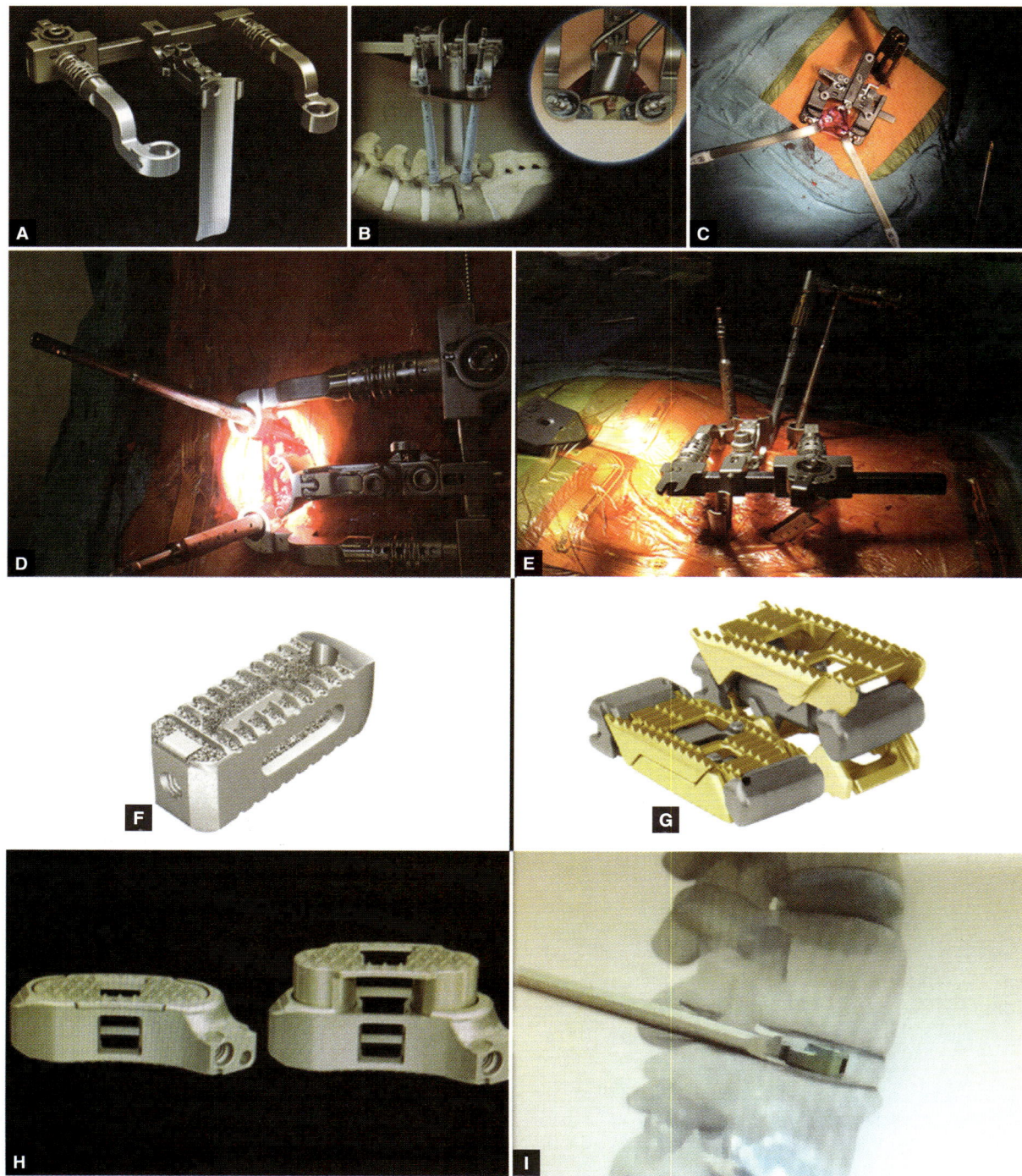

Fig. 22.14A to I: Steps of TLIF and PLIF cage insertion

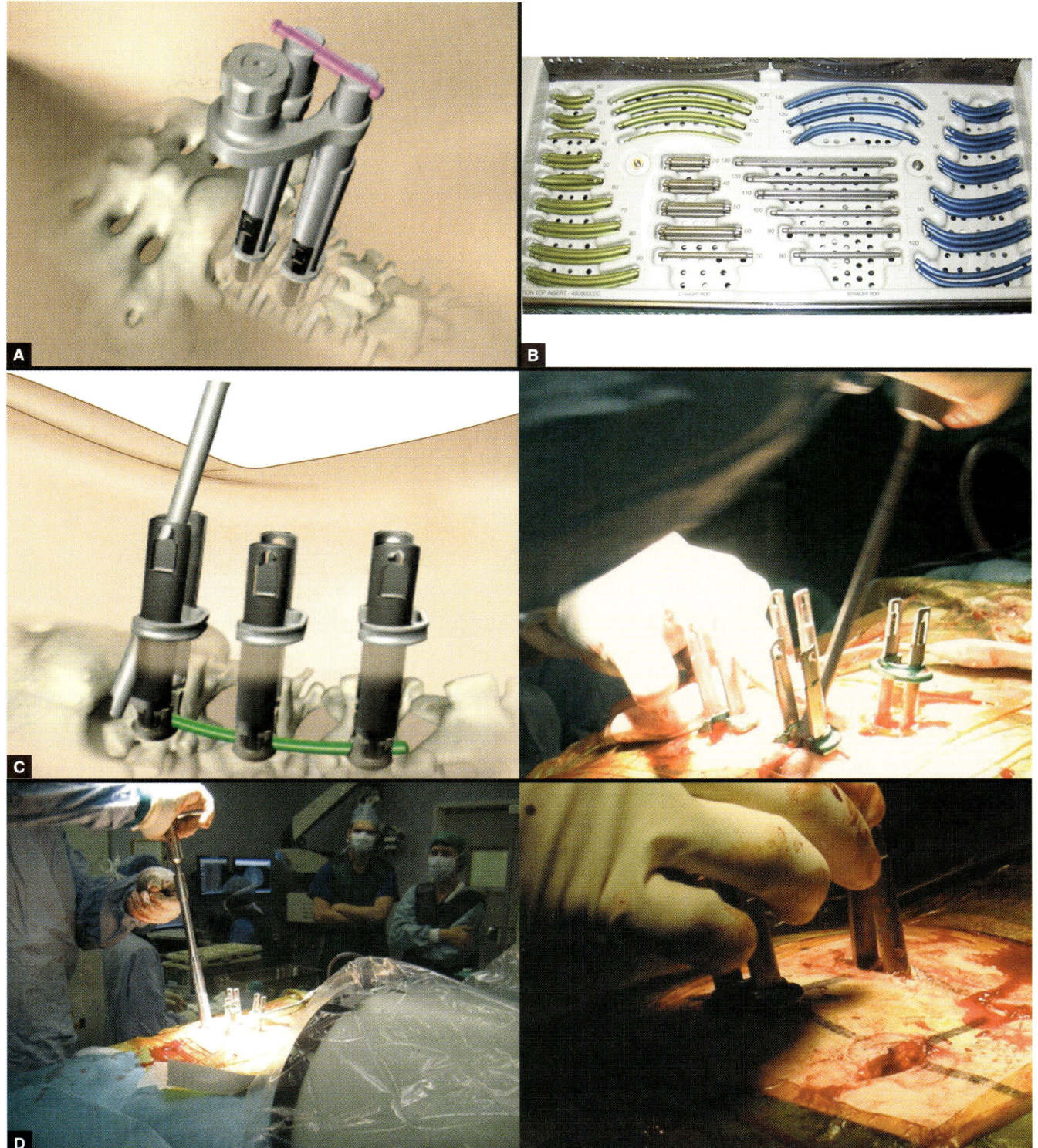

Fig. 22.15A to D: Steps of rod insertion: (A) Rod contouring shafts and measurement of rod; (B) Various sizes and shapes of rods; (C) Rod insertion using rod inserter; (D) Final screw tightening and removal of blades and green rings

Postoperative Management

Apart from general care, patients are mobilised early due to less pain. We routinely do postoperative CT scans to check the position of screws and cages (Fig. 22.16A to C). This is not required when navigation system is used as positions of the screws and cages are rechecked intraoperatively when the patient is on the operation table.

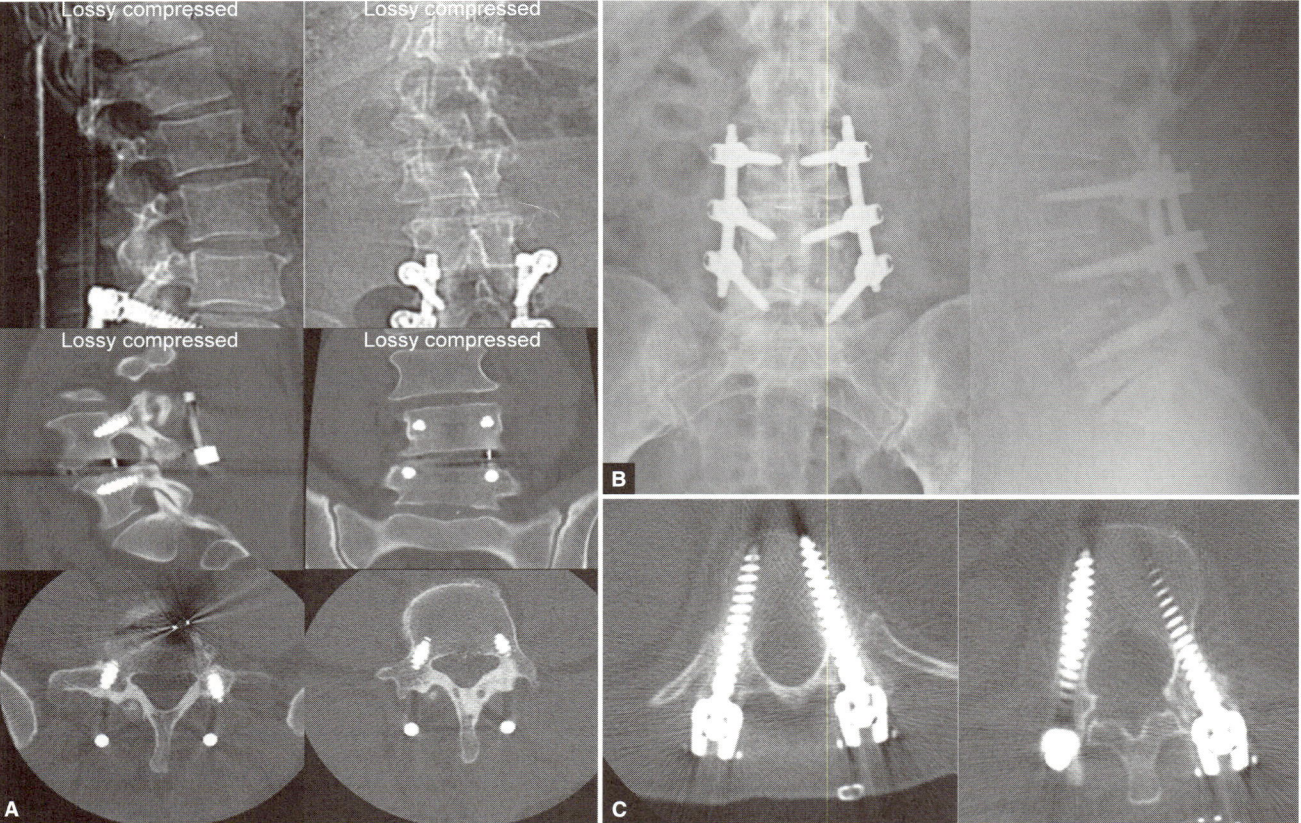

Fig. 22.16 A to C: Postoperative images of PS done by MISS techniques: (A) Percutaneous MIS TLIF L4/5; (B) Percutaneous MIS TLIF L3/4, L4/5; (C) Postoperative CT scans showing precisely positioned screws in pedicles

Complications

Though very rare, one may come across the following complications
1. Malpositioning of screws and rods
2. Neural injury
3. Infection
4. Pneumothorax
5. Pulmonary embolism

Conclusion

Percutaneous pedicle screw and rod fixation is a promising and minimally invasive procedure for spinal stabilisation. It clearly has more advantages over the open technique which involves extensive muscle dissection and blood loss.

REFERENCES

1. AO spine manual—principles and techniques, Vol 1, Thoracic spine, p.173–92.
2. Dick W, Kluger P, Magerl F, Worsdorfer O, Zach G. A new device for internal fixation of thoracolumbar and lumbar spine fractures: the "fixature interne." Paraplegia 1985;23:225–32.
3. Foley KT, Gupta SK. Percutaneous pedicle screw fixation of the lumbar spine: preliminary clinical results. J Neurosurgery (Spine 1) 2002;97:7–12.
4. Greenberg MS, Handbook of Neurosurgery, 6th ed., 2006.
5. Lowery GL, Kulkarni SS. Posterior percutaneous spine instrumentation. Eur Spine J 2000;9:S126–S130.
6. Magerl F: External skeletal fixation of the lower thoracic and the lumbar Spine in Uhtoff HK, Stahl E: Current Concepts of External Fixation of Fractures. Berlin: Springer-Verlag, 1982, pp 353–66.
7. Mathews HH, Long BH: Endoscopy assisted percutaneous anterior interbody fusion with subcutaneous supra-fascial internal fixation: evolution, techniques and surgical considerations. Orthop Int Ed 1995;3:496–500.
8. Panjabi MM et al. Complexity of the thoracic spine pedicle anatomy. Euro spine 1997;6:19–24.

23 Combination of Percutaneous Stabilization and Endoscopic Surgery in the Surgical Management of Lumbar Canal Stenosis

Yoshitaka Hirano

INTRODUCTION

Pedicle screw fixation of lumbar spine is a widely used procedure for lumbar stabilization in patients with unstable lumbar spine. Pedicle screw systems have the advantage of engaging all the three columns of the spine to resist motion in all planes. Open pedicle screw fixation requires extensive tissue dissection to expose the entry points to provide a lateromedial approach for the optimal screw trajectory.[1,3] Consequently, percutaneous pedicle screw system has been developed to achieve good results with less surgical invasiveness. The technique was first described by Foley et al in 2001[1], and since then there has been several changes in the technique. Such percutaneous techniques are described as minimally invasive spinal stabilization (MISS), and the indications for MISS are essentially the same as those for conventional open fixation. MISS techniques are designed to preserve soft tissue and allow for safe and effective insertion of the implants into the lumbar spine. In this technique, following insertion of the needle to the optimal position the guidewire is then inserted along the track and the screw which in this system is always cannulated is threaded into the pedicle over the guidewire.[1,3]

MISS technique allows approach to the disc space where tubular retractors are used for insertion of the interbody cages. Thus combining the two techniques of percutaneous and endoscopic procedures. Given below is an example of my daily practice with a report of an illustrative case.

Patients and Methods

A total of 117 patients with degenerative spondylolisthesis with instability were treated with transforaminal lumbar interbody fusion (TLIF) or posterior lumbar interbody fusion (PLIF). For the patients requiring bilateral decompression (IDSS), the procedure was followed by PLIF or TLIF. Following decompression through tubular retractors (quadrant; Medtronic Sofamor Danek, Memphis, Tennessee, USA) Polyetheretherketone (PEEK) cages are widely used for interbody stabilization. It has been my observation in my earlier cases that cystic degeneration occurred in most patients treated with interbody PEEK cages, which is rarely seen with titanium cages. The reliability of the PEEK material as the lumbar interbody implant is now considered to be questionable due to its lower rigidity compared to titanium, so I have changed my practice to use titanium implants in recent times.[2] My recent mainstream of implants for the interbody fixation is the Contact Fusion Cage (DePuy-Synthes Spine, Raynham, Massachusetts, USA) together with artificial bone compound made of hydroxyapatite and collagen fibers (Refit; Hoya Technosurgical, Tokyo, Japan).

Following interbody stabilization with titanium cages, percutaneous pedicle screw fixation was carried out. Indwelling a needle to the ideal trajectory is the first step of this procedure. Regarding the pedicle as a column, the entry point should be the lateral edge of the upper surface, and the exit point should be the center of the base (Fig. 23.1). For the elderly patients with some restrictions in daily activities, pedicle screws were inserted through the cortical bone trajectory (CBT). Even with the CBT technique, I follow the same procedure using confidence needle (MISS-CBT). 2 For the percutaneous pedicle screw fixation, I usually use VIPER X-tab (DePuy Synthes Spine) or Voyager (Medtronic Sofamor Danek) systems, and for cortical bone trajectory (CBT technique) I use the Matrix system (DePuy Synthes Spine).

Illustrative Case

A 63-year-old man, who runs a bedding store, suffered from low back pain and right-dominant dysesthetic

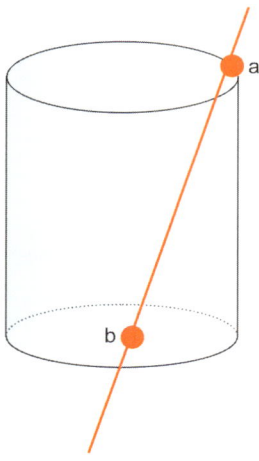

Fig. 23.1: A schematic drawing to show the ideal trajectory of the needle insertion to the pedicle. Regarding the pedicle as a column, the entry point (a) should be the lateral edge of the upper surface, and the exit point (b) should be the center of the base

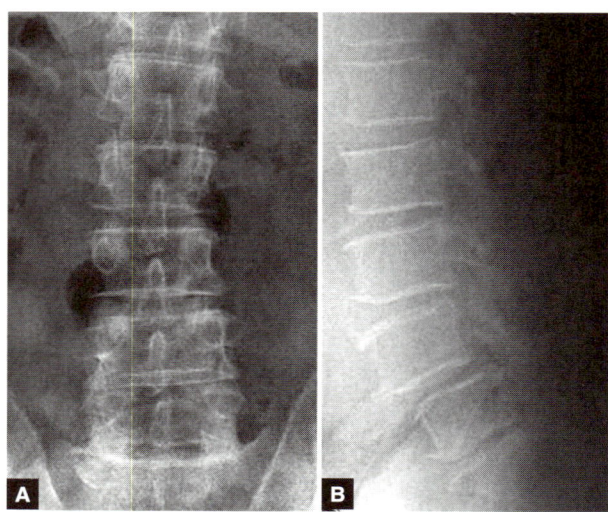

Fig. 23.2: Standing lumbar radiographs (A: posteroanterior, B: lateral flexion) showing degenerative spondylolisthesis (grade 1) at the L4–5 level

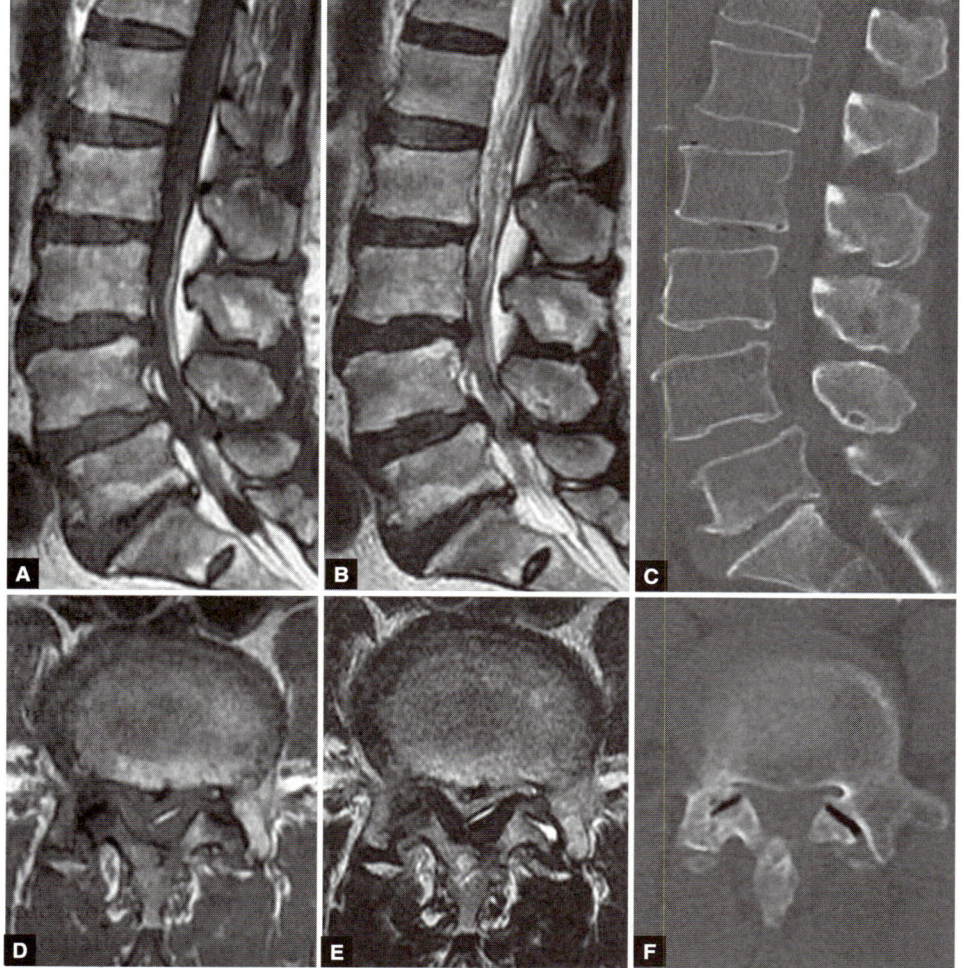

Fig. 23.3: Magnetic resonance study (A: T1-weighted mid-sagittal section, B: T1-weighted axial section at the L4–L5 level, C: T2-weighted mid-sagittal section, and D: T2-weighted axial section at the L4–L5 level) showing right-dominant spinal canal stenosis due to degenerative spondylolisthesis at the L4–L5 level. Computerized tomographic scan (E: reconstructed mid-sagittal section, and F: reconstructed axial section at the L4–L5 level) revealed degenerative spondylolisthesis with significant facet degeneration and vacuum phenomenon

pain of his legs for 3 years. He visited a local orthopedic service but conservative treatment did not solve his symptoms. The patient was too busy with his work to see his doctor regularly, and his symptoms aggravated gradually. He visited our clinic after developing difficulty in walking with aggravated low back pain in motion. Neurological examination revealed slight muscle weakness of the extensor hallucis longus on the right side and decreased Achilles tendon reflex bilaterally. Standing lumbar radiographs (Fig. 23.2) showed degenerative spondylolisthesis (grade 1) with instability at the L4–5 level, and magnetic resonance study (Fig. 23.3A to D) revealed right-dominant spinal canal stenosis. Computerized tomographic scan (Fig. 23.3E and F) showed right-dominant facet degeneration with vacuum phenomenon. Due to the significant impairment of his daily activities, the patient opted for surgical treatment.

A skin incision of 4.5 cm length was taken at 3.5 cm from the midline to the right side and the quadrant retractor of 6 cm depth was introduced at L4–5 level (Fig. 23.4). Right L4 inferior articulate process was removed with osteotome, and lateral recess was widened. After discectomy and curettage of the end plates, autologous local bone chips were abundantly implanted in the L4–5 disc space. TLIF was completed with a cylindrical titanium cage of 12 mm diameter and 25 mm length (INTERFIX: Medtronic Sofamor Danek) under fluoroscopic observation.

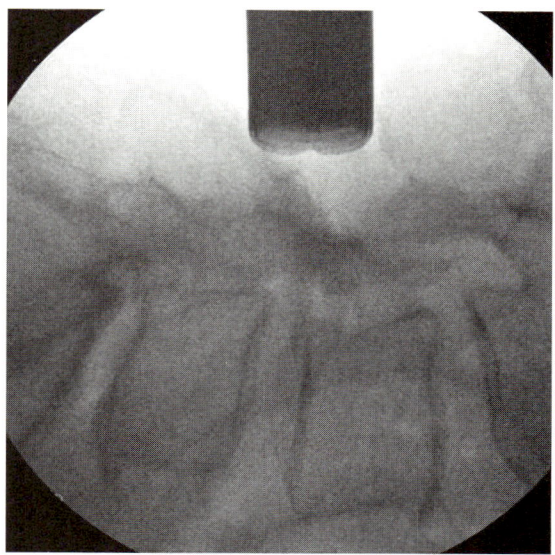

Fig. 23.4: Intraoperative fluoroscopy showing appropriately placed quadrant retractor (Medtronic Spfamor Danek) of 6 cm depth at the L4–L5 level

The procedure was followed by percutaneous pedicle screw fixation with Voyager system (Medtronic Sofamor Danek). On the right side the screws were inserted from the same original skin incision and individual skin incisions of 1.8 cm length were made for screw insertion on the left side. The subfascial rods were connected and the operation was completed with reduction and compression. Figure 23.5 demonstrates

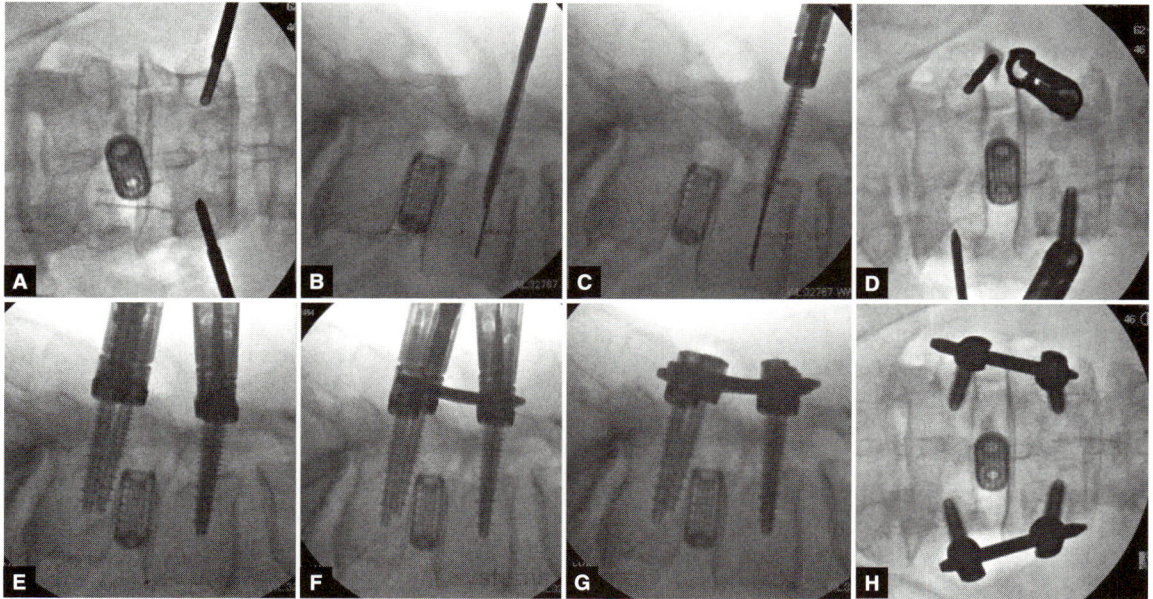

Fig. 25.5: Intraoperative fluoroscopic images showing the surgical procedure of percutaneous pedicle screw fixation with VOY-AGER system (Medtronic Sofamor Danek), step by step. PAK needles are indwelled to the bilateral L4 pedicles at the appropriate trajectory (A) followed by insertion of the guide wire, (B) Screw is inserted through the guide wire, (C) after completion of the L4 procedures, PAK needles are indwelled to the bilateral L5 pedicle, (D) screws are inserted with the same procedure, (E) then an interconnecting rod is percutaneously inserted through the subfascial trajectory, (F) Final lateral,(G) anteroposterior and (H) images confirm appropriate completion of the procedure

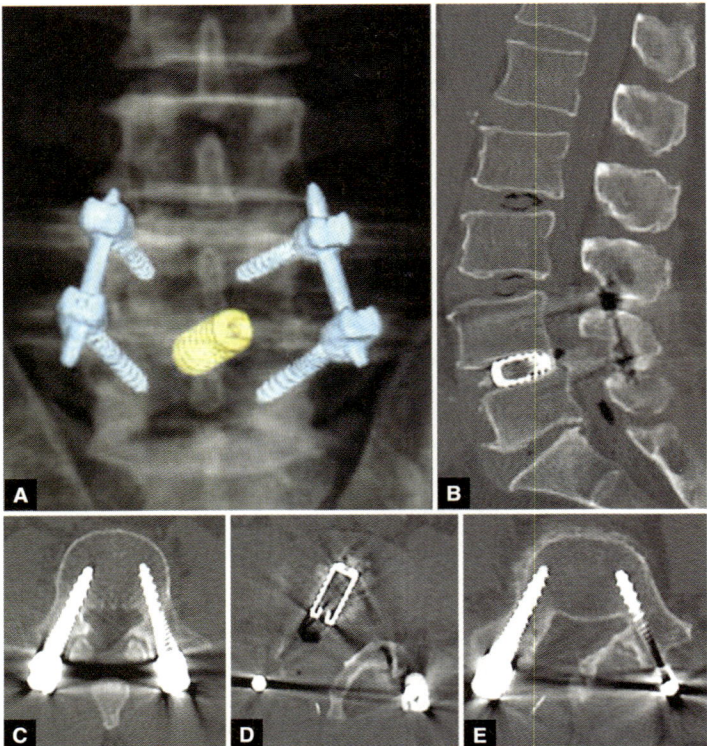

Fig. 23.6: Postoperative CT scan (A: Volume rendering image, B: Reconstructed mid-sagittal section, and reconstructed axial sections at C: L4, D: L4–L5, and E: L5 levels) showing appropriately placed implants with corrected spinal alignment

the procedure of percutaneous pedicle screw fixation with the Voyager system, step by step.

Patient felt immediate relief from his disabling symptoms and he was discharged home 10 days after the operation. The patient resumed his daily activities and returned to work and even succeeded in weight reduction by adopting physical training. Postoperative studies (Fig. 23.6) revealed appropriately placed implants with corrected spinal alignment.

Conclusions

The MISS techniques, including various percutaneous procedures and endoscopic interbody fusion are considered beneficial for stabilization of the lumbar spine in lumbar canal stenosis giving better surgical results with minimum invasiveness. With the progress of techniques and tools it may be possible in future to improve the invasiveness of the procedure.

Disclosure

No conflict of interest.

REFERENCES

1. Foley KT, Gupta SK, Justis JR, Sherman MC: Percutaneous pedicle screw fixation of the lumbar spine. Neurosurg Focus 2001; 10(4):E10.
2. Hirano Y, Bansil R, Maddala S, Itoh Y, Numazawa S, Matsuoka H, Mizuno J, Watanabe S, Watanabe K: Application of minimally invasive spine stabilization techniques to posterior lumbar fusion with the cortical bone trajectory. In: Batoe HS (ed.) Progress in Spinal Surgery 2017, Jay Dee Services Inc.; 2017:51–61.
3. Khoo LT, Palmer S, Laich DT, Fessler RG: Minimally invasive percutaneous posterior lumbar interbody fusion. Neurosurgery 2002;51(5 Suppl): S166-S181.

Management of Adjacent Segment Disease in Lumbar Canal Stenosis—The Role of Minimally Invasive Surgery

Mazda Turel, Mena G Kerolus, Brian T David, Richard G Fessler

INTRODUCTION

An increasing number of lumbar spine operations is being performed over the decades. As a result of which, the incidence of adjacent segment disease (ASD) continues to become more relevant and concerning, resulting in higher reoperation rates, longer fusion constructs, and increased morbidity.[38] The prevalence of symptomatic ASD requiring surgery is variable and ranges from 5 to 16% at 5 years, and 10 to 36% at 10 years.[14,48,49] Reoperation rates for laminectomy alone and laminectomy with non-instrumented fusion vary from 1.3 to 5.6%, whereas reoperation rates for ASD after instrumented posterior lumbar interbody fusion have been reported as high as 80% at 5 postoperative years.[12] A recent meta-analysis concluded that patients undergoing minimally invasive spine surgery (MIS) may have a lower incidence of ASD than patients undergoing open surgery.[23] The evidence supporting the efficacy of motion-sparing techniques in reducing adjacent level pathology remains inconclusive.[11,31] Potential risk factors for developing ASD include age >60 years, body mass index >25 kg/m^2, preexisting disc and facet degeneration, and number of levels fused in the lumbar spine.[21,45,48]

The treatment strategy for management of ASD of the lumbar spine often involves open revision surgery with replacement, revision, or extension of existing hardware. These procedures are associated with longer operative duration, an increase in blood loss, a longer hospital stay, and a higher incidence of postoperative complications.[37,50] The operative morbidity of revision surgery and the increasing health care costs related to their management further burden society.[1] To mitigate the complexity of open revision lumbar spine surgery for ASD, various instrumented and noninstrumented MIS techniques can be performed.

Pathophysiology of Adjacent Segment Disease

The pathophysiology of adjacent segment disease is multifactorial. Literature is still confounded about the fact if this may indeed be related to previous fusion surgery rather than the natural history of the underlying degenerative disease.[18] Disc degeneration at the adjacent segment is the most common abnormal finding. Biomechanical changes consisting of increased intradiscal pressure, increased facet loading, and increased mobility occur after fusion and have additionally been implicated.[32] Several risk factors contribute to ASD following the application of instrumentation; fusion length (especially three or more levels), preoperative sagittal malalignment, facet breach, advanced age, increased body mass index (BMI), and preoperative documentation of cephalad degenerative disease (e.g., disc disease, stenosis).[11] Hence, potentially modifiable risk factors for the development of adjacent segment disease include fusion without instrumentation, protecting the facet joint of the adjacent segment during placement of pedicle screws, fusion length, and sagittal balance.

The rate of symptomatic ASD in the lumbar spine after decompression and stabilization is approximately 2–3% per year. This can be addressed with a number of different surgical techniques while providing long-term improvement in low-back pain, disability, and quality of life.[2,34] It is important to subdivide ASD into adjacent segment stenosis and adjacent level instability to determine if decompression alone versus an extension of fusion is necessary.[10] Minimally invasive surgical techniques for decompression, stabilization, and fusion of the spinal column have become increasingly popular over the past decade.[46] MIS techniques limit the disruption of the paraspinal muscles and ligamentous structures. When surgery is done open, this disruption may potentially compromise lumbar stability and lead to further ASD.[4] Other advantages include diminished blood loss, shorter hospital stays, and decreased postoperative pain.[13] The utility of MIS techniques continues to expand and the surgical indications now include a wider spectrum of pathologies. With increasing familiarity and experience, these techniques can be used for the management of ASD (Table 24.1).

Table 24.1: Various MIS techniques used for the management of adjacent segment disease
1. Non-instrumented; foraminotomy, discectomy, laminectomy
2. ALIF; stand alone with integrated screws/plates, +/– percutaneous posterior fixation, +/– facet fusion
3. TLIF; (traditional pedicle screws or cortical bone trajectory) with removal, addition or extension of rods; +/– interspinous device or dynamic stabilization device
4. LLIF; stand alone +/– percutaneous posterior fixation with pedicle/ facet screws, +/– removal or extension of rods
5. Minimally invasive extension of a previous lumbosacral fusion to the pelvis

Non-instrumented MIS Techniques

Although the standard surgical paradigm involves extending a prior fusion, in patients who are symptomatic from unilateral foraminal disease or stenosis secondary to foraminal narrowing or disc encroachment, an MIS discectomy or foraminotomy may suffice even in the presence of a prior fusion[36] (Fig. 24.1).

This should be done in select patients in whom decompression can be achieved without significant violation of the facet joint, which may eventually result in instability.[16] Phillips et al[35] reported a 58% improvement in back and leg pain after MIS tubular decompression alone, while Schlegel et al[42] showed a 64% improvement in a similar cohort.

Percutaneous microendoscopic discectomy (PED) or foraminotomy, offers an advantage by providing direct visualization of the compression and adequate decompression at the desired level.[39] Indistinct anatomic alterations and perineural scarring makes revision spinal surgery more challenging than the primary one, not only at the initial level, but also at adjacent levels. However, the endoscope provides excellent visualization in delineating these structures to accomplish the goals of surgery. This procedure can also be performed under local anesthesia with sedation. The incidence of an intraoperative dural tear was reported to be lower in endoscopic discectomy alone when compared to fusion procedures.[25]

Telfian et al[43] reported their experience performing a PED adjacent to the level of fusion and found that while all patients had significant improvement in back and leg pain scores postoperatively, 3 of their 9 patients (33%) eventually required a fusion by their 2 year follow-up. This technique may be a useful procedure in elderly patients who do not wish to undergo an instrumented fusion.

Anterior Lumbar Interbody Fusion (ALIF)

The ALIF procedure, either with a stand-alone cage or with an integrated screw and/or plate system, serves as an excellent MIS option in patients with lumbosacral ASD[19,26] (Fig. 24.2).

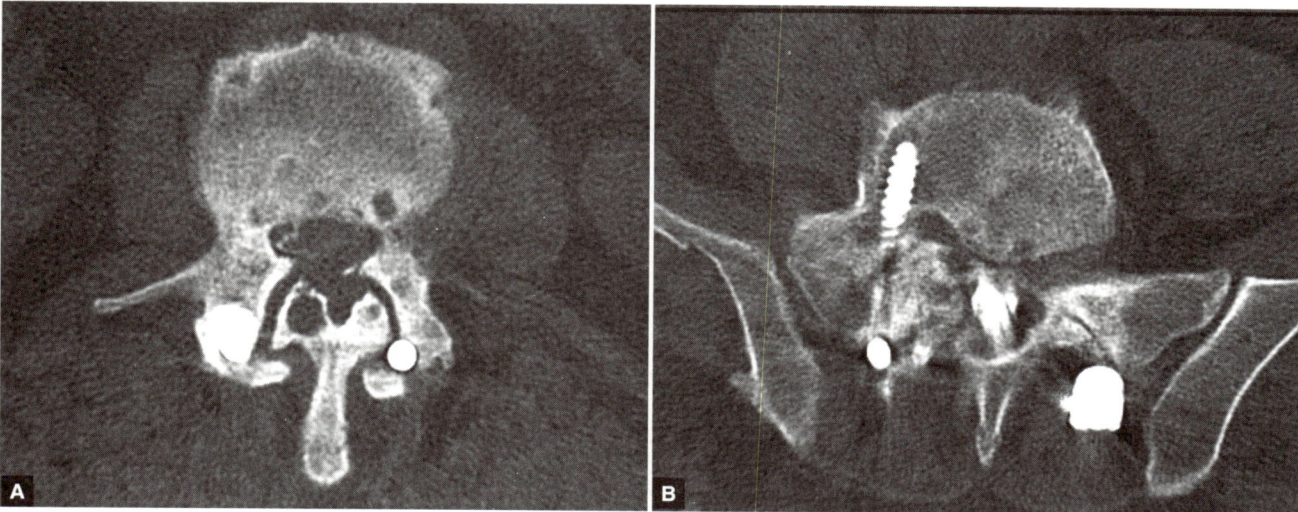

Fig. 24.1: Axial CT scan demonstrating stenosis at L1–2: (A) Right L5–S1 stenosis; (B) after a prior L1–S1 fusion. The patient underwent a successful MIS L1–2 laminectomy and right L5–S1 foraminotomy with excellent outcome without the need for any further instrumentation

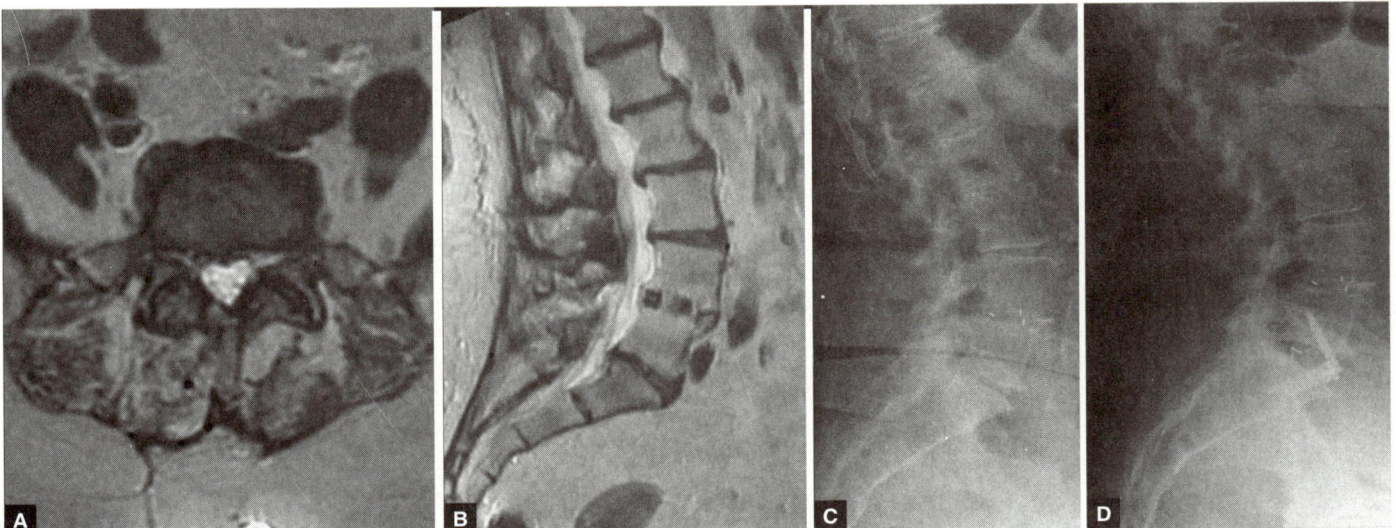

Fig. 24.2: Axial (A) and sagittal (B). T2-W MRI of a patient who underwent a prior L4–5 discectomy and TLIF with removal of implants followed by an ALIF, presented with a degenerated disc and L5–S1 stenosis. Lateral lumbosacral spine radiographs demonstrated an adequate fusion across L4–5 but a collapsed L5–S1 disc space (C). The patient subsequently underwent an L5–S1 ALIF; (D) with resolution of symptoms

This clearly avoids all the complications of a posterior approach such as a durotomy, nerve root injury, and secondary damage to posterior muscular and ligamentous structures. ALIF offers direct anterior column support, restores lordosis, increases fusion rates (due to a large surface area for grafting and placement of a graft under direct compression), shortens operative time, and expedites patient recovery. It can be performed on up to 3 levels within the same incision, with a short operative time and minimal blood loss. The addition of percutaneous posterior fixation, either with or without facet fusions, can be done if there is instability or significant deformity.

Rao et al[40] performed this procedure in 5 patients with ASD with a fusion rate of 80%. Mamuti et al[27] successfully used this approach in 35 patients with recurrent disc herniation who had undergone prior discectomy and posterior instrumentation. All patients showed clinical improvement; postoperative CT scans at 1 and 2 years demonstrated bony fusion, normal position, and morphology of the fusion cage in all patients. In cases of disc herniation, resection of the extruded disc fragments can be accomplished by opening the posterior longitudinal ligament by doing a direct decompression rather than an indirect decompression, as is often the case with an ALIF.[44] The most commonly reported complications are retrograde ejaculation, vascular injury, superficial infection, urological injury, and abdominal muscle damage.[19]

Sacroiliac fusion and instrumentation extension for correction of failed lumbosacral fusions traditionally requires a long revision surgery, especially if they have already had an ALIF and the only option left is to extend the fusion down to the pelvis. Reopening of the prior surgical incision to expose the prior instrumentation requires a large incision with increased blood loss, increased operative time, increased risk of infection and longer hospitalization times. We have described (in press) a series of cases using a minimally invasive surgical (MIS) sacroiliac screw technique for extension of a prior fusion to the pelvis. Using two small 3 cm para median incision on each side, we are able to obtain autologous iliac crest bone graft, place the sacroiliac screw minimally invasive, perform an arthrodesis, and connect the prior surgical hardware to the sacroiliac screw safely. The technique utilizes paramedian incisions with sub-fascial exposure of the facet and transverse process. The iliac crest screws are inserted under fluroscopic guided direct vision. Side to side connectors and a short adjunct rod connect the new screw to the existing rod, obviating the need for removal of the previous instrumentation. The exposure of the facet and transverse process allows for bone graft material to be layered promoting fusion at the fixation site (Fig. 24.3).

Transforaminal Lumbar Interbody Fusion (TLIF)

TLIF is a very versatile operation and is the workhorse of posterior lumbar fusion.[6,7,15] Using MIS techniques, it is easy to perform at a level adjacent to a previous fusion. Rods can be removed, connected, or extended (Fig. 24.4).

In patients with a prior TLIF Lee et al[22] reported that the cost effectiveness for revision extension surgery

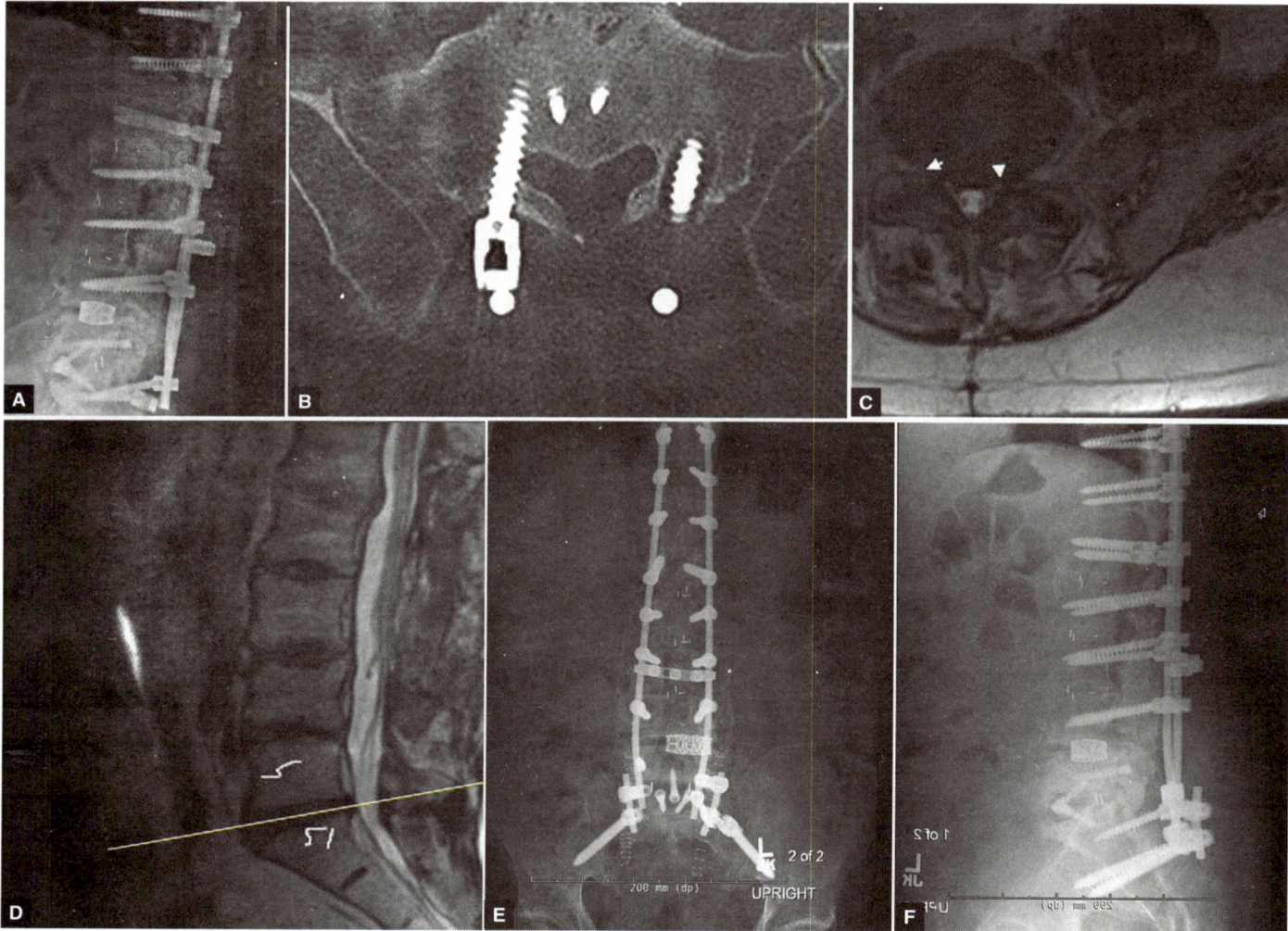

Fig. 24.3: (A) Lateral radiograph; and (B) axial CT of a patient with a previous long-segment lumbosacral fusion with pseudoarthrosis as evidenced by the left S1 screw lucency. (C) Axial and (D) sagittal MRI showing residual foraminal stenosis at L5–S1. (E) AP and (F) lateral postoperative radiograph after minimally invasive extension of the fusion to the pelvis

for ASD reusing the pedicle screws extracted from the fused segments resulted in excellent clinical and radiological outcomes. The fusion rates, too, were comparable to those when new screws were used. The perioperative complication rate is approximately 15%, with the most common complication being a durotomy.[47]

TLIF can be considered an effective, reliable, and safe alternative procedure for the treatment of recurrent lumbar disc herniation, either at the same or adjacent level.[24] The posterior instrumentation can be done either using unilateral or bilateral pedicle screws, translaminar facet screws, or a combination of these.[5] Whether an interbody is required or just a posterolateral extension of fusion would suffice to treat the adjacent segment continues to be a matter of debate. One has to be extremely vigilant while placing percutaneous screws adjacent to a previous fusion. Park et al[33] retrospectively

reviewed their series of 184 pedicle screws placed using a MIS fluoroscopic technique in 92 patients with ASD and found a surprisingly high and unexpected incidence of cranial facet joint violation (50% of all patients and 32% of all screws). The clincial implication of this has yet to be determined.

Some authors have described the use of navigation guided mini-open cortical bone trajectory screws in cases with ASD, which allows for placement of pedicle screws in a previously instrumented pedicle.[41] Since the entry point is at the lateral aspect of the pars inter-articularis, this procedure avoids extensive tissue dissection by limiting the surgical corridor to the levels adjacent to the existing hardware, thus eliminating the need to expose, remove, or extend the hardware with the anticipated benefits of reduced operative time, blood loss, and dissection.

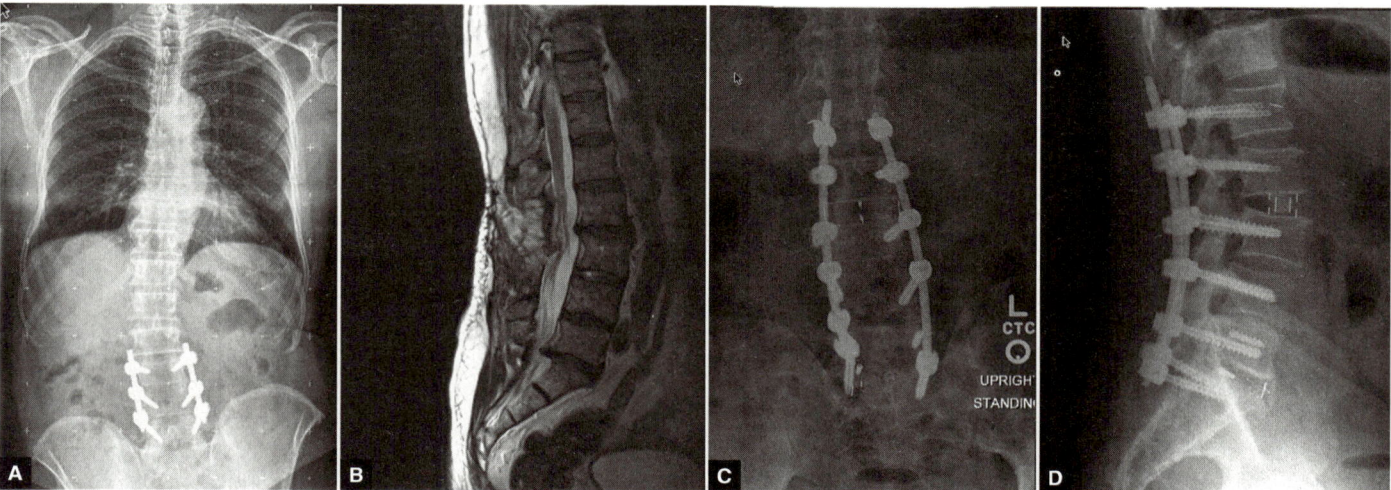

Fig. 24.4: Preoperative anteroposterior radiograph (A) and sagittal T2-W MRI (B); of a patient who underwent a prior L3–5 postero-lateral fusion now presenting with symptomatic disc degeneration at L3–4 and L5–S1. He underwent an MIS L3–4 LLIF with restoration of disc height, followed by an L5–S1 MIS TLIF, L1–2 facet fusion, and L1–S1 percutaneous fixation, as seen on anteroposterior; (C) lateral and (D) radiographs with remarkable recovery

In certain cases of multilevel ASD, a TLIF can be combined with an interspinous or hybrid stabilization device at the cranial segment (topping off technique) to further reduce the incidence of future ASD.[8,9] Other dynamic stabilization devices have also been used in isolation to connect to a previous fusion.[28] Posterior dynamic stabilization, in which pedicle screw fixation is coupled with a flexible longitudinal connecting system, presumably allows for the normalization of intersegmental motion. This stands in contrast to traditional fusion surgery, in which the goal is the complete and immediate elimination of motion and, ultimately, arthrodesis. These devices theoretically avoid an abrupt transfer of stress from a rigid construct to the neighboring segments and thereby potentially diminish further ASD.[51]

Lateral Lumbar Interbody Fusion (LLIF)

LLIF is also an effective surgical treatment option for ASD in regards to both clinical and radiographic outcomes.[3,30,46] Given the widespread use of electro-physiology and the tubular retractor technology, the lateral approach has gained further popularity. Although a stand-alone LLIF is associated with a narrower spectrum of adverse effects compared to circumferential fusion, posterior instrumentation, either in the form of pedicle screws and rods (unilateral or bilateral) or facet screws alone, may be necessary to increase segmental stability in certain cases 3 (Fig. 24.5).

Biomechanical studies have shown that the addition of a lateral interbody device super-adjacent to a 2-level fusion significantly reduces motion in flexion, extension, and lateral bending. Supplementing with a lateral plate further reduces motion during lateral bending and torsion. The addition of posterior cortical screws provided the most stable LLIF construct, demonstrating range of motion comparable to a traditional 3-level TLIF.[29]

The LLIF has the advantage of providing an indirect decompression while using a large footprint interbody device. It provides an alternate route for decompression and may be helpful by avoiding a dissection through a prior laminectomy defect or scar tissue. It also provides the added benefit of avoiding ligamentous disruption, which has been hypothesized to exacerbate ASD.[17]

In patients with ASD, the LLIF results in an improvement in back and leg pain due to an increase in disc height, increase in segmental lordosis, and decrease in coronal segmental angulation.[3] However, Aichmair et al[3] showed that the reoperation rate after LLIF for ASD was 21.2%, with a trend towards a higher fusion rate in patients who underwent circumferential fusion compared to the stand-alone sub-group (87.5% vs. 53.8%; p=0.173). On the other hand, in their series of 21 patients, Wang et al[46] described only 1 patient that had further ASD requiring posterior revision surgery. Cage subsidence rates were also lower when the LLIF was used in patients with ASD, probably due to presence of pedicle screws in the caudal vertebral body.[46] In addition, if one desires not to handle the previous fusion caudally, posterior fixation can be achieved with facet screws alone that achieve comparable results to pedicle screw fixation[20] (Fig. 24.6).

The frequent development of transient thigh pain, weakness, numbness, or dysesthesias is a limiting factor of this method, but can be minimized with increased

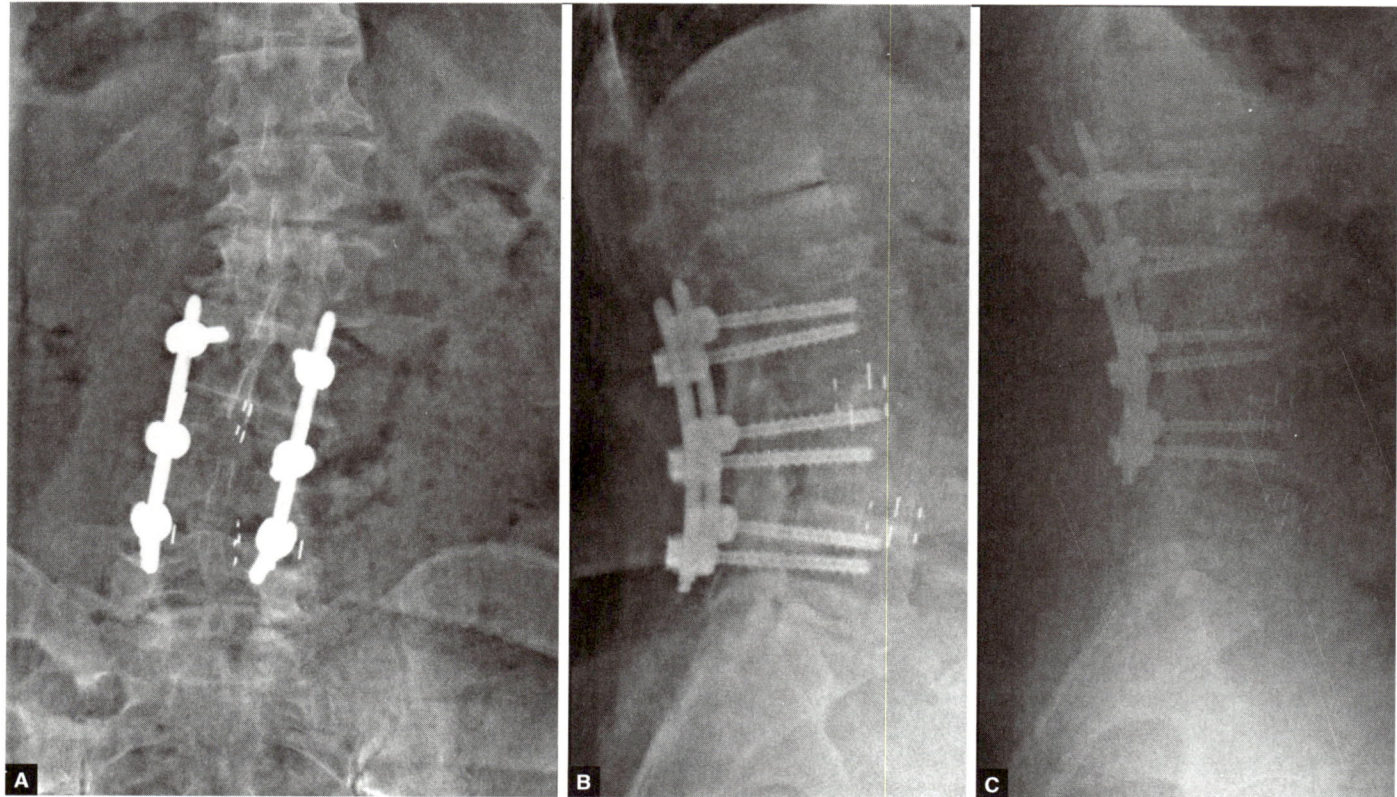

Fig. 24.5: Coronal standing radiographs (A) in a patient with adult degenerative scoliosis who underwent a prior L3–5 posterior fusion. Postoperative lumbosacral spine lateral radiographs (B) demonstrated an adequate fusion at those levels with collapsed discs at L1–2 and L2–3 for which the patient was symptomatic. Postoperative lateral lumbosacral spine radiograph; (C) after an L1–2 and L2–3 LLIF with revision of posterior instrumentation

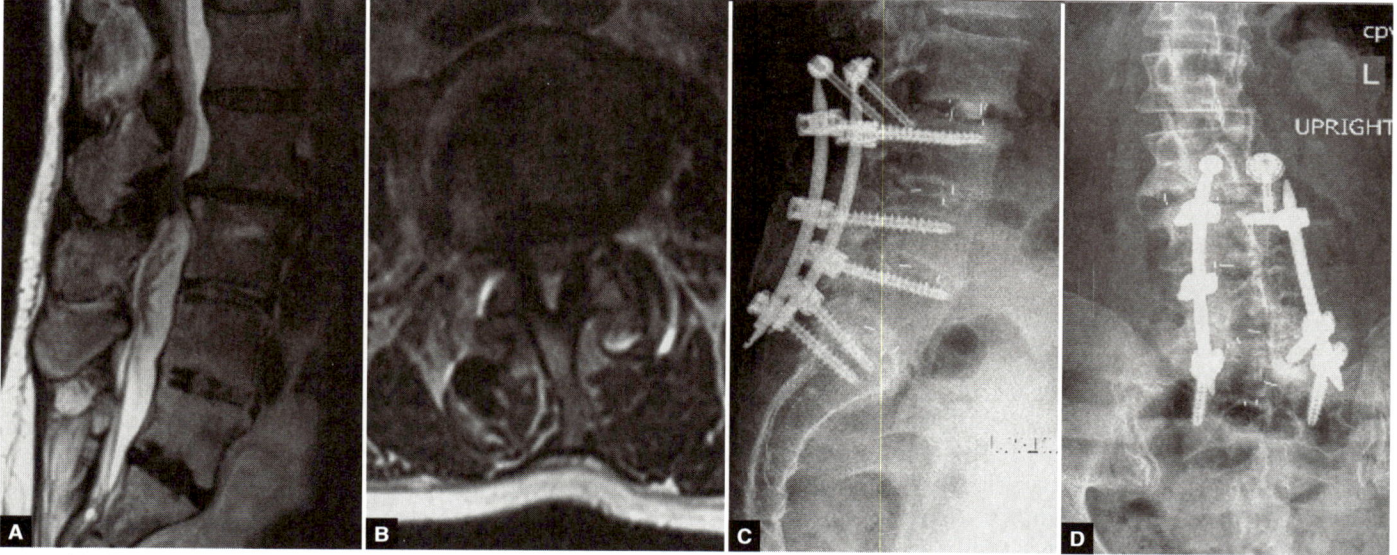

Fig. 24.6: Preoperative sagittal (A) and axial (B) T2-W MRI of a 57-year-old female patient who underwent a prior L3–S1 fusion done over eleven years ago. The patient eventually began experiencing low back pain and posterior thigh pain, predominantly with the right greater the left. Her neurologic examination was normal. She underwent conservative treatment with minimal relief. An MRI of the lumbar spine demonstrated near complete collapse of L2/3 disc space from adjacent segment disease. After discussion with the patient, she underwent a left L2/3 lateral interbody fusion followed by L2/3 facet screws. On one-year follow-up her pain was completely resolved. Lateral (C) and anteroposterior (D); radiographs showed good fusion

familiarity with this approach. These complications seem to be lower when an oblique trajectory is used as opposed to a direct lateral one.

Conclusions

MIS techniques to address ASD after a prior lumbar fusion provide decompression of the neural elements, stabilization, and fusion. As familiarity and comfort with MIS increases, this surgical technique can treat ASD while limiting posterior soft tissue disruption and increased surgical morbidity from open surgery with excellent clinical and radiological outcomes.

Disclosures

Dr. Fessler receives royalties from DePuy, Stryker, and Medtronic. He has an ownership interest in In Queue Innovations.The other authors report no conflict of interest concerning the materials or methods used in this study or the findings specified in this paper.

REFERENCES

1. Adogwa O, Owens R, Karikari I, Agarwal V, Gottfried ON, Bagley CA, et al. Revision lumbar surgery in elderly patients with symptomatic pseudarthrosis, adjacent-segment disease, or same-level recurrent stenosis. Part 2. A cost-effectiveness analysis: clinical article. J Neurosurg Spine 2013;18:147–53.
2. Adogwa O, Parker SL, Shau D, Mendelhall SK, Cheng J, Aaronson O, et al. Long-term outcomes of revision fusion for lumbar pseudarthrosis: clinical article. J Neurosurg Spine 2011;15:393–8.
3. Aichmair A, Alimi M, Hughes AP, Sama AA, Du JY, Härtl R, et al. Single-level Lateral Lumbar Interbody Fusion for the Treatment of Adjacent Segment Disease: A Retrospective Two-center Study. Spine:2016
4. Bresnahan LE, Smith JS, Ogden AT, Quinn S, Cybulski GR, Simonian N, et al. Assessment of Paraspinal Muscle Cross-sectional Area After Lumbar Decompression: Minimally Invasive Versus Open Approaches. Clin Spine Surg 30:E162-E168, 2017.
5. Cao Y, Chen Z, Jiang C, Wan S, Jiang X, Feng Z. The combined use of unilateral pedicle screw and contralateral facet joint screw fixation in transforaminal lumbar interbody fusion. Eur Spine J Off Publ Eur Spine Soc Eur Spinal Deform Soc Eur Sect Cerv Spine Res Soc 2015;24:2607–13.
6. Chandra VVR, Prasad BCM, Jagadeesh MA, Jayachandar V, Kumar SA, Kumar R. Segmental polymethylmethacrylate-augmented fenestrated pedicle screw fixation for lumbar spondylolisthesis in patients with osteoporosis-A case series and review of literature. Neurol India 2017;65:89–95.
7. Chandra Vemula VR, Prasad BC, Jagadeesh MA, Vuttarkar J, Akula SK: Minimally invasive transforaminal lumbar interbody fusion using bone cement-augmented pedicle screws for lumbar spondylolisthesis in patients with osteoporosis. Case series and review of literature. Neurol India 2018;66:118–5.
8. Chen X-L, Guan L, Liu Y-Z, Yang J-C, Wang W-L, Hai Y. Interspinous dynamic stabilization adjacent to fusion versus double-segment fusion for treatment of lumbar degenerative disease with a minimum follow-up of three years. Int Orthop 2016;40:1275–1283.
9. Chou P-H, Lin H-H, An HS, Liu K-Y, Su W-R, Lin C-L: Could the Topping-Off Technique Be the Preventive Strategy against Adjacent Segment Disease after Pedicle Screw-Based Fusion in Lumbar Degenerative Diseases? A Systematic Review. BioMed Res Int 2017:4385620.
10. Drysch A, Ajiboye RM, Sharma A, Li J, Reza T, Harley D, et al. Effectiveness of Reoperations for Adjacent Segment Disease Following Lumbar Spinal Fusion. Orthopedics 2017;1–7.
11. Epstein NE. Adjacent level disease following lumbar spine surgery: A review. Surg Neurol Int 2015;6:S591–599.
12. Epstein NE. A review: Reduced reoperation rate for multilevel lumbar laminectomies with noninstrumented versus instrumented fusions. Surg Neurol Int 2016;7:S337–346.
13. Fessler RG, Smith ZA, Slimack N, Smith JS, Parkinson RJ. Current advances and evidence in minimally invasive spine surgery. Minim Invasive Surg 2012:508415.
14. Ghiselli G, Wang JC, Bhatia NN, Hsu WK, Dawson EG. Adjacent segment degeneration in the lumbar spine. J Bone Joint Surg Am 2004;86-A:1497–1503.
15. Hari A, Krishna M, Rajagandhi S, Rajakumar DV. Minimally invasive transforaminal lumbar interbody fusion-indications and clinical experience. Neurol India 2016;64:444–54.
16. Hari A, Krishna M, Rajagandhi S, Sharma A, Deshpande RV. Minimally invasive lateral foraminotomy with partial lateral facetectomy for lumbar radiculopathy—An evaluation of facet integrity and description of the procedure. Neurol India 2017; 65:1358–65.
17. Helgeson MD, Bevevino AJ, Hilibrand AS: Update on the evidence for adjacent segment degeneration and disease. Spine J Off J North Am Spine Soc 2013;13:342–51.
18. Hilibrand AS, Robbins M. Adjacent segment degeneration and adjacent segment disease: the consequences of spinal fusion? Spine J Off J North Am Spine Soc 2004;4:190S–194S.
19. Kerolus M, Turel MK, Tan L, Deutsch H. Stand-alone anterior lumbar interbody fusion: indications, techniques, surgical outcomes and complications. Expert Rev Med Devices 2016;13:1127–1136.
20. Kretzer RM, Molina C, Hu N, Umekoji H. Baaj AA, Serhan H, et al. A Comparative Biomechanical Analysis of Stand Alone Versus Facet Screw and Pedicle Screw Augmented Lateral Interbody Arthrodesis: An In Vitro Human Cadaveric Model. Clin Spine Surg 2016;29:E336–343.
21. Lee CS, Hwang CJ, Lee S-W, Ahn Y-J, Kim Y-T, Lee D-H, et al. Risk factors for adjacent segment disease after lumbar fusion. Eur Spine J Off Publ Eur Spine Soc Eur Spinal Deform Soc Eur Sect Cerv Spine Res Soc 2009;18:1637–43.
22. Lee JK, Jo Y-H, Kang C-N: Cost-effectiveness Analysis of Existing Pedicle Screws Reusing Technique in Extension Revision Operation for Adjacent Segmental Stenosis After Lumbar Posterolateral Fusion. Spine 2016;41:E785–790.
23. Li X-C, Huang C-M, Zhong C-F, Liang R-W, Luo S-J: Minimally invasive procedure reduces adjacent segment degeneration and disease: New benefit-based global meta-analysis. PloS One 2017;12:e0171546.
24. Li Z, Tang J, Hou S, Ren D, Li L, Lu X, et al. Four-year follow-up results of transforaminal lumbar interbody fusion as revision surgery for recurrent lumbar disc herniation after conventional discectomy. J Clin Neurosci Off J Neurosurg Soc Australas 2015; 22:331–37.
25. Liu C, Zhou Y: Percutaneous Endoscopic Lumbar Diskectomy and Minimally Invasive Transforaminal Lumbar Interbody Fusion for Recurrent Lumbar Disk Herniation. World Neurosurg 2017;98:14–20.
26. Ma J, Fan S, Zhao F, Fang X. Minimally invasive anterior lumbar interbody fusion for adjacent segment disease after posterior lumbar fusion. Orthop Surg 2014;6:78–9.
27. Mamuti M, Fan S, Liu J, Shan Z, Wang C, Li S, et al. Mini-open Anterior Lumbar Interbody Fusion for Recurrent Lumbar Disc Herniation Following Posterior Instrumentation. Spine 2016;41:E1104–14.
28. Mashaly H, Paschel EE, Khattar NK, Goldschmidt E, Gerszten PC. Posterior lumbar dynamic stabilization instead of arthrodesis for

symptomatic adjacent-segment degenerative stenosis: description of a novel technique. Neurosurg Focus 2016;40:E5.

29. Metzger MF, Robinson ST, Maldonado RC, Rawlinson J, Liu J, Acosta FL. Biomechanical analysis of lateral interbody fusion strategies for adjacent segment degeneration in the lumbar spine. Spine J Off J North Am Spine Soc. 2017.

30. Palejwala SK, Sheen WA, Walter CM, Dunn JH, Baaj AA. Minimally invasive lateral transpsoas interbody fusion using a stand-alone construct for the treatment of adjacent segment disease of the lumbar spine: review of the literature and report of three cases. Clin Neurol Neurosurg 2014;124:90–6.

31. Pan A, Hai Y, Yang J, Zhou L, Chen X, Guo H. Adjacent segment degeneration after lumbar spinal fusion compared with motion-preservation procedures: a meta-analysis. Eur Spine J Off Publ Eur Spine Soc Eur Spinal Deform Soc Eur Sect Cerv Spine Res Soc 2016;25:1522–32.

32. Park P, Garton HJ, Gala VC, Hoff JT, McGillicuddy JE: Adjacent segment disease after lumbar or lumbosacral fusion: review of the literature. Spine 2004;29:1938–44.

33. Park Y, Ha JW, Lee YT, Sung NY. Cranial facet joint violations by percutaneously placed pedicle screws adjacent to a minimally invasive lumbar spinal fusion. Spine J Off J North Am Spine Soc 2011;11:295–302.

34. Parker SL, Adogwa O, Mendenhall SK, Shau DN, Anderson WN, Cheng JS, et al. Determination of minimum clinically important difference (MCID) in pain, disability, and quality of life after revision fusion for symptomatic pseudoarthrosis. Spine J Off J North Am Spine Soc 2012;12:1122–28.

35. Phillips FM, Carlson GD, Bohlman HH, Hughes SS. Results of surgery for spinal stenosis adjacent to previous lumbar fusion. J Spinal Disord 2000;13:432–37.

36. Prasad BCM, Ramesh Chandra VV, Devi BV, Chivukula SS, Pundarikakshaiah K. Clinical, radiological, and functional evaluation of surgical treatment in degenerative lumbar canal stenosis. Neurol India 2016;64:677–83.

37. Proietti L, Scaramuzzo L, Schiro' GR, Sessa S, Logroscino CA. Complications in lumbar spine surgery: A retrospective analysis. Indian J Orthop 2013;47:340–45.

38. Rajaee SS, Kanim LEA, Bae HW. National trends in revision spinal fusion in the USA: patient characteristics and complications. Bone Jt J 2014;96-B:807–16.

39. Ranjan A, Lath R. Microendoscopic discectomy for prolapsed lumbar intervertebral disc. Neurol India 2006;54:190–4.

40. Rao PJ, Loganathan A, Yeung V, Mobbs RJ. Outcomes of anterior lumbar interbody fusion surgery based on indication: a prospective study. Neurosurgery 76:7–23; discussion 2015;23–24.

41. Rodriguez A, Neal MT, Liu A, Somasundaram A, Hsu W, Branch CL. Novel placement of cortical bone trajectory screws in previously instrumented pedicles for adjacent-segment lumbar disease using CT image-guided navigation. Neurosurg Focus 2014;36:E9.

42. Schlegel JD, Smith JA, Schleusener RL. Lumbar motion segment pathology adjacent to thoracolumbar, lumbar, and lumbosacral fusions. Spine 1996;21:970–81.

43. Telfeian AE. Transforaminal Endoscopic Surgery for Adjacent Segment Disease After Lumbar Fusion. World Neurosurg 2017;97:231–5.

44. Vishteh AG, Dickman CA. Anterior lumbar microdiscectomy and interbody fusion for the treatment of recurrent disc herniation. Neurosurgery 48:334–337; discussion 2001;338.

45. Wang H, Ma L, Yang D, Wang T, Liu S, Yang S, et al. Incidence and risk factors of adjacent segment disease following posterior decompression and instrumented fusion for degenerative lumbar disorders. Medicine (Baltimore) 2017;96:e6032.

46. Wang MY, Vasudevan R, Mindea SA. Minimally invasive lateral interbody fusion for the treatment of rostral adjacent-segment lumbar degenerative stenosis without supplemental pedicle screw fixation. J Neurosurg Spine 2014;21:861–66.

47. Wong AP, Smith ZA, Nixon AT, Lawton CD, Dahdaleh NS, Wong RH, et al. Intraoperative and perioperative complications in minimally invasive transforaminal lumbar interbody fusion: a review of 513 patients. J Neurosurg Spine 2015;22:487–95.

48. Xia X-P, Chen H-L, Cheng H-B. Prevalence of adjacent segment degeneration after spine surgery: a systematic review and meta-analysis. Spine 2013;38:597–608.

49. Zhang C, Berven SH, Fortin M, Weber MH. Adjacent Segment Degeneration Versus Disease After Lumbar Spine Fusion for Degenerative Pathology: A Systematic Review With Meta-Analysis of the Literature. Clin Spine Surg 2016;29:21–9.

50. Zheng F, Cammisa FP, Sandhu HS, Girardi FP, Khan SN. Factors predicting hospital stay, operative time, blood loss, and transfusion in patients undergoing revision posterior lumbar spine decompression, fusion, and segmental instrumentation. Spine 2002;27:818–24.

51. Zhou Z-J, Xia P, Zhao X, Fang X-Q, Zhao F-D, Fan S-W. Can posterior dynamic stabilization reduce the risk of adjacent segment deterioration? Turk Neurosurg 2013;23:579–89.

Complications in Surgery on Lumbar Spine for Lumbar Canal Stenosis

Kumar Abhinav, PS Ramani

INTRODUCTION

Although the words "complication" and "adverse event" have significantly different meaning, they are often used interchangeably. Presently, there is no clear or consistent definition of a complication in the surgical literature. Complication is defined as "a morbid process or event occurring during a disease that is not an essential part of the disease, although it may result from it or from independent causes." To be precise, any unexpected or undesirable event resulting from an intervention, regardless of consequence is the literal meaning of complication.

The awareness of adverse events and development of preventative measures are obviously the best ways for preventing or minimizing the incidence of complications. Improved patient safety in surgery for lumbar canal stenosis can only be maximized by the development of methods to record prospectively adverse event data, so that enhanced clinical protocols can be developed in an evidence-based manner.

SURGICAL SITE INFECTION (SSI)

Surgical site infection (SSI) is quite common in spine surgery and can lead to devastating consequences, including pseudarthrosis, neurological deficit, sepsis, and occasionally death. A multifaceted approach to management is crucial, including risk stratification, early diagnosis, and effective treatment. When assessing risk factors for SSI, it is important to consider factors relating to the patient, the pathology, and the procedure. Patient-related factors include medical comorbidities, such as diabetes, obesity, heart ailments, hypertension and nutritional status.

A number of regression-based SSI prediction risk models have been developed to identify statistically significant risk factors.[1] In terms of spine pathology:

Deformity has a higher rate of SSI when compared with standard degenerative surgery (4.2% *vs* 1.4%), spinal trauma compared with elective spinal surgery (9.4% vs 2.3%), and surgery for spinal cord injury when compared with elective spine surgery (9.4% *vs* 3.3%).[4]

All these factors lead to increased rate of infection. There are other surgical risk factors, e.g. surgical case order in the day's list has an impact on SSI. A posterior lumbar decompression performed later in the operating list is more likely to get an SSI than the first case of the day.[5]

Three factors are important in the pathogenesis:
1. Endogenous pathogens
2. Exogenous pathogens, and
3. The host's immune status: Endogenous pathogens include the host's flora and a seedling from a distant focus. Exogenous pathogens are from surgical personnel, the operating environment or equipment, and materials being used.

Although the pathogenesis is multifactorial, SSI usually occurs as a result of direct inoculation or contamination at the time of surgery. This contamination is often by endogenous skin flora. Coagulase-negative *Staphylococcus*, *Propionibacterium acnes*, and *Corynebacterium* are the most common bacteria. *Staphylococcus aureus* accounts for 50% of SSI. *Staphylococcus epidermidis* is often involved in cases involving spinal instrumentation. Gram-negative bacteria (e.g. *Enterococcus* , *E. coli*, *Peptostreptococcus*) because of proximity to the perianal area and bowel and bladder incontinence are risk factors.

There are no universally accepted diagnostic criteria for SSI. It is often a combination of clinical, laboratory, and radiological parameters. Wound drainage on postoperative day 10 to 14 is the most common early clinical sign. C-reactive protein (CRP) is elevated in over 98% of cases following surgery on the spine.[6]

Intraoperative cultures are often negative. CRP accuracy does vary. It is the second postoperative peak or failure to decrease postoperative peak is suggestive of SSI.[20,21] Usually WBC, ESR, and CRP tend to normalize by 7th postoperative day. Serum amyloid A has been assessed as a marker of SSI in a prospective study of 106 patients following PLIF surgery.[23]

CRP levels in the SSI group both decreased on postoperative day 7 and then dramatically increased on 13th postoperative day.

Procalcitonin (PCT) is another serological marker that has been assessed in the screening of SSI. PCT and CRP significantly correlated with SSI.

MRI is an useful tool to demonstrate SSI. The "pedicle screw sign," essentially 5 mm of high signal around the screw head on axial MRI, has been demonstrated to have 88% sensitivity for deep SSI in patients without wound discharge. PET/CT may have a role in evaluating suspected deep infections in patients with spinal instrumentation.

Prevention

Surgical gowns may carry significant contamination.[7] The C-arm machine needs close attention. In one study swab samples of 25 draped C-Arms used for spine cases demonstrated that the top and upper front of the C-arm receiver were the most contaminated areas.[8] Surgeons should avoid personally moving the C-arm near the sterile field. Similar practices need to be considered when using a microscope. A study of sterile culture swabs from 25 microscope drapes used in spine operations, demonstrated contamination to be most common around optic eyepieces, from inadvertent touching.[9] The surgeon should change the gloves after adjusting the eyepiece. Spinal implants can also be a source of contamination. A recent study has highlighted that cultures from covered implants demonstrated a 9.5% contamination rate, compared with cultures from uncovered implants having a 16.7% contamination rate.[10] Covering each implant separately was found to significantly reduce implant contamination (P = 0.016).[11] Implant trays should be covered with sterile towels until they are being used.

The time a tray was left open, implant type and the number of implants used and the number of scrubbed personnel was not associated with contamination. A retrospective cohort study of 389 lumbar spine fusions, with control (n = 179) and treatment (n = 210) groups, who initially double gloved, then removed their outer gloves before handling instrumentation, demonstrated a statistically significant reduction in SSI from 3.35 to 0.48% at 1 year.[12] Allograft may also be associated with contamination. In a study, 9.4% demonstrated

positive cultures, yet none led to antibiotic treatment or revision surgery at 1 year.[13] There was no difference in the SSI rate at 1 year for irradiated autograft or allograft.

Use of allogeneic blood transfusion is another risk for SSI. Allogeneic blood transfusion should be used judiciously. Povidone-iodine irrigation (PVP-I) is the only solution demonstrated to have a positive impact on minimizing SSI rates in spine surgery.[14,15] In a study where the surgical site was soaked with dilute PVP-I for 3 minutes, then copiously irrigated with normal saline, prior to bone decortication, there was a reported SSI Rate of 0%. A recent retrospective cohort study, compared the efficacy of a povidone iodine intra-operative irrigation and gentamicin antibiotic irrigation and adjunctive local vancomycin powder to reduce the SSI rate.[16] The SSI rate for both superficial and deep infections was higher with gentamicin regimen (26.7%) than with the povidone iodine irrigation (7.0%) and vancomycin powder use (6.3%). The SSI rates for povidone-iodine and vancomycin regimens were deemed comparable. Administration of local vancomycin powder has become a common practice among spine surgeons, though the evidence supporting its use remains somewhat controversial.[17] Furthermore, direct application of vancomycin powder to human dura mater tissue induced cell death and inhibited dural growth. Local vancomycin powder has an inhibitory effect on dural healing when durotomy is done.[18] There is also concern that application of vancomycin may increase the risk of development of antibiotic resistance among infectious organisms.

Conclusion

Surgical intervention is usually reserved for infections resistant to medical management. The multifaceted approach along with early diagnosis and effective treatment, is essential for successful prevention and effective treatment.

DURAL TEAR

Spinal dural tear is common in spinal surgery. Previous studies have shown that potentially serious problems, such as pseudomeningocele, external CSF fistula, meningitis and arachnoiditis with subsequent chronic pain are possible sequalae of dural tears and CSF leakage after spinal surgery. Suturing of the dura,[28–30] strict bedrest,[28,29,31,32] fibrin glue,[31,32] and lumbar drainage[30,32,33] have been used to treat intraoperative dural tears to prevent spinal CSF fistula. The morbidity associated with spinal CSF fistula due to primary dural tears accomplished with microsurgery alone,[29] or bedrest and spinal lumbar drain insertion have been minimal. The outcome of dural tear management, however, is based on CSF fistulas rates from studies of different types of spinal procedures.[28–30,32–39] There is lack of consensus in the literature and the potentially serious nature of this complication needs to evaluate its management. Actual size of the lesion, as well as location of the tear is often the most important to determine the time of the procedure.

Incidence

Durotomy occurs in four different anatomical spinal areas.

1. The caudal margin of the cranial lamina.
2. Cranial margin of the caudal lamina
3. Herniated disc level, and
4. Medial aspect of the facet joint adjacent to the insertion of the hypertrophic ligamentum flavum.[32] They reported an overall incidence of 4%. The incidence of dural tear was significantly higher in women (5.6%) than in men (3%). The incidence of dural tear was 2% in patient with LCS and 9% with degenerative spondylolisthesis, and almost 20% with juxtafacet cysts, still, the overall incidence of dural tears, based on national databases,[33,37] was higher in lumbar stenosis than in discectomy as in our cases. Furthermore, the effect of incidental durotomy on in-hospital Spinal stenosis is seen more in older people, while disc herniation is seen in younger population. Older age, previous surgery and smoking were risk factors for having dural tears, which, however, did not affect the 1 year outcome negatively.[35,40] Another factor that may contribute to dural tearing is the presence of residual bone spikes after bony decompression.[41,42]

Pathogenesis

According to study by Galarza et al

Type I dural tear consisted of disruption of the dura, with clean borders, minimal or no breach of the arachnoid, and exit of a few drops of CSF.

Type II dural tear consisted of disruption of the dura, with clean borders, evident breach of the arachnoid, and exit of multiple drops or a single line of CSF.

Type III dural tear consisted of disruption of the dura, with more than one border, gross breach of the arachnoid sometimes with protrusion of the rootlets or nerve roots. Dural tears located at the nerve root shoulder, or axilla, however, these treatment options are less appealing because they are associated with a higher morbidity rate.[43]

Fibrin glue alone in simple cases of dural tears, that is Type I cases is sufficient. In all Type II dural tears, tissue-glue coated collagen sponge application was found to be useful. In more complex cases, as in Type III dural tears repair, polypropylene stitches, in a combination of the two previous agents was found to be useful. We routinely use collagen matrix patch with tissel solution to cover the defect in the dura.

Implant Related Complications

In PLIF surgery , pedicle screw misplacement has been classified into five categories:

1. Medial cortical perforation (MCP),
2. Lateral cortical perforation (LCP),
3. Anterior cortical perforation of vertebral body (ACP),
4. Endplate perforation (EPP), and
5. Entering into the neural foramen (FP).

Screw misplacement is considered positive, if its misplacement is greater than 2 mm, dangerous injury nerve root if it is 5 mm and negative if screw is fully contained into the pedicle.[44]

Screw entering the vertebral foramen could have serious consequence, if it damages the nerve root. Similarly screw just breaching the medial cortex can brush against the nerve root and cause pain, much to the discomfort of the patient and the surgeon.

During follow-up period the presence of a radiolucent rim of 1 mm or more surrounding the screw surrounded by radio-optic dense bone "double halo signal" is considered as screw loosening.[45]

In the interspinous implant patients, particularly with C0-Flex device the metal and bone contact surfaces between metallic blades and spinous process can cause erosion and fracture of spinous process. The device can get dislocated. Fortunately such incidences have no bearing on the outcome of patient even if the implant is removed.

During the second follow-up at one year or later, repeat X-ray may show breakage of one of the pedicle screws due to bio-mechanical mismatch. Removal of such a screw is not mandatory as bony fusion takes over making the role of screws redundant. As a matter of fact the screw breaks at its junction with the cortex of the vertebral body and attempting to remove the broken piece from the vertebra is the most difficult task.

Kidney-shaped interbody cages are known to have ruptured through the anterior longitudinal ligament or come out partially through the entry track. Fortunately, in both situations the neural elements are quite far away to be irritated causing pain. Removal and correct placement of cage is mandatory. In osteoporotic patients cages are know to have sunk into the vertebral bodies causing reduction in disc space. However, clinical satisfaction of the patient does not warrant taking action against such happenings.

REOPERATION

Based on the timing, reoperations are classified as early or late. Early reoperations are caused by an acute complication (<1 year). Indications for reoperation 1 year or more after surgery may be, persistent pain or recurrence of symptoms or adjacent segment pathology (ASP).[13,14]

According to population-based analysis, cumulative reoperation rates accounting for any unplanned surgery, including both decompression or fusion surgery are 12.5–14.0% at 4 years.[13,15] The Finnish National Hospital Discharge Register studies show 20% cumulative risk for reoperation within 15 years after spinal fusion.[13] The length of the fusion influences the reoperation rate. Howe, et al.[16] reported a reoperation rate as high as 35% during a mean 26-month follow-up of instrumented fusions from the thoracic spine to the pelvis.

OTHER MISCELLANEOUS COMPLICATIONS (DVT AND OBESITY)

Body mass index (BMI) >30 kg/m^2],[1] secondary medical complications associated with obesity, including metabolic and musculoskeletal problems, can be extensive and significantly limit a person's ability to function and participate in life.[2] High prevalence of obese patients who elect to have lumbar surgery, despite the potential negative influence obesity may have on surgical outcomes.[3–6] Obesity has the potential to affect outcomes of lumbar spine surgery in a number of ways, including intraoperative challenges, health-related comorbidities and because of the long-term effect of stresses due to excessive body weight. Immediate intraoperative challenges include the need for a larger incision and soft tissue retraction due to excess subcutaneous tissue, which may increase blood loss, operative time, and risk of intraoperative complications. Health-related effects of chronic obesity may increase the incidence of medical complications after surgery, including deep surgical site infection (deep infection), deep vein thrombosis (DVT), all-cause mortality, acute myocardial infarction (MI), pneumonia, pulmonary embolism (PE), and respiratory failure. Over time, excessive body weight can impose undue stress on the surgical implants, adjacent soft tissue, and joints, increasing risk for long-term surgical complications including reoperation and adjacent segment disease (ASD).

Patients undergoing posterolateral fusion surgery, obesity was associated with increased blood loss but there was no difference in rates of epidural hematomas.[13] Similarly, McGuire et al reported a relationship between obesity, classified as a BMI of ≥35,

and increased operative time and blood loss, but not with intraoperative complications for a sample of patients with spondylolisthesis.[14] Peng et al reported longer operative times, but no differences in blood loss or intra-complications in patients with and without obesity.[12] Most prior investigators also have reported that obesity increases risk of deep surgical site infection in a variety of patient samples.[13,14,21] Radcliff et al reported no effect of BMI on reoperation rates in patients treated with a posterior decompression or fusion for spinal stenosis.[7] Fu et al reported no difference in ASD or revision surgeries in obese and non-obese patients treated with lumbar fusion.[10] However, investigators only divided patients into normal, overweight, and obese categories, with no stratification of obesity severity. Min et al also reported no difference in BMI between patients with and without ASD treated with instrumented lumbar fusion.[23]

Intraoperative Excessive Bleeding

Intraoperative excesive bleeding is reported to cause a decrease in hemostatic and anticoagulant factors, leading to clotting disorder. Increased loss of blood results in decreased antithrombin and prolonged half-lives of thrombin and activated factor X (Xa), thereby increasing thrombogenic tendency and contributing to the development of DVT.[11] This mechanism may explain the significantly high incidence of DVT postoperatively. Augmented coagulation cascade associated with excessive bleeding is responsible for DVT. Anticoagulant therapy was recently introduced into spinal surgery, and there are reports stating that the use of unfractionated or low-molecular-weight heparin reduces the occurrence of DVT by 40 to 50%.[15]

Increasing obesity and BMI was associated with a statistically significant increase in the length of surgery, EBL, deep infection, DVT, and rate of re-operation. This information is of value when discussing surgical risk with obese patients who elect to undergo instrumented lumbar spine surgery. These findings are also of value in perioperative management for these patients, including medical optimization prior to surgery, utilization of alternative surgical approaches and techniques, and comprehensive postoperative management. Future study is needed to determine the impact of obesity and increasing BMI on patient-centered outcomes and costs of care.

VISCERAL AND VASCULAR INJURIES

Vascular Injury

Although, a catastrophic occurrence, it is one that may not be mentioned in obtaining an informed consent because of its rarity, or because the surgeon has just not considered it at the time of counseling the patient. The first described vascular complication secondary to intervertebral disc surgery (L4/5) was an arteriovenous fistula between the right iliac artery and the inferior vena cava reported by Linton and White in 1945. Weber is credited[40] with having reported the first case of an isolated venous injury, i.e. a laceration of the inferior vena cava.

DeSaussure (1959)[20] reported, however, that in less than 50% of the cases he reviewed, arterial bleeding from the disc space was seen. Jarstfer and Rich (1976) in their review of the literature of 68 cases of arteriovenous fistulae, to which they added another five cases, found an incidence of 28.3% with bleeding from the disc space. In those cases in which hypotension was reported (22.7%), bleeding was seen from the disc space in 8.8% and no bleeding from the disc space was seen in 13%.

The most common vascular injury is a tear of the left common iliac artery, which is immediately anterior to the L4/5 lumbar disc space[7] (Fig 25.1). Other injuries include the right iliac artery, the aorta, the inferior vena cava, iliac veins, branches of the iliac vessels and bridging veins, and formation of arteriovenous fistulae.

Perforation of the ALL may not be noted by the surgeon unless there is a resistance and then give-away, which the surgeon appreciates as a puncture of the ALL. It is the injury to the vessel with blood briskly issuing from the disc space, sudden unexplained hypotension, or the finding of a piece of vessel wall (or viscera) within the rongeur/forceps that would alert the surgeon to the injury. Bleeding into the retroperitoneal space and peritoneal cavity may not be obvious to the surgeon, leading to a delay in diagnosis. Hypotension may be delayed or not present until the patient has been turned supine, or may be delayed until the patient is in the recovery room. Abdominal distention and discomfort associated with nausea and vomiting, are the cardinal symptoms. An absent pulse, pallor, and decreased

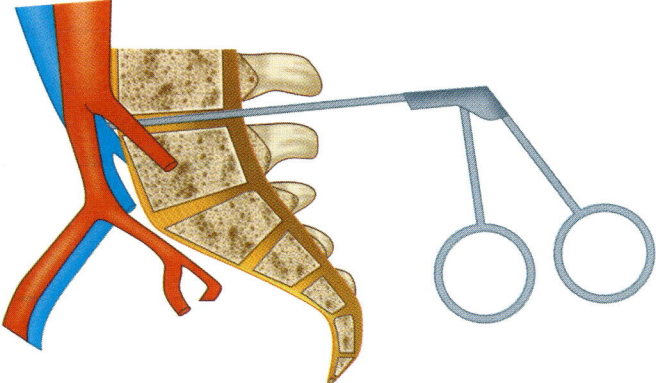

Fig. 25.1: Injury to the common iliac vessel

temperature in a lower extremity may be present, suggesting damage to a major artery.[7]

Swelling and engorgement of the lower extremities misinterpreted as a "thrombophlebitis syndrome," which is actually a manifestation of an arteriovenous fistula leading to a delay in diagnosis has been described.[7,45] The most common fistula found was between the common iliac artery and inferior vena cava.[45] The most common discectomy level associated with an arteriovenous fistula was at L4/5.[45] One review of "Iatrogenic Arteriovenous Fistulas," noted that discectomy was the most common surgical cause. Angiography may be indicated in the acute stages when the diagnosis is in question.

Visceral Injury

Epidemiology

The first indication of injury to an abdominal viscera may be the finding of mucosa or fat in the surgical specimen.[8,42] Harbison (1954)[42] reported the first reference to an intestinal injury. Other reported complications have included abdominal/pelvic abscesses and enterocutaneous fistulae. The majority of cases followed surgery at the L5/S1 level. Cases of discitis after visceral injuries have been reported by various authors. When bowel organisms are grown from the infection in the spine, it is a strong indication that the bowel is injured during discectomy. Smith and Hanigan has reported that there is no need to suspect bowel injury in the presence of bowel infection when abdominal signs are absent.

Ureter injury: Injury to the ureter is a possibility. Diagnosis is difficult because of lack of specific diagnostic signs. Usually, ureter injury can occur during L4–L5 discectomy. Smith and Hanigan recommended careful attention to the tissue specimen submitted, which may avoid delays in diagnosis. However, if one accepts Boutin and Hogshead's[11] recommendation that "routine examination of surgically removed disc material by the pathologists is not essential to the quality of care," then it may not be possible to examine the removed specimen.

REFERENCES

1. Radcliff KE, Neusner AD, Millhouse PW, et al. What is new in the diagnosis and prevention of spine surgical site infections. Spine J 2015;15:336–47.
2. Smith JS, Shaffrey CI, Sansur CA, et al. Rates of infection after spine surgery based on 108,419 procedures: a report from the Scoliosis Research Society Morbidity and Mortality Committee. Spine (Phila Pa 1976) 2011;36:556–63.
3. Lonjon G, Dauzac C, Fourniols E, et al. Early surgical site infections in adult spinal trauma: a prospective, multicentre study of infection rates and risk factors. OrthopTraumatolSurg Res 2012;98:788–94.

4. Blam OG, Vaccaro AR, Vanichkachorn JS, et al. Risk factors for surgical site infection in the patient with spinal injury. Spine (Phila Pa 1976) 2003;28:1475–80.

5. Gruskay J, Kepler C, Smith J, et al. Is surgical case order associated with increased infection rate after spine surgery? Spine (Phila Pa 1976) 2012;37:1170–4.

6. Pull terGunne AF, Hosman AJ, Cohen DB, et al. A methodological systematic review on surgical site infections following spinal surgery: Part 1: risk factors. Spine (Phila Pa 1976) 2012;37:2017–33.

7. Bible JE, Biswas D, Whang PG, et al. Which regions of the operating gown should be considered most sterile? Clin OrthopRelat Res 2009;467:825–30.

8. Biswas D, Bible JE, Whang PG, et al. Sterility of C-arm fluoroscopy during spinal surgery. Spine (Phila Pa 1976) 2008;33:1913–7.

9. Bible JE, O'Neill KR, Crosby CG, et al. Microscope sterility during spine surgery. Spine (Phila Pa 1976) 2012;37:623–27.

10. Waked WR, Simpson AK, Miller CP, et al. Sterilization wrap inspections do not adequately evaluate instrument sterility. Clin OrthopRelat Res 2007;462:207–11.

11. Bible JE, O'Neill KR, Crosby CG, et al. Implant contamination during spine surgery. Spine J 2013;13:637–40.

12. Rehman A, Rehman AU, Rehman TU, et al. Removing outer gloves as a method to reduce spinal surgery infection. J Spinal Disord Tech 2015;28:E343–6.

13. Couture J, Cabana F. Irradiated allograft bone in spine surgery: to culture or not? A single center retrospective study. Spine (Phila Pa 1976) 2013;38:558–63.

14. Chang FY, ChangMC,Wang ST, et al. Can povidone-iodine solution be used safely in a spinal surgery? Eur Spine J 2006;15:1005–14.

15. Cheng MT, Chang MC, Wang ST, et al. Efficacy of dilute betadine solution irrigation in the prevention of postoperative infection of spinal surgery. Spine (Phila Pa 1976) 2005;30:1689–93.

16. van Herwijnen B, Evans NR, Dare CJ, et al. An intraoperative irrigation regimen to reduce the surgical site infection rate following adolescent idiopathic scoliosis surgery. Ann R Coll Surg Engl 2016;98:320–23.

17. Eder C, Schenk S, Trifinopoulos J, et al. Does intrawound application of vancomycin influence bone healing in spinal surgery? Eur Spine J 2016;25:1021–8.

18. Goldschmidt E, Rasmussen J, Chabot JD, et al. The effect of vancomycin powder on human dural fibroblast culture and its implications for dural repair during spine surgery. J Neurosurg Spine 2016;25:665–70.

19. Scott CP, Higham PA, Dumbleton JH. Effectiveness of bone cement containing tobramycin. An in vitro susceptibility study of 99 organisms found in infected joint arthroplasty. J Bone Joint Surg Br 1999;81:440–3.

20. Lall RR, Wong AP, Lall RR, et al. Evidence-based management of deep wound infection after spinal instrumentation. J Clin Neurosci 2015;22:238–42.

21. Kowalski TJ, Berbari EF, Huddleston PM, et al. The management and outcome of spinal implant infections: contemporary retrospective cohort study. Clin Infect Dis 2007;44:913–20.

22. Zwolak P, König MA, Osterhoff G, et al. Therapy of acute and delayed spinal infections after spinal surgery treated with negative pressure wound therapy in adult patients. Orthop Rev (Pavia) 2013;5:e30.

23. Rohmiller MT, Akbarnia BA, Raiszadeh K, et al. Closed suction irrigation for the treatment of postoperative wound infections following posterior spinal fusion and instrumentation. Spine (Phila Pa 1976) 2010;35:642–46.

24. Mitra A, Mitra A, Harlin S. Treatment of massive thoracolumbar wounds and vertebral osteomyelitis following scoliosis surgery. Plast Reconstr Surg 2004;113:206–13.

25. Mericli AF, Tarola NA, Moore JH Jr, et al. Paraspinous muscle flap reconstruction of complex midline back wounds: risk factors and postreconstruction complications. Ann Plast Surg 2010;65:219–24.

26. Mericli AF, Mirzabeigi MN, Moore JH Jr, et al. Reconstruction of complex posterior cervical spine wounds using the paraspinous muscle flap. PlastReconstr Surg 2011;128:148–53.

27. Diapaola CP, Saravanja DD, Boriani L, et al. Postoperative infection treatment score for the spine (PITSS): construction and validation of a predictive model to define need for single versus multiple irrigation and debridement for spinal surgical site infection. Spine J 2012;12:218–30.

28. Camissa FP, Girardi FP, Sangani PK. Incidental durotomy in spine surgery. Spine 2000;25(20):2663–7.

29. Desai A, Ball PA, Bekelis K, Lurie JD, Mirza SK, Tosteson TD, et al. Outcomes after incidental durotomy during first-time lumbar discectomy. J Neurosurg Spine 2011;14(5):647–53.

30. Stolke D, Sollmann W, Seifert V. Intra- and postoperative complications in lumbar disc surgery. Spine 1989;14:56–9.

31. Jankowitz BT, Atteberry DS, Gerszten PC, Karausky P, Cheng BC, Faught R, et al. Effect of fibrin glue on the prevention of persistent cerebral spinal fluid leakage after incidental durotomy during lumbar spinal surgery. Eur Spine J 2009;18:1169-74.

32. Takahashi Y, Sato T, Hyodo H, Kawamata T, Takahashi E, Miyatake N, Tokunaga M. Incidental durotomy during lumbar spine surgery: risk factors and anatomic locations: clinical article. J Neurosurg Spine 2013;8(2):165–9.

33. Yoshihara H, Yoneoka D. Incidental dural tear in lumbar spinal decompression and discectomy: analysis of a nationwide database. Arch Orthop Trauma Surg 2013;11:1501–8.

34. Goodkin R, Laska LL. Unintended "incidental" durotomy during surgery of the lumbar spine: medicolegal implications. SurgNeurol 1995;43:4–12.

35. Bosacco SJ, Gardner MJ, Guille JT. Evaluation and treatment of dural tears in lumbar spine surgery: a review. Clin OrthopRelat Res 2001;389:238–47.

36. Wang JC, Bohlman HH, Riew KD. Dural tears secondary to operations on the lumbar spine: management and results after a two-year minimum follow-up of eighty-eight patients. J Bone Joint Surg Am 1998;80:1728–32.

37. Strömqvist F, Jönsson B, Strömqvist B. Swedish Society of Spinal Surgeons. Dural lesions in decompression for lumbar spinal stenosis: incidence, risk factors and effect on outcome. Eur Spine J 2012;21(5):825–8.

38. Hodges SD, Humphreys SC, Eck JC, Covington LA. Management of incidental durotomy without mandatory bedrest. A retrospective review of 20 cases. Spine (Phila Pa 1976) 1999;24:2062–4.

39. Ghobrial GM, Theofanis T, Darden BV, Arnold P, Fehlings MG, Harrop JS. Unintended durotomy in lumbar degenerative spinal surgery: a 10-year systematic review of the literature. Neurosurg Focus 2015 Oct;39(4):E8.

40. Deyo RA, Mirza SK, Martin BI, Kreuter W, Goodman DC, Jarvik JG. Trends, major medical complications, and charges associated with surgery for lumbar spinal stenosis in older adults. JAMA 2011;303(13):1259–65.

41. Chen Z, Shao P, Sun Q, Zhao D. Risk factors for incidental durotomy during lumbar surgery: a retrospective study by multivariate analysis. Clin Neurol Neurosurg 2015;130:101–4.

42. Smorgick Y, Baker KC, Herkowitz H, Montgomery D, Badve SA, Bachison C, et al. Predisposing factors for dural tear in patients undergoing lumbar spine surgery. J Neurosurg Spine 2015;22:483–6.

43. Kitchel SH, Eismont FJ, Green BA. Closed subarachnoid drainage for management of cerebrospinal fluid leakage after an operation on the spine. J Bone Joint Surg Am 1989;71:984–7.

44. Gelalis ID, Paschos NK, Pakos EE, et al. Accuracy of pedicle screw placement: a systematic review of prospective *in vivo* studies comparing free hand, fluoroscopy guidance and navigation techniques. Eur Spine J. 2012;21:247–55. doi: 10.1007/s00586-011-2011-3.

45. Dakhil-Jerew F, Jadeja H, Cohen A, et al. Inter-observer reliability of detecting Dynesys pedicle screw using plain X-rays: a study on 50 post-operative patients. Eur Spine J. 2009;18:1486–93. doi: 10.1007/s00586-009-1071-0.

Long-Term Outcome in Lumbar Canal Stenosis

Sudhendoo Babhulkar, PS Ramani

INTRODUCTION

Verbiest[31] was one of the first to define lumbar canal stenosis. He defined congenital stenosis. But being the first it was not possible for him to define outcome. His main intention was relief from suffering. One must judiciously evaluate the patients with degenerative lumbar canal stenosis before choosing the line of treatment although all such patients undergo a period of conservative treatment in the beginning. Generally all patients with sciatic pain or neurological deficit should be given the surgical option. Several modalities like only decompression, decompression and fusion, IDSS and PDS are the three main groups and the surgeon must choose the one where he has familiarity. Other point to be considered is open versus minimally invasive techniques. The surgeon must have experience in the latter techniques. The third point to be considered is the use of tools for assistance like neuro navigation. Solid bony fusion should be the goal for treatment of instability. Just like verbiest the long-term outcome of minimally invasive surgery or IDSS with PDS are not available. Today's practice believes in high quality evidence which is still lacking in spite of the fact that more than sixty years have passed since the understanding of lumbar canal stenosis. There is a reason for this. We have passed through a period of technological boom which has resulted in emergence of newer instrumentation, newer techniques and newer operative procedures. Life goes on and so is the advance. A single cohort study becomes impossible and long-term outcomes become confused (Fig. 26.1).

Nonsurgical versus Surgical Management

A section of patients with spinal stenosis can be managed conservatively without surgery. Both young and old patients with severe comorbidities that may preclude risky surgical intervention even if MRI and

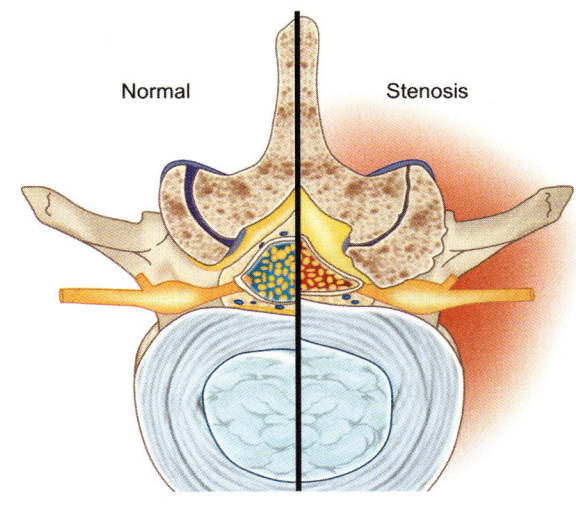

Normal   Stenosis

Spinal Stenosis

Fig. 26.1: Schematic representation showing comparison between normal spine and stenotic spine

CT document severe stenosis may benefit from treatment at multimodality pain centers. In one study the Oswestry Disability Index[12] (ODI) and surgeons' clinical assessment were used to compare outcomes for 50 patients with lumbar canal stenosis treated nonoperatively versus with laminectomy showed no significant difference in the outcome.

Other studied have documented the superiority of surgery for lumbar canal stenosis including decompression or decompression with fusion over nonsurgical alternatives. In a study conducted by Atlas et al[1,2] at 10 years follow-up, low back pain and patient's satisfaction were similar among the two groups. However surgically treated patients reported greater improvement in leg symptoms than nonsurgically treated patients.

In a study conducted by Weinstein et al[34-36] combining the randomized and observational cohorts of patients with spinal stenosis those treated surgically showed significant improvement in pain, function and satisfaction compared to patients treated nonsurgically.

Based on Roland Morris questionnaires to assess outcomes, patients undergoing surgery exhibited higher scores than those treated conservatively.[13] In another study patients with stenosis from 13 centers were randomly enrolled on two treatment groups. They were evaluated with SF-36 and a modified ODI score at 1, 3, 6, 12 and 24 months postoperatively. The study demonstrated substantial gains in pain relief and function following decompressive laminectomy with or without fusion. They were evaluated with SF-36 and a modified ODI score at 1,3,6,12 and 24 months postoperatively.

In a randomized control trial, Malmivaara[22] found that patients with surgical management maintained better outcomes compared with nonoperative patients at 4 years follow-up.

Minimally Invasive Surgery

Older Patients

In our study of a series of 50 patients with mean age of 60 years were assessed before and after internal decompression of spinal stenosis (IDSS) procedures using the visual analog scale (VAS) and ODI score. The postoperative scores improved significantly in these patients. It was concluded that minimally invasive procedures were safe and effective in managing spinal stenosis inelderly population. However, there is one drawback in these patients as stenosis increase the risk of cerebrospinal fluid (CSF) leaks and formation of fistulas, neural damage and possibility of incomplete decompression in these minimally invasive procedures.

Younger Patients

Younger patients undergoing minimally invasive procedures for spinal stenosis may be at a greater risk of developing stress fractures (secondary to ligamentous laxity) or facet joint degeneration in absence of degenerative disease.

PDS or Posterior Dynamic Procedures

In an attempt to prevent adjacent segment degeneration as seen in rigid fixation the posterior dynamic stabilization devices were introduced. Various interspinous process spacers (like X-Stop, Device for Intervertebral Assisted Motion (DIAM), Interspinous Posterior Device (IPD), Coflex, etc.) or pedicle-based systems (like PercuDyn, or Dynesys) have been introduced in this category.

X-stop Interspinous Spacer

X-stop devices are used to treat one to two level lumbar canal stenosis. The device theoretically "opens" the spinal canal thereby relieving the symptoms of stenosis. In an initial randomized multicentre trial involving 190 patients with lumbar stenosis, implantation of the X-Stop[38] device resulted in a 73% satisfaction rate compared with only 37% satisfaction rate among those managed nonsurgically.

In-space Interspinous Device

'In-space' works on a similar principal by opening up the spinal canal and relieving the symptoms of stenosis.[23] In a study of 50 patients the percutaneous insertion of in space was augmented with IDSS 3. Preoperatively we observed that the average ODI score for the study group preoperatively was 45.43% and postoperatively at 10 days, 3 months and 6 months were 33.37%, 18.68% and 10.58 % respectively. The ODI decreased by 34.85 percentage points, an improvement by 77.44% at 6 months as compared to preoperatively (Fig. 26.2 and Graph 26.1).

Preoperative the average VAS score was 4.86 points before the surgery and 5.86, 2.86 and 1.22 at the 10 days, 3 months and 6 months respectively. The VAS score decreased by 3.64 points, an improvement by 74.89% at 6 months compared to preoperatively (Graph 26.2).

'Co-flex' Interlaminar Device

Co-flex is an interspinous device used in the surgical management of patients with lumbar canal stenosis.[27] (Fig. 26.3).

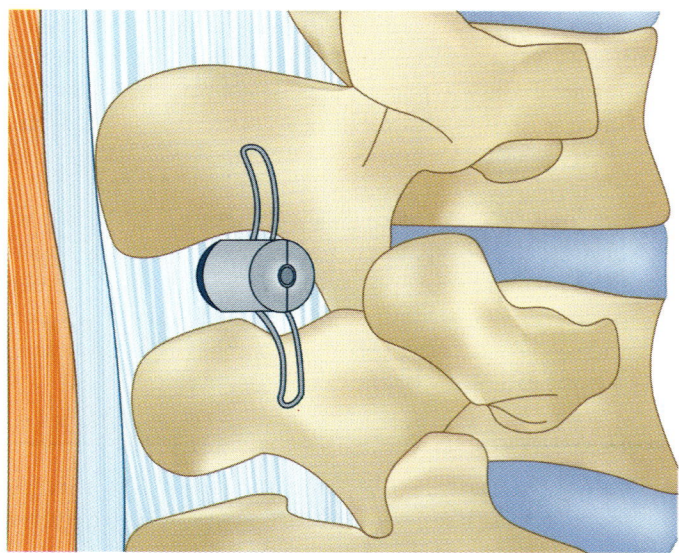

Fig. 26.2: *In situ* deployment of in-space

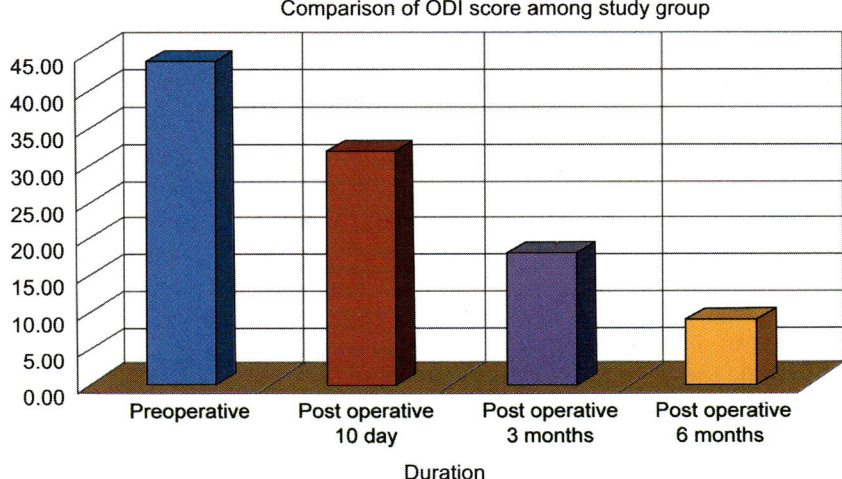

Graph 26.1: ODI score of patients in the series

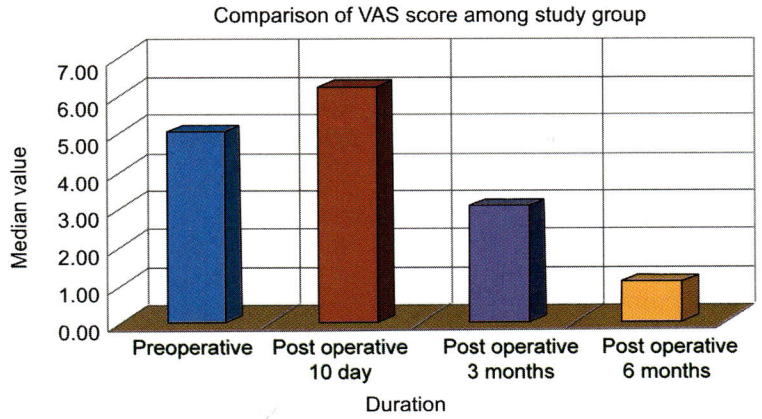

Graph 26.2: Comparison of VAS score in the series

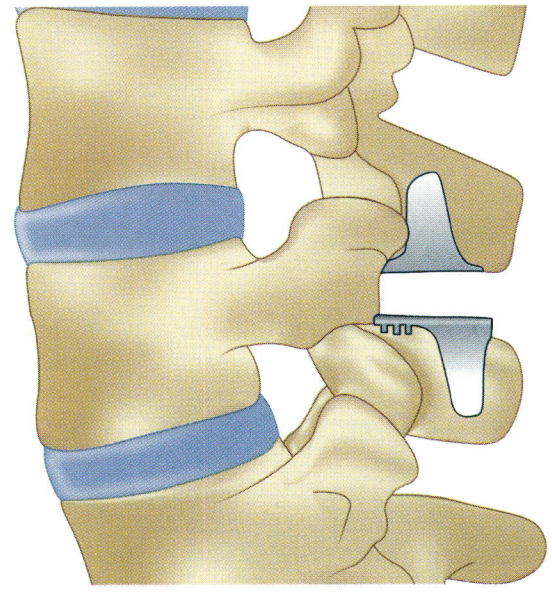

Fig. 26.3: *In situ* placement of co-flex

Endoscopic Decompression

Endoscopic modalities have been used in recent times more frequently to decompress the lumbar canal. In one series of 10 patients undergoing endoscopic facetectomy 15 to treat severe lumbar canal stenosis, dynamic radiographs showed no postoperative instability when compared with control patients.

Open Decompression Procedures

Laminotomy

In a study when 100 patients undergone unilateral laminotomy as an alternative for decompression were followed for 5 years, remained improved showing excellent results.[33]

Bilateral IDSS

For patients with moderate rather than severe central stenosis fenestration approaches defined as IDSS[28, 29] can be considered. In one series bilateral IDSS provided symptomatic relief for up to 5 postoperative years. In another study bilateral IDSS adequately decompressed nerve roots and preserved stability yielded 70% good results on surgeon based outcomes and 76% on patient based questionnaires. In a series of 267 cases, 147 cases had 100% improvement in pain while 80 cases had 75% and 40 cases had 50% reduction in pain.[30]

Lumbar Laminectomy without Fusion

The canal has three distinct areas of potential compression: the central canal, the lateral recess and the neural foramen. Decompressive surgery must address each of these regions at all involved levels.

The number of surgical levels undergoing decompression should be based on full assessment of radiographic, MRI and CT evaluations to avoid the most common pitfall leading to failed lumbar stenosis surgery (Fig. 26.4).

Success rates associated with laminectomy for stenosis ranges from 80 to 90%. Other studies have quoted nearly comparable 80–84% success rates following decompression alone for stenosis without fusion.

In a study by Silvers and associates,[32] performed 258 laminectomies, observed a 75% incidence of good and excellent over and average of 5 years following surgery. Deyo and colleagues[8] documented comparable outcomes morbidity, mortality, for patients undergoing laminectomy with or without fusion.

Outcome

Comparison of the outcome of surgery to those of conservative treatment for lumbar canal stenosis

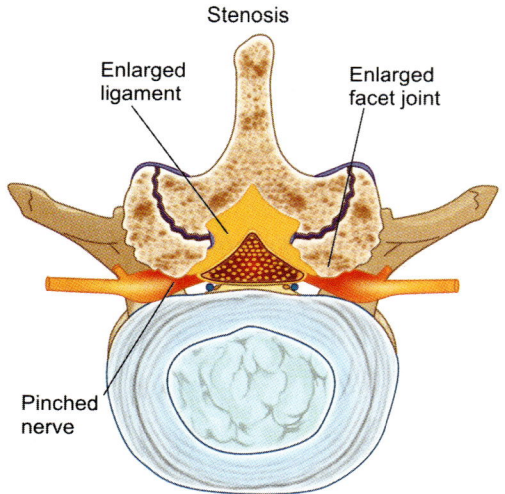

Fig. 26.4: Neural elements can be compressed due to protruding disc, ligamentum hypertrophy, facetal arthritis, canal stenosis or foraminal stenosis

suggests surgery provides greater symptomatic improvement.

There are primarily two types of outcome measures:
1. Surgeon based and
2. Patient based questionnaires.

A surgeon based outcome study demonstrated significant relief of leg pain and back pain over an average of 42 months.

The patient based ODI administered and average of 4 years after lumbar laminectomy for stenosis revealed only 62% women and 57% men experienced good and excellent outcomes. The maine lumbar spine study[1-2] (MLSS) reported that surgery may increase a patient's relative odds of definite improvement by up to 2.6 times when compared with nonsurgical treatment. But the four year and ten year surgeon based outcomes reveal a decline in the incidence of the surgical patients. A recent randomized trial[37] found that patients with spinal stenosis who presented with greater leg pain than back pain were more likely to benefit from the surgery than nonoperative management.

Non-instrumented Fusion

In a series of Katz and co-workers[20] patients undergoing non-instrumented fusions demonstrated better symptomatic relief at 6 and 24 months follow-up postoperatively compared with those having laminectomy alone or instrumented fusion.

In McCulloch's study the overall satisfaction rate for patients undergoing single level non-instrumented fusion for stenosis was 86%.[24]

Instrumented Lumbar Fusion

In one study of 50 patients with stenosis and listhesis treated with laminectomy alone versus laminectomy with fusion, better results were observed in the latter at an average of 3 years postoperatively.[14] In another study of 28 patients[37] with spinal stenosis without spondylolisthesis, average four level laminectomy and one or two level instrumented fusion yielded an 85% incidence of good or excellent outcomes.

Adjunctive Demineralized Bone Matrix (DBM)

Adequate fusion rates and outcomes were observed following one or two level posterolateral fusion (PLF) using lamina autograft supplemented with demineralized bone matrix in 50–50 mix. SF-36 outcomes[11] and the frequency of fusion were both evaluated following multilevel laminectomies and one or two levels instrumented pedicle rod screw fusions. One year later, patients in both fusion groups comparably improved on six of eight SF-36 health scales. Dyanamic radiographs showed 98% fusion rates.

Adjunctive β-tricalcium Phosphate (TCP)

Fusion rates and outcomes were initially evaluated following multilevel laminectomy and one or two level posterolateral instrumented fusion using lamina autograft supplemented with β-TCP. A subsequent analysis of patients undergoing instrumented posterolateral fusion with lamina autograft and β-TCP revealed that 88% showed complete fusions within first postoperative year.

Instrumented Fusion for Lumbar Stenosis with Spondylolisthesis or Spondylosis

In one series good or excellent outcomes were achieved in patients undergoing instrumented fusion for grade I and grade II listhesis.[14]

Second Surgery or Re-exploration

In one series, ODI results revealed good to excellent outcomes in 67% of patients undergoing first procedure but it declined to 46% after re-exploration surgery. When patients answered questionnaires, significantly better outcomes were demonstrated for those undergoing one surgery rather than two surgeries especially when the time interval was short between the two surgeries. Re-exploration surgery especially within short-time (1 year) does give satisfaction to the patient but it is not as good as the first surgery. In fact this observation is recorded by several senior surgeons.

Recurrent Stenosis

Recurrent stenosis does occur but the incidence varies from series to series. Not all need surgery but some patients do require it. As said above one cannot expect as good results in second surgery as it was during first surgery. This is true even if the surgery is done both times by the same surgeon. Surgeon's experience and astute judgment is extremely important. The incidence varies from 9 to 28%.

In one series of 100 patients which were followed for less than 5 years, 16% demonstrated recurrent stenosis at or above previously decompressed levels but not all required re-exploration surgery. In another series of 108 patients followed for an average of 7 years, 19.3% required surgery a second time for recurrent stenosis. Katz and co-workers[20] reported 6% repeat surgery for recurrent stenosis or instability at 1 year and 15% at 3 years.

Discussion

Degenerative lumbar stenosis is a slowly progressive ailment that is often managed conservatively in many patients. A significant number of these patients will progress to pain and discomfort that markedly affect their quality of life. Once deemed medically suitable, such patients are the candidates for lumbar decompressive surgery. Reported results and studies show immediate improvement from the surgery compared with nonsurgical treatment.

In a study by Atlas, et al.[1,2] evaluating long-term outcomes of lumbar canal stenosis, surgically treated patients reported greater improvement in leg symptoms and back related functional status than conservatively treated patients. But over the period of 10 year follow-up, long-term outcomes did not differ for those treated surgically or nonsurgically. The reason being the ongoing degenerative process causes recurrent symptomatic stenosis. The graph of improvement slowly comes down as time passes. It is significantly influences by comorbidities like obesity, diabetes, smoking and most importantly lack of exercise.

Regardless of significant variation in outcome, there is considerable variation in the percentage of individuals reporting long-term benefits from the treatment. This message must be clearly understood.

Message

Lumbar canal stenosis is a relentless ongoing degenerative process.

A majority of patients improve with conservative treatment.

A proportion of patient needs surgical intervention. Preferably, the decision to perform surgery must be endorsed by a senior experienced surgeon.

Although outcome results at 10 years follow-up show no difference between two groups, patients with sciatic pain, neurological deficit, bladder and bowel involvement, paresthesiae in the legs should be operated upon.

Patients with any grade of instability should be fused.

Bony fusion should be achieved. Additional supplements like DBM or TCP when available and when patient can afford to pay should be used to enhance the fusion rate.

MISS should be encouraged.

Even without obvious instability the presence of degenerative lumbar scoliosis of kyphosis should be corrected by instrumentation to maintain proper sagittal balance.

All patients should be encouraged to do regular exercise to achieve mobility, strength and toning of muscles.

Patients should be made aware of side effects of co-morbidities.

REFERENCES

1. Atlas SJ, Keller RB, Robson D, Deyo RA, Singer DE. Surgical and nonsurgical management of lumbar spinal stenosis: four-year outcomes from the Maine lumbar spine study. Spine 2000;25:556–62.

2. Atlas SJ, Keller RB, Wu YA, Deyo RA, Singer DE. Long-term outcomes of surgical and nonsurgical management of lumbar spinal stenosis: 8 to 10 year results from the Maine Lumbar Spine Study. Spine 2005;30:936–43.

3. Babhulkar SS, Ramani PS. Evaluation of clinical outcome in patients treated with Interspinous distraction and stabilization with In Space with Moderate instability in Lumar Spine. 2014

4. Carrino JA, Lurie JD, Tosteson ANA, et al. Lumbar spine: reliability of MR imaging findings. Radiology 2009;249(3):161–70.

5. Chou R, Baisden J, Carragee EJ, Resnick DK, Schaffer WO, Loeser JD. Surgery for low back pain. A review of the evidence for an American pain society clinical practice guideline. Spine 2009; 10:1094–109.

6. Ciol MA, Deyo RA, Howell E, et al. An assessment of surgery for spinal stenosis: time trends, geographic variations, complications, and reoperations. J Am GeriatrSoc 1996;44:285–90.

7. Cornefjord M, Byrod G, Brisby H, Rydevik B. A long-term (4- to 12-year) follow-up study of surgical treatment of lumbar spinal stenosis. Eur Spine J 2000;9:563–70.

8. Deyo R, Gray D, Kreuter W, et al. United States trends in lumbar fusion surgery for degenerative conditions. Spine 2005;30:1441–5.

9. Diaz R, Berbeo M, Esteban E. Clinical and radiological results of minimal invasive percutaneous interspinous device (In Space) in the management of degenerative lumbar spinal stenosis. 18 months follow up study. AO Global Spine Congress San Fransico, California USA, 2009: 23–6.

10. Drew B, Bhandari M, Kulkarni AV, Louw D, Reddy K, Dunlop B. Reliability in grading the severity of lumbar spinal stenosis 2000;13:253–8.

11. Epstein NE. SF-36 Outcomes and fusion rates following multilevel laminectomies and 1-2 level posterolateral fusions using lamina autograft and demineralized bone matrix. J. Spinal Discord tec. 2007;20:380–6.

12. Fairbank J, Couper J, Davies J, O'Brien JP. The Oswestry low back pain disability questionnaire. Physiotherapy 1980;8:271–3.

13. F Zaina, C Tonkins-Lane, E Carragee, S Negrini. Surgical versus nonsurgical treatment for lumbar spinal stenosis Spine (Phila Pa 1976), 41 (2016), pp. E857–68.

14. Försth P, Ólafsson G, Carlsson T, et al. A Randomized, Controlled Trial of Fusion Surgery for Lumbar Spinal Stenosis. N Engl J Med 2016;374:1413–23. 10.1056/NEJMoa1513721

15. Hansraj KK, O'Leary PF, Cammisa FP Jr, Hall JC, Fras CI, Cohen MS, Dorey FJ. Decompressive surgery for typical lumbar spinal stenosis. ClinOrthop 2001;384:10–7.

16. Hyeun SungKim1ByapakPaudel1Ji SooJang1Seong HoonOh2Sol Lee3Jae EunPark3Il TaeJang3. Percutaneous Full Endoscopic Bilateral Lumbar Decompression of Spinal Stenosis Through Uniportal-Contralateral Approach: Techniques and Preliminary Results. wneu.2017.03.130

17. Jansson K-Å, Németh G, Granath F, Jönsson B, Blomqvist P. Health-related quality of life (EG-5D) before and one year after surgery for lumbar spinal stenosis. J Bone JtSurg (Br) 2009;91-B:211–6.

18. Johnsson KE, Rosen I, Uden A. The natural course of lumbar spinal stenosis. ClinOrthop 1992;279:82–6.

19. Jönsson B, Annertz M, Sjöberg C, Strömqvist B. A prospective and consecutive study of surgically treated lumbar spinal stenosis. Spine 1997;22:2938–44.

20. Katz JN, Lipson SJ, Chang LC, Levine SA, Fossel AH, Liang MH. Seven- to 10-year outcome of decompressive surgery for degenerative lumbar spinal stenosis. Spine 1996;21:92–8.

21. Lohman CM, Tallroth K, Kettunen J, Lindgren KA. Comparison of radiologic signs and clinical symptoms of spinal stenosis. Spine 2006;31:1834–40.

22. Malmivaara A, Slätis P, Heliövaara M, Sainio P, Kinnunen H, Kankare J, Dalin-Hirvonen N, Seitsalo S, Herno A, Kortekangas P, Niinimaki T, Rönty H, Tallroth K, Turunen V, Knekt P, Härkänen T, Hurri H. Finnish Lumbar Spinal Research Group. Surgical or nonoperative treatment for lumbar spinal stenosis? A randomized controlled trial. Spine 2007;32:1–8.

23. Mayer HM, Zentz F, Siepe C, Korge A: Percutaneous interspinous distraction for the treatment of dynamic lumbar spinal stenosis and low back pain. 2010 Nov;22(5-6):495–511.

24. McCulloch JA. Microsurgical spinal laminotomies, in Frymoyer JW(ed): The Adult Spine: Priciples and practice. New York: Raven Press, Ltd,1991, 1821–31.

25. Mirza SK, Deyo RA. Systematic review of randomized trials comparing lumbar fusion surgery to nonoperative care for treatment of chronic back pain. Spine 2007;32:816–23.

26. Ogikubo O, Forsberg L, Hansson T. The relationship between the cross-sectional area of the cauda equina and the preoperative symptoms in central lumbar spinal stenosis. Spine 2007;32:1423–8.

27. Pawar SG, Dhar A, Prasad A, Munjal S, Ramani PS. Internal decompression for spinal stenosis (IDSS) for decompression and use of interlaminar dynamic device (CoflexTM) for stabilization in the surgical management of degenerative lumbar canal stenosis with or without mild segmental instability: our initial results. Neurol Res. 2017;Apr;39(4):305–10.

28. Ramani PS, Maheshwari S. Surgical technique of internal decompression for spinal stenosis (IDSS). J Spinal Surg. 2011;2(4):566–9.

29. Ramani PS, Singh A, Cahyadi A, Babhulkar SS, Pawar SG. Use of technological advance in surgical management of Internal Decompression for Spinal Stenosis (IDSS) in lumbar canal stenosis J. Spinal Surg. 2012;4(3): 992–5.

30. Ramani PS. Texbook of Spinal Surgery; Vol 2. Pg. 607–15.

31. Schönström N, Hansson T. Pressure changes following constriction of the cauda equina Spine 1988;13:385–8.

32. Silvers HR, Lewis PJ. Decompressive lumbar laminectomy for spinal stenosis. J. Neurosurg, 1993;78:695–701.

33. Verbiest H. A radicular syndrome from developmental narrowing of the lumbar vertebral canal. J Bone Joint Surg Br 1954;36-B:230–7.

34. Weinstein JN, Lurie JD, Tosteson TD, Hanscom B, Tosteson AN, Blood EA, Birkmeyer NJ, Hilibrand AS, Herkowitz H, Cammisa FP, Albert TJ, Emery SE, Lenke LG, Abdu WA, Longley M, Errico TJ, Hu SS. Surgical versus nonsurgical treatment for lumbar degenerative spondylolisthesis. N Engl J Med 2007;356:2257–70.

35. Weinstein JN, Tosteson TD, Lurie JD, Tosteson AN, Blood E, Hanscom B, Cammisa F, Albert T, Boden SD, Hilibrand A, Goldberg H, Berven S, An H. SPORT Investigators. Surgical versus nonsurgical therapy for lumbar spinal stenosis. N Engl J Med 2008;358:794–810.

36. Weinstein JN, Lurie JD, Tosteson TD, Zhao W, Blood EA, Tosteson AN, Birkmeyer N, Herkowitz H, Longley M, Lenke L, Emery S, Hu SS. Surgical compared with nonoperative treatment for lumbar degenerative spondylolisthesis. Four-year results in the spine patient outcomes research trial (SPORT) randomized and observational cohorts. J Bone Joint Surg [Am] 2009;91:1295–1304.

37. Yaman O, Ozdemir N, Dagli AT, Acar E, Dalbayrak S, Temiz C. A comparison of bilateral decompression via unilateral approach and classic laminectomy in patients with lumbar spinal stenosis: a retrospective clinical study. Turk Neurosurg. 2015;25:239–45.

38. Zucherman JF, Hartjen, et al. A multicenter, prospective, randomized trial evaluating the X STOP interspinous process decompression system for the treatment of neurogenic intermittent claudication: two year follow up results. Spine. 2005;30(12):1351–8.

Epilogue

PS Ramani

Lumbar canal stenosis is a degenerative disease of the aging spine. Spinal surgery is not even 100 years old. Its attention was drawn to the spinal surgeons by RB Cloward in 1944. The attention to lumbar canal stenosis was drawn by Verbiest in 1954. Since then a lot of water has flown under the bridge in rapid succession and within a short period there has been tremendous advance in understanding the pathophysiology and epidemiology and biomechanics of the disease. But the fast evolving technology made a tremendous difference to the management. Lumbar decompression laminectomy was a standard surgical procedure of the past. Undoubtedly it has stood the test of time and long-term follow-up results are available to say that it helps in more than 50% of the patients. Surging technological advance helped to introduce fusion techniques with pedicle screws. The open technique has been quickly replaced by minimally invasive microscopic, endoscopic and percutaneous techniques in rapid succession.

Certainly life has been more comfortable to the patients increasing their mobility and agility and PDS techniques has been a boon to the elderly patients getting quick relief from back pain and sciatic pain and increasing their mobility.

The greatest advantage has been the power of patients going back to the original job that he was doing before surgery. In the present era of rapidly moving society it is of utmost importance to go back quickly to the original job. Modern spinal surgery and in particular surgery for lumbar canal stenosis has been very successful in achieving this marvellous success.

We are spinal surgeons from third world country where patients are loathe to come to the surgery early. They will try all sorts of conservative measures until due to relentless degenerative process the pain and disability cripples the patient and like a gullible he begs with the spinal surgeon for help. Sometimes, it is too late as degeneration has progressed beyond limits. Help does come but it has limited value and can produce several restrictions in life.

The question that arises is with the present progress in technology and its application to patients with lumbar canal stenosis has helped surgeons to halt the progress of degeneration. The answer is perhaps negative. LCS is a problem of elderly patients who are already afflicted with several co-morbidities. In spite of good help from spinal surgeons the expectations of patients are not fulfilled.

Perhaps education and training the population could be the answer to this waxing problem. Right from childhood if people indulge in good exercise, balanced diet, stress on nutrition and training mental activities towards positive thinking may help the body to be preserved in good shape with good strength and agility with preserved spinal balance, then the incidence of degenerative lumbar canal stenosis could be brought down. But it is a massive project to change at first the attitude of the people living in a society. Moreover, they are heavily influenced by aggressive marketing of junk food and most unfortunately addicting the young school going mind of the younger breed.

Being not able to be useful to the society in the latter issues the spinal surgeon of tomorrow will concentrate on evolving yet less and less invasive spinal procedures and transform fully the spinal surgery into day care surgery or even outpatient procedures. Everything in life has a price tag and spinal surgery which is afflicting more the poorer section in the society particularly dock and mine workers and farm labourers. Will the modern spinal surgery be out of reach for them reverting their attitude once again to more conservative measure. What we as spinal surgeons cannot think more clearly for the future, will time alone walking side by side with development of science can answer such waxing questions? We as elderly spinal surgeons may not be there and the younger breed might be able to see a new day in their life in managing patients with lumbar canal stenosis.